Contemporary Gynecology:
An Integrated
Chinese-Western Approach

Lifang Liang

Published by:
BLUE POPPY PRESS
A Division of Blue Poppy Enterprises, Inc.
1990 57th Court North, Unit A
BOULDER, CO 80301

First Edition, March, 2010
Second printing, October, 2010
Third printing, January, 2013
Fourth printing, January, 2016

ISBN 1-891845-50-0
ISBN 978-1-891845-50-5
LCCN # 2010922504

10 9 8 7 6 5 4

Printed at Frederic Printing, Aurora, CO
on acid free paper and soy inks

Contemporary Gynecology:

An Integrated
Chinese-Western Approach

Lifang Liang

Table of Contents

Letters and Testimonials vii

Acknowledgements xvii

Preface xix

Chapter 1   Overview of Female Reproductive Anatomy
            and Physiology 1

Chapter 2   Introduction to TCM Gynecology 15

Chapter 3   Irregular Menstruation 23

Chapter 4   Amenorrhea. 39

Chapter 5   Abnormal Uterine Bleeding 57

Chapter 6   Premenstrual Syndrome (PMS) 71

Chapter 7   Dysmenorrhea 83

Chapter 8   Menopausal Syndrome 103

Chapter 9   Vomiting in Pregnancy. 117

Chapter 10 Prevention of Miscarriage 125

Chapter 11 Ectopic Pregnancy 143

Chapter 12 Postpartum Hemorrhage 155

Chapter 13 Insufficient Lactation. 163

Chapter 14 Vaginal Itching. 177

Chapter 15 Abnormal Vaginal Discharge 185

Chapter 16 Pelvic Masses. 201

Chapter 17 Infertility 217

            Formula List 261

            Chinese Herbs for Gynecological Teatment 279

            TCM Nutrition 293

            Recipes 299

            General Index 303

            Formula Index. 309

Letters and Testimonials

Good health results when a body is in balance. The conflicting forces of growth and development, and repair and decline, battle to maintain a thriving individual. When these forces are out of balance, health declines, and when balance is restored, health returns.

Western medicine has developed phenomenal treatments based on diagnosis and treatment of specific disorders. By focusing on individual problems, specific disorders can be cured. Consideration of individual problems, though, ignores consideration of the whole individual.

Dr. Liang has much to teach us about balance. Her advice on treatment of gynecological disorders focuses on restoring body forces that are out of balance. We in Western medicine have much to learn about what practitioners of Eastern medicine have long practiced. Her practical strategies and case examples serve as a model for balancing Eastern and Western medical care.

My congratulations on Dr. Liang's achievement – an excellent book.

Philip E. Chenette, MD
Pacific Fertility Center
San Francisco, CA

Dr. Lifang Liang has done it again. In her first book she shared with us many intensely personal and life altering events that led her to become a healer and a nurturer rather than an engineer. That book focused on acupuncture and IVF, and now, with *Contemporary Gynecology: An Integrated Chinese-Western Approach* she has turned her attention to general gynecology. Her training in gynecology, both Western as well as Traditional, gives her unique insight into both modalities, and allows her to combine the best of both worlds in delivering care to her patients.

Practitioners of Western medicine have long been skeptical about alternative therapies, mainly out of ignorance of the exact nature of the theory and the practice and also out of fear of competition and possible loss of livelihood. Dr. Liang very eloquently outlines the complementary nature of the Eastern and the Western approaches and explains in detail the concepts of the yin and the yang, the vital substances of qi, blood, essence and body fluids along with the five phases and their interaction. In this book she provides a means for Westerners, both medical practitioners and patients, of understanding the basis of therapies that have evolved over more than 4,000 years, while also providing details of acupuncture and herbal therapies which will enable other practitioners of TCM to compare protocols and communicate and collaborate to further improve outcomes.

Christo Zouves, MD
Medical Director, Zouves Fertility Center
Author: "Expecting Miracles"

I have had the pleasure of collaborating with Dr. Lifang Liang for nearly 15 years. She has been an invaluable clinical resource for me and my patients. I remain impressed by her unwavering enthusiasm and passion for her work. Dr. Liang has blessed us with another wonderful resource for Western and Eastern clinicians alike. In this comprehensive text, Dr. Liang shares her medical knowledge in the often daunting challenge of women's reproductive medicine. She thoroughly reviews each major gynecologic diagnosis and treatment with the thoughtful expertise that only 35 years of practice can provide. Many of my patients have benefitted from the combined benefits of Traditional Chinese Medicine and Western Medicine.

It is with great honor that I present Dr. Liang's latest labor of love.

Katherine T. Hsiao, MD
Board Certified Fellow, American College of Obstetricians and Gynecologists
San Francisco, CA

Testimonials

My husband and I wanted to start trying for a baby soon after we were married. Since my husband had had testicular cancer in his 20s, we scheduled an appointment with his doctor. In the appointment, we found out that he had a zero sperm count. The doctor suggested that we do IVF with his banked sperm and for my husband to get a procedure called a vericocele. The vericocele might help his natural production of sperm but would never increase it to the point where we could get pregnant naturally. We would use his sperm for IUI if it did improve. After two failed IVFs, I decided to take matters into my own hands. I started seeing Dr. Liang. After the very first month, she had my cycle on a 28 day cycle consistently. I also had my husband see her to help his sperm production. After three months, my husband checked in with his doctor and his sperm count had risen to 18 million. The doctor said we could start trying naturally and that he couldn't believe the results of the procedure! We got pregnant that very next month. I continued to see Dr. Liang until I was 8 months pregnant.

Shannon and Scott

After four recurrent miscarriages and a diagnosis of "unexplained infertility" I was beginning to feel quite hopeless about the prospect of having another child. My husband and I started trying for a second child when our daughter turned two years old, we hadn't had any previous losses or any issues with that pregnancy. I was consumed with wanting to get pregnant right away so that she would have a sibling right away. A friend who had a similar experience could see how stressed out I was and referred me to Dr. Liang. She was very sympathetic and always confident that we would succeed in having another baby. Dr. Liang convinced me that I needed to reduce my stress and prepare my body for a good pregnancy, she prescribed a once a week acupuncture for me and my husband as well as herbs twice daily for at least 3 months before trying again. As much as I didn't want to wait it was the right thing to do, not only did it help me physically but it really benefitted me emotionally. Being a busy working mother, it became my special time each week to relax or focus on my wellness. I did suffer an additional miscarriage but continued with treatment and made sure to give myself the adequate time to build up my blood flow. I could tell it was working, I no longer had cold hands and feet all the time. With the help of Dr. Liang and her staff, I'm happy to say that I am almost six months pregnant with twin boys! We are the fourth couple we know who have been treated by Dr. Liang and have healthy children to show for it. We are convinced that the acupuncture treatments and herbs were instrumental in increasing our fertility. We are very grateful to Dr. Liang for helping us on our journey. For other couples who are struggling with infertility and recurrent miscarriage, acupuncture is a wonderful option.

Ambra Wellbeloved

My journey to pregnancy started with a variety of tests, as commonly suggested by obstetricians and gynecologists. I did the blood test on Day 3 levels of FSH, LH and estradiol, the Clomiphene Citrate Challenge test, and the Hysterosalpingogram. I also had Laparoscopy and Hysteroscopy. My husband did the semen analysis test. All the test results came out fine. In fact, my FSH is as low as 6.0IU/ml, a number most commonly seen in 20-30 year olds. Despite the encouraging test results, however, our own efforts and further clinical treatments did not achieve conception. I was told that at age 39, I was in a game with very low odds to win.

Coming from China, I have a general understanding of traditional Chinese medicine, the harmony of Qi and the balance of Yin and Yang. I especially like the idea of a holistic approach. However, Chinese medicine is often regarded as a black box because it often lacks the laboratory tests and quantifying methods that modern medicine is known for. This lack of standardization makes the role of the physician very important in traditional Chinese medicine treatment: choosing different physicians can have different, if not opposite, diagnosis and treatment results. So I went for it as a last resort with my expectations set low.

When we first visited Dr. Liang, she explained to us how Chinese medicine can improve the body's circulation, therefore the function of the reproductive organs. Her training in both traditional Chinese medicine and Western medicine and years of practice as an obstetrician and gynecologist in China and an acupuncturist in America, gave her an edge in this field and and a more integrated view toward the problem. By the time we finished our first visit, Dr. Liang had removed our initial reservations and we knew that we had come to the right place. So when Dr. Liang suggested treatments for both my husband and me, we started treatments right away. It is herb tea twice a day and acupuncture once a week.

One month into our treatment, I was pregnant! At age 41, I was pregnant naturally! We were estatic. However, two weeks later, I had light spotting. Dr. Liang changed herbs accordingly. After another 2 weeks, the spotting stopped. Ever since then, it was a smooth sail. I kept on treatments for 6 months. During the period of pregnancy, I was able to go to work and take a one hour walk every day. I had a good appetite and slept well. It was surprisingly uneventful. I am now a believer in Dr. Liang and her work-wonder herbs and acupuncture.

I had a cesarean section delivery. My son was born 8lb-4oz, strong and healthy. But I lost 1,500mL of blood during the surgery and my blood count dropped to 7.8mg. I was very weak and in anemic condition which made the postpartum recovery even harder. I was told it could take months to get the blood count to normal. I went to Dr. Liang and was on the treatment again. In a month, my blood count was back to normal 12mg, and so did my health condition. My obstetrician and gynecologist were surprised at my quick recovery. What they did not know is I have Dr. Liang on my side and her herbs and acupuncture worked wonders again.

Now my son is seven months old. He is happy, healthy and active, and he is the joy of our lives. I thank Dr. Liang for making this possible for us.

Grace Cheng

To: Dr. Lifang Liang and staff

Hello from Shanghai! I wanted to let you know that we gave birth to a healthy baby girl on April 27, 2007. She weighed 7 lbs 15 oz and was 20 inches long. We named her Angelina Wu. Big sister Isabella and parents are all well and enjoying the addition to our family.

I want to thank you and your team for helping us make our little miracle. We had all but given up hope of having a second child after five unsuccessful rounds of IVF. In fact, my expensive fertility doctors had told me that we had less than 1% chance of conceiving naturally. We were encouraged to consider donor eggs if we really wanted to have another baby. I was so discouraged and sad.

It was at that point I decided to try Dr. Liang and alternative medicine after hearing a glowing testimonial from a friend. I admit I was skeptical at first. But after our initial consultation with Dr. Liang, I actually started to have hope again. When I found out I was pregnant after just two months of treatment, I couldn't believe it. I kept waiting for something "bad" to happen – either another miscarriage or for the OB to tell me the fetus wasn't growing properly or something. Instead, I had a smooth, uneventful pregnancy and delivered a beautiful, chubby, healthy baby girl! We couldn't be more thrilled.

Your work made a tremendous difference to my family. Thank you so much. We'll be visiting the Bay area next month – we hope to get a chance to introduce you to Angelina.

Julie and Jerry Wu

My wife and I have both long wished to be parents, but after a series of surgeries beginning in childhood and continuing through young adulthood, at the age of 36 my wife had only a part of 1 ovary remaining and was ovulating at best every other month. Her FSH levels were extremely high, and understanding the odds, we began working with a highly recommended fertility specialist, who, along with a steady, reassuring approach, was also thankfully blunt. He urged beginning IUI immediately, which we did, but after a few months of failed efforts, he also reluctantly advised giving up on the idea of conceiving.

In an early consultation, the specialist had also encouraged us to contact Dr. Liang. The specialist, a classically-trained straight shooter, suggested that although it is not well understood by Western doctors, in some circumstances acupuncture can improve the odds, so in parallel with his efforts both of us began to see Dr. Liang weekly.

I am the son of an academic cardiologist, and my wife is Chinese-American, and despite profound differences in our ways of thinking about things, in Dr. Liang we each found someone who gave us a deep and steady sense that we were in the hands of someone wise. Dr. Liang reached out to us with compassion and a quiet confidence. She said that she believes it is good to work with both the father and the mother whatever the presenting issues because she believes in balance, so each of us visited her weekly for acupuncture sessions and daily made tea from herbs that she gave us.

Meanwhile, when we were advised by our fertility specialist that the data was so compellingly disheartening that it was time to give up, we stopped the injections. We understood that parenting is a deeply fulfilling experience regardless of how the family comes together. We took some time to mourn and spoke with friends who are adoptive parents and began to explore both adoption and egg donation. It will of course also sound like denial, but at the same time, we each also felt that Dr. Liang's confidence was based on something powerful, and without really talking about why, we continued to see her for a few more months. Seeing her had become a reassuring and calming part of what was a very difficult time, and with the thought that we would face things directly, but still leave open the possibility of unexpected things, we continued our visits.

A short time later, my wife became pregnant, and we are convinced that Dr. Liang made a difference. Dr. Liang is, in the best sense of the word, a healer, and as soon as we became pregnant, Dr. Liang guided us through more unexpected tough times (in the second month of the pregnancy, there was a lot of unanticipated bleeding for several weeks), and throughout the pregnancy and afterwards, she has continued to offer care and wisdom. Our fertility specialist and gynecologist have both used the word "miracle" to describe the pregnancy. We feel fortunate to have received assistance from such a fine group of doctors, all of whom appreciate the others' skill and orientation. Dr. Liang has played a special role in our becoming pregnant, and in our lives, and we will forever be grateful to her.

Anonymous

Pain. I am still at odds when I think how easy it was for me to get used to live with pain. It became a normal and justified condition in my life especially since I found, pretty much by accident, that I had developed endometriosis, and that by the time I discovered it, it was already grade IV, the most severe.

My periods always came accompanied by mild cramps that were considered "normal" by the doctors whom I have seen over time. Five years ago, those cramps started to be increasingly painful but there was no apparent cause to explain why. After several years of living abroad, I paired a transoceanic move back to my native Mexico with a pause in my intake of contraceptive pills. Soon I found that my menstrual cramps were almost unbearable. I had to lie down for most of the first day, and I started experiencing severe PMS.

Once settled back home, I looked for the OB doctor that I used to see before I moved away. He suggested a number of tests and concluded that I was fine and advised me to be back to the pill. And while the pill was indeed very helpful, the pain continued with an unusual intensity every time I had my period. Follow-up check ups suggested no major issues. In one of my consultations I asked the doctor if there were chances that I had developed endometriosis—my best friend suffered from it and thanks to her I had read quite a bit about its symptoms. The doctor answered back with a funky lecture on the relation between an overdose of internet information and hypochondria.

Few months later he was the one who moved, so I had to find a new OB for my routine check-ups. This is how on my first appointment, a new doctor suggested that I should undergo a series of new tests because he had the impression my right ovary was way bigger than the left one. "It is not urgent—he said—but get the tests done sooner rather than later." It took me more than three weeks to finally get a final ultrasound test done. During the test, I saw my uterus shaped like a horseshoe, and some blood from my period that was still trapped in its upper part. The blood could not go out because the uterus was bent. The doctor who performed the test said that the horseshoe shape suggested a huge ovarian cyst. To her, the most worrisome situation was the trapped blood in my uterus, which could very easily cause a bad infection. My new OB phoned that same afternoon, and we met next day in the morning. He was also really concerned about the trapped blood and a laparoscopy was scheduled four days later. It was then when my new doctor realized that I had endometriosis. I had endometrial tissue spread all over my abdominal cavity, and a huge ovarian chocolate cyst. Right on the surgery spot, doctors decided to perform a laparotomy to facilitate the removal of endometrial tissue. My right ovary was so affected that it burst open when it was being cleaned. Bouncing back from the surgery was hard, especially due to the hormonal treatment that I had to undergo to help the absorption of the endometrial tissue that could not be removed during the surgery. I was on Lupron for a year, living a quite disturbing artificial menopause. When my periods resumed, they were less painful, but still very uncomfortable. I also had severe digestion problems, which were attributed to the hormones I was taking. A year later, another string of tests came, and as a result a second surgery was scheduled. Doctors found that endometrial tissue formed scars that pulled my intestines behind my uterus. However, the endometriosis seemed somehow under control, and the advice I got was to consider getting pregnant rather soon to avoid jeopardizing my chances to be a mother. Doctors warned me about the high risk to have the endometriosis back.
It was as a result of that piece of advice that I discovered the relation between acupuncture and fertility. I found some medical papers on the internet covering the

issue, and found a reference to Dr. Liang's book on acupuncture and IVF. What I found out was fascinating, and I started looking for a good acupuncturist in Mexico City. She does not work with herbal medicine, but I started having acupuncture sessions twice a week. I had a better recovery from the second surgery thanks to acupuncture. My periods kept on being painful though, and I was still being prescribed contraceptive pills. My local acupuncturist suggested I should stop taking the pill, but I was dubious about it. One day, when I was about to travel to Menlo Park, California for business reasons, I googled Dr. Liang and I found that her clinic is in San Francisco. I immediately made an appointment and that is how we met. It was really interesting to me that she also suggested that I should quit the pill and start taking four different combinations of herbs to help my body normalize its hormonal functions, my periods, and help ease the pain. By that time I had already been dealing with endometriosis and severe pain for almost three years, had two surgeries and had blindly followed my doctors' prescriptions and advice. So I decided to quit the pill and give the herbs (from Dr. Liang), the needles (from my local acupuncturist), and myself a chance. I came back home with half a suitcase filled with jars of powdered herbs. I brought enough for four months, until my next trip to California. After taking the herbs for a month, in combination with two acupuncture sessions per week, the first thing I noticed was that my period was punctual at 28 days for the first time in my life. But the big surprise was to realize that my menstrual pain was much less intense than usual. Months went by and my periods kept their new-normal punctuality, flew better and became pain free!! I could spend a lot of time just observing myself and realizing that I had no pain at all. It was such an unbelievable feeling! My local OB doctor accepted my decision to stop with the pill—under my responsibility of course—but he had really hard time accepting that "herbs and needles" were actually more effective than synthetic hormones. At some point I gave him a copy of Dr. Liang's book. It was interesting that he started sending patients out to look for acupuncturists, even knowing that they won't be able to provide the herbal medicine that Dr. Liang prepares for me... And I eventually stopped seeing that doctor.

It has been almost two years since I met Dr. Liang. I always take advantage of my work trips to Menlo Park to pass by her clinic, say hi, get some acupuncture from her gentle hands, as well as jars of powdered herbs, that I carry around to take every morning and every evening wherever I am. When my body recovered its balance –it was so noticeable, especially due to the total absence of menstrual cramps- Dr. Liang's herbs accompanied me and my husband in the process of getting pregnant. I had a normal, very enjoyable pregnancy and to support it, Dr. Liang has prepared herbal mixes to nourish my baby while in my womb. My daughter was born on April 14, 2008. It was an amazingly quick delivery—I left my office around 4:00 pm that day, and my baby was born at 6:29 pm. My Little Angel is a healthy baby that was born on week 39. I had no drugs during labor. Today I can tell that natural childbirth is the most amazing mix of inner strength and animal instinct that women can experience. I am deeply grateful at the chance of living such a miracle of life. To help me recover from delivery, I have been taking some herbs that Dr. Liang and her team prepared for me last time we met. My postpartum bleeding has been minimal, had almost no blood-clots, have a great deal of energy for a nursing mom, and most importantly, I have enough milk to feed my hungry two-week old! I could not be more grateful to Dr. Liang and I am certain that I will continue visiting her for as long as I am able to. I really want to keep my endometriosis under control, and to continue to live a healthy, pain free life!

Guadalupe Mendoza

Acknowledgements

It is with great pleasure and with a multitude of thanks that I acknowledge the many kind people who have helped me in the writing of this book.

Beginning with the core of my professional training, in China at the Guangzhou University of Chinese Medicine and in the USA at the University of Texas Medical School and the American Global University, I would like to express my sincere appreciation to these institutions. I am deeply indebted to the directors, teachers, and staff members for their care and patience in sharing their profound knowledge with me.

And to my professor, the late Dr. Huan-shen Wu, I am also greatly indebted for sharing his 40 years of clinical experience in the treatment of infertility. To Dr. Robert Schenken, MD, of the University of Texas Health Science Center, I would like to convey my genuine gratitude for training me in IVF techniques.

I would also like to acknowledge my appreciation to the following Western physicians for their wealth of knowledge, support, and collaboration: Dr. Katherine T. Hsiao, Dr. Christo G. Zouves, and Dr. Seth L. Feigenbaum; Dr. Philip E. Chenette, Dr. Carolyn R. Givens, Dr. Carl M. Herbert, Dr. Isabelle P. Ryan, and Dr. Eldon D. Schriock of the Pacific Fertility Center; Dr. Marcelle I. Cedars, Dr. Victor Y. Fujimoto of the University of California, at San Francisco; Dr. Amin A. Milki of Stanford University; and Dr. Michelle L. Bourgault, Dr. Cynthia A. Farner, and Dr. Frederica S. Lofquist.

And especially to my students, Adria Amenti, Candace Bartholomay, Jennifer Everett, Jennifer French, Sean Gee, Eun-hye Kim, Amy Kisslinger, Susan Ko, Jennifer Little, Melissa Margolis, Lorraine Mock, Showing On, Bonnie Trach, and Merissa Tsang from the American College of Traditional Chinese Medicine, and Yee Man Mo, thank you for your genuine interest in the medicine and in learning from me as well as for your generous assistance in the creation of this book.

Thank you also to my patients for your support and important feedback in the generation of this book.

Finally, I must acknowledge that without the constant support and inspiration of my loving husband, Mr. Yiwang Xie, I could not have accomplished this work. And to my son, Min Xie, I am also appreciative for his help in writing this book even while he was busy with his post-graduate work at Stanford University.

Preface

For the past 35 years, I have had the honor and privilege of practicing Traditional Chinese Medicine (TCM) as a gynecological specialist. During this time, it has become apparent to me that the most effective way for me to help my patients is to combine TCM and Western medicine. In China, such a combination is called *zhong xi yi jie he* (中西医结合), integrated Chinese-Western medicine. As a gynecologist in China, I personally felt the deep sadness of so many couples who were unable to conceive. Because of that heart-felt suffering, I made a conscious commitment to improving my clinical outcomes. Based on that commitment, I began exploring the advantages of combining Chinese and Western medicines in the treatment of gynecological complaints, and I continue this exploration to this day. Therefore, in this book, I would like to share my experiences using such an integrated approach and, in particular, the specific clinical protocols I have developed for the treatment of a variety of gynecological diseases and conditions.

In my previous book, *Acupuncture and IVF*, I described ways in which Chinese and Western medicines can work together to achieve the greatest possible success rates in the treatment of infertility. My belief in this style of integrative treatment is based on my many years of working closely with leading Western physicians of infertility clinics across the San Francisco Bay area. Since *Acupuncture and IVF* covers the treatment of female infertility (and male sterility) in depth, readers specifically interested in that aspect of gynecology should see that book.

Now in my new book, *Contemporary Gynecology*, I am delighted to extend this integrated approach to gynecology as a whole. Through my years of practice, both in China and in the U.S., I have seen so many women suffering from a variety of gynecological issues. These diseases can not only impede their ability to conceive, but can affect all aspects of their lives. Working closely with OBGYNs to culminate the results of Western medical tests, examinations and procedures with Traditional Chinese Medicine; we have helped countless women to achieve optimum gynecological heath.

Each style of medicine (traditional Chinese and modern Western) is very strong on its own and can treat conditions the other cannot. In some cases, Western medicine or surgery may be the preferred option. In others, TCM alone is effective. This is especially true in certain situations for which Western medicine has no answers. My experience in combining the two treatment methods has shown me that the strength of one balances the weaknesses of the other. Thus, in a joint approach, the patient will enjoy a better outcome than if either medicine were used alone.

Hence, I would like this book to serve as a reference guide for both professional practitioners of acupuncture and Chinese herbal medicine and MDs. As we better understand each other's medicines, we can work together to prepare more effective treatment plans and coordinate our efforts to achieve the best possible results for our patients. In short, I believe that "two hands are better than one."

Book Organization

The gynecological diseases described in this book are categorized according to classical Chinese medical thought. Diseases are discussed according to the symptoms they cause. For, example, endometriosis often leads to painful periods. Therefore, endometriosis is discussed under the category of dysmenorrhea.

Each chapter contains the following:

• Western Medical View: Brief summary of the current Western medical view of etiology, signs and symptoms, risk factors, diagnosis and treatment methods

• Traditional Chinese Medical View: Summary of the classical TCM view, including differential diagnosis, signs and symptoms, tongue and pulse, treatment principles, herbal and acupuncture treatments

• Clinical Treatment: My personal clinical experience, detailing the methodology and power of combining Eastern and Western Medicines

• Case Study: Case studies that illustrate how the integrative methods work in practice

My highest priority is good results for all patients. My dream is for TCM practitioners and Western physicians to communicate and educate each other about their practices. Together, I believe we can create a better medicine for the future.

Dr. Lifang Liang
San Francisco, CA

1

Overview of Female Reproductive Anatomy and Physiology

We begin our discussion of integrated Chinese-Western gynecology with an overview of female anatomy and physiology from the point of view of modern biomedicine. This is because this is the dominant conceptual system in the world today, and all professional health care practitioners must be conversant with this model.

Female Reproductive Anatomy

The uterus consists of the cervix and uterine corpus or body and is joined by the isthmus. The isthmus is a transitional area where cervical epithelium gradually turns into endometrial lining. The uterus is an inverted pear-shaped muscular organ that lies under the bladder and above the rectum. Generally speaking, the size and weight of the uterus depends on previous pregnancies. The endometrial lining normally ranges from 2-10 millimeters in thickness depending on the stage of the menstrual cycle. The uterus of a woman who has never carried a fetus to full term is approximately eight centimeters long, five centimeters wide, 2.5 centimeters thick, and weighs 40-50 grams. After a woman has had a baby, each measurement is about 1.2 centimeters larger and the uterus is 20-30 grams heavier. The uterus at full-term pregnancy can be 10-20 times its normal weight. Other factors can increase the size and weight of the uterus, such as uterine fibroids or leiomyomas. Fibroids begin as small seedlings that spread throughout the muscular walls of the uterus. They can be so tiny that one needs a microscope to see them. However, they can also grow very large. They may fill the entire uterus and may weigh several pounds. Although it is possible for just one fibroid to develop, usually there is more than one.

The fallopian tubes are 10-14 centimeters in length and about one centimeter in diameter as measured from the exterior. They are light grey to pearly white in color and are lined internally with ciliated epithelium that is folded. The cilia are impor-

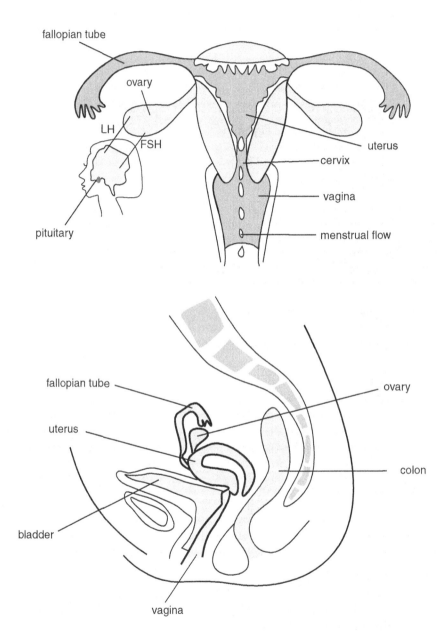

Pelvic Organs

tant for helping the egg or zygote traverse the length of the tube to the uterus. The tubes extend outward from the superolateral part of the uterus and surround each ovary in a funnel-shape fashion without actually touching the ovaries. The end of the tube has finger-shaped projections called fimbria that assist the capture of the egg into the tube at the time of ovulation.

The ovaries are oval in shape and measure about three centimeters by 1.5 centimeters by 1.5 centimeters. During reproductive years, they can be a little larger than that, sometimes reaching five centimeters in length. Enlargement beyond five centimeters is considered abnormal. The ovaries contain 1-2 million oocytes (immature ova) at the time of birth. During a women's reproductive lifetime, about 8,000 follicles are recruited for development, but only about 300 eggs are eventually released. If an ovarian follicle fails to rupture in the course of follicular development and ovulation, a cyst may develop. A cyst may also develop if the corpus luteum fails to respond to ovulatory signals to be reabsorbed promptly. Typically, these cysts are called "functional cysts" and may be three centimeters or larger. As menopause sets in, it is normal for the ovaries to atrophy to a size where they cannot be easily palpated during a pelvic exam.

The Menstrual Cycle

A woman's reproductive years begin when she enters puberty. On average, this occurs at 10 years of age. The first signs that a girl is entering puberty occur when secondary sex characteristics begin to develop, such as the development of breasts (breast budding), broadening of the hips, and growth of pubic and underarm hair. The time interval from breast budding to the first menstrual period (menarche) is usually about two years. During this time, a girl's body will go through a growth spurt and her percentage of body fat will increase. Once menstruation arrives, usually between 11-13 years of age, the growth spurt slows dramatically. By 14-16 years of age, a woman is usually mature in the reproductive sense and will continue menstruating until menopause sets in.

The menstrual cycle is regulated by the continuous interaction of the hormones estrogen and progesterone which are released from the ovaries. Follicle-stimulating hormone (FSH) and luteinizing hormone (LH) are released by the pituitary gland in response to gonadotropin-releasing hormone (GnRH) from the hypothalamus. There are three phases of the menstrual cycle: the follicular phase, the ovulatory phase (more of an event than a phase), and the luteal or secretory phase. The follicular phase begins on the first day of the menses, which is also counted as day one of the menstrual cycle.

The hormones involved:

- Estrogen
- Progesterone
- Follicle-stimulating hormone (FSH)
- Luteinizing hormone (LH)
- Gonadotropin-releasing hormone (GnRH)
- Human chorionic gonadotropin hormone (HCG)

The main organs involved:

- Hypothalamus
- Pituitary gland
- Ovaries

The cycle length is counted from the first day of one period to the first day of the next. The average length of the menstrual cycle is 28 days, but each woman is different and what may be normal for one woman may be abnormal for another. A "normal" cycle can vary from anywhere between 21-35 days. It is important that the number of days between menses stays about the same. If there is variation of more than eight days, then there may be concern that the periods are becoming irregular. In an average cycle, most women experience their LH surge around day 12, with ovulation occurring anywhere between day 13-14. A woman is most likely to get pregnant the three days before and the day of ovulation. Typically, once ovulation occurs and fertilization does not occur, it will be another 14 days before menses begins. Again, this number can vary among women but should remain about the same each month for each individual.

The follicular phase

Day one of the menstrual cycle starts on the first day of the menstrual flow or shedding of the endometrial lining. It usually lasts from 3-7 days. The average blood loss during menstruation is 35 milliliters, with 10-80 milliliters considered normal. Released from the influence of high progesterone levels, the hypothalamus secretes gonadotropin-releasing hormone (GnRH) to the pituitary gland, stimulating the secretion of follicle-stimulating hormone (FSH). FSH causes the ovaries to recruit 3-20 candidate follicles for maturation. Under the influence of several hormones, all but one of these follicles will undergo atresia, while one (sometimes two) dominant follicles will continue on to maturity. The maturing follicle secretes estrogen in increasing amounts which stimulates the uterine lining to thicken. The estrogen also stimulates the production of fertile cervical mucus.

The ovulatory phase

As the follicle reaches maturity, it secretes enough estradiol (a form of estrogen) to trigger a spike in the levels of luteinizing hormone (LH) and follicle-stimulating hormone (FSH) from the pituitary gland. It is this spike in LH and FSH that stimulates the follicle to release the egg. The release of LH helps to weaken the wall of the follicle and release the mature egg. Ovulation typically occurs 16 to 44 hours after the onset of the LH surge. The egg is swept into the fallopian tube by the fimbria (defined on page 3) that surround the opening of the fallopian tube. It is the movement of the fimbria that pulls the egg into the fallopian tube. After ovulation, the ruptured follicle closes. The egg moves down the fallopian tube to the uterus. If fertilization occurs, it will usually happen within the fallopian tube. Increasing levels of estrogen right before ovulation also change the consistency of the cervical mucus, making it more fluid and stretchy to help ease the sperm into the uterus.

The luteal phase

After ovulation, the ruptured follicle turns into the corpus luteum under the influence of LH. During the luteal phase, the levels of FSH drop and the corpus luteum secretes increasing amounts of progesterone. Along with estrogen, progesterone prepares the lining of the uterus for implantation of the fertilized egg, an embryo. Estrogen thickens the endometrial lining whereas progesterone makes the lining rich with glycogen, mucus, and other substances that will support the embryo during the initial stages of implantation. Progesterone will also increase the body temperature by 0.25-0.5°C (0.5-1.0°F). If fertilization does occur, the embryo will travel from the fallopian tube to the uterine cavity and will usually implant itself 6-12 days after ovulation. Once implantation has occurred, the embryo signals the corpus luteum that pregnancy has occurred by secreting the hormone human chorionic gonadotropin (HCG). This causes the corpus luteum to continue to secrete progesterone to maintain the pregnancy. If fertilization does not occur, there will be no HCG secretion and the corpus luteum will start to disintegrate. As the corpus luteum disintegrates, it no longer produces the same levels of estrogen and progesterone. As the levels of both of these hormones start to decline, the uterine lining is no longer supported and nourished and it begins to shed. This shedding is the menses and marks the beginning of another menstrual cycle. Once estrogen drops below a certain level, it signals the hypothalamus to release gonadotropin-releasing-hormone (GnRH), which then causes the pituitary gland to release more FSH to mature a new ovum for the next cycle.

Pregnancy

The length of a pregnancy is officially dated from the first day of the last menstrual period. Since conception cannot occur until a woman ovulates, which is typically about two weeks after the menstrual period begins, the age of the embryo is usually about two weeks younger than the length of the pregnancy. On average, a pregnancy lasts about 38 weeks from the time of conception or 40 weeks from the first day of the last menstrual period. Most women give birth within one or sometimes two weeks of the calculated delivery date. Pregnancy is usually divided into three trimesters. The first trimester is week one through week 12; the second trimester is week 13 to week 25; and the third trimester is week 25 to delivery.

Conception

Pregnancy begins at the moment of conception when the sperm fertilizes the egg. Fertilization usually occurs within the fallopian tube and then the zygote (or fertilized egg) continues to divide as it moves down the fallopian tube to the uterus. It usually takes 3-5 days for the zygote to reach the uterus, at which time the zygote becomes a blastocyst. A blastocyst is a hollow ball of dividing cells that is only one cell thick except for one area that is 3-4 cells thick.

Implantation

Implantation of the blastocyst into the uterine wall usually begins 5-12 days after fertilization. The blastocyst should implant near the top of the uterus. The thin outer part of the blastocyst that implants into the wall of the uterus will develop into the placenta, while the thicker inner part of the blastocyst develops into the embryo. The developing placenta forms tiny projections into the uterine wall that make intricate branches to increase the surface area of contact between the mother and embryo. This allows nutrients, oxygen, and waste to be exchanged easily. It is also responsible for producing the hormones essential for maintaining pregnancy. However, the major source of progesterone is still the ovary until to the sixth or seventh week of pregnancy. Thereafter, the placenta begins to produce progesterone. The process of implantation is usually complete 9-10 days after fertilization, but the placenta continues to form until about 18 weeks after fertilization.

The first trimester

The cells of the blastocyst begin to differentiate by day eight following fertilization. At day 10, the amniotic cavity forms with the yolk sac, placenta, and growing embryo inside. The yolk sac helps to nourish the embryo as the placenta is forming. By day 16 or 17, the brain and spinal cord have started to form and the heart and major blood vessels take shape. The cardiovascular system is the first system to function in the embryo. Usually by day 20, the cardiac cells begin to beat for the first time. The pharangeal arches begin to form which will become the future face, neck, mouth, and nose. During the next three weeks, the development of all organ systems occurs, so that by week 12 all of the anatomic organs are fully developed except for the brain and lungs. The embryonic period is very important because this is the time when all internal and external structures develop in the embryo. During this critical period, the exposure of an embryo to certain agents may cause major congenital malformations. By the end of the first trimester, the fetus is about three inches long.

The second trimester

During the second trimester, the pregnancy begins to show and the chance of miscarriage decreases drastically. The baby continues to grow rapidly so that, by the end of week 25, the baby will weigh approximately two and a half to three pounds and be about 11 inches long. The mother will be able to feel the baby moving around inside of her at this time. The brain continues to develop rapidly, especially in the frontal cortex where all of the higher brain functioning occurs. About halfway through the second trimester, the doctor may be able to determine the sex of the baby through an ultrasound. Four to six ounces of amniotic fluid surrounds the fetus at this time. This allows the doctor to do an amniocentesis if needed. Many of the early symptoms from the first trimester, such as nausea, begin to decrease as hormone levels even out. The mother should also experience an increase of energy during this time.

The third trimester

The last stage of pregnancy is the third trimester. Things start to get very crowded for the baby (and mother) and the baby will take on the typical fetal position. It is a time for organ finalization and for the baby to grow strong enough to survive on its own after birth. By the middle of the third trimester the lungs become fully formed, although the baby will not need them until the moment of birth. The brain is still developing in complexity, and each section of the brain becomes more differentiated and specialized. The eyes actually open during this time too. Near the middle of the ninth month, the baby will move into the position it will take during delivery. Commonly this is where the head moves down into the pelvic area and is facing the mother's back. When the head moves down into the mother's pelvis, the mother will be able to breathe much easier but may have more difficulty with sitting or walking. In the days before labor begins, there can be tightening of the uterus which may cause discomfort. Labor begins when the mother begins to feel uterine contractions at regular intervals. The contractions increase in frequency and intensity as labor progresses. When the baby finally enters the world, he or she will weigh, on average, 6-9 pounds and measure 17-22 inches.

The Physiological Changes of Pregnancy

All of the body's hormones and organ systems are affected by pregnancy. The placenta itself produces hormones to help maintain the pregnancy, namely HCG. Its role is to prevent the disintegration of the corpus luteum thereby maintaining the progesterone production that is critical for pregnancy. The high levels of progesterone prevent the maturation of a new egg, while LH and HCG stimulate the ovaries to produce higher levels of estrogen and progesterone to continue to maintain the pregnancy. The placenta also produces a hormone that increases adrenal hormone levels, such as aldosterone and cortisol, which, along with progesterone, contribute to edema. This increase in adrenal hormones can cause insulin resistance and an increased need for insulin. This is one reason why diabetics need to be especially careful during pregnancy and also why doctors look out for gestational diabetes. In addition, the placenta also produces a hormone that causes the thyroid gland to become more active which can lead to mood swings, increased sweating, heart palpitations, and, sometimes, an enlarged thyroid.

The digestive system is also another area of the body that undergoes a lot of change. Constipation is very common as the pregnancy progresses as the growing uterus puts pressure on the rectum and the lower part of the intestine. In addition, the higher levels of progesterone cause the muscular contractions of the intestinal wall to slow down so food moves more slowly through the intestines. This also causes food to remain in the stomach a little longer, increasing belching and heartburn. The heartburn is not due to an increase in stomach acid, as stomach acid production tends to decrease during pregnancy, but is instead due to relaxing of the sphincter between the stomach and esophagus.

During pregnancy, the heart needs to work much harder to meet the demands of the growing fetus. The heart rate increases from the normal 70 beats per minute to 80-90 beats per minute. The amount of blood pumped per minute (cardiac output) also increases by 30-50%. The volume of blood and the number of red blood cells also increase during pregnancy. This increases the requirements for iron by the mother which can be met by iron supplements. By week eight, the uterus is receiving one-fifth of the entire blood supply of the mother. This increase in the volume of blood required by pregnancy increases the demand on the kidneys to filter that blood. Urination becomes more frequent and urgent as the uterus grows and presses on the bladder and the kidneys filter more blood.

As the fetus grows, the enlarging uterus will change how the lungs expand and raise the resting position of the diaphragm. This decreases the functional residual air capacity of the lungs. Oxygen consumption needs to increase by about 15-20% to meet the metabolic needs of the growing fetus as well as to meet the increased cardiac and renal work. The respiratory rate does not increase to meet these needs. Rather the tidal volume increases (the volume of air inspired and expired with each breath). Also, increased progesterone levels signal to the brain that carbon dioxide (CO_2) levels in the blood need to decrease. This is done by increasing cardiac output and alveolar ventilation to a level that supercedes oxygen requirements by the body, thereby decreasing the total partial pressure of CO_2 within the blood.

Labor and delivery

The exact trigger which leads to labor is unclear to doctors. It is believed to be caused by the release of oxytocin from the pituitary gland which then causes the uterus to contract. The length of time labor lasts can vary among women and depends on whether or not they have had a baby before. Usually, labor lasts anywhere from 6-14 hours.

There are three stages that occur during labor: early labor, active labor, and transtion.

During early labor, the cervix dilates 3-4 centimeters and contractions occur lasting 30-60 seconds and come at regular but increasing intervals. There may also be a backache or cramps. The mother's water will break as a gush or a trickle, and there will be a discharge that is bloody or brown called the "bloody show."

During active labor, the cervix will dilate to seven centimeters, and the contractions become stronger, more frequent, and longer in duration. Pain usually becomes intense at this point, and pain medication is often given. The mother is usually encouraged not to push until she is fully dilated. Pushing too soon may cause the cervix to tear.

The last phase of labor is the transition phase. This is when the cervix dilates from 7-10 centimeters leading up to the delivery. Here the contractions reach peak intensity, last longer, and become so frequent that there may not be much time in between to breathe. Once fully dilated, it is time to push.

There are many different positions the mother can take while pushing. The most common is lying in a semi-upright position in the birthing bed. Squatting or sitting can also work well for some. When about two inches of the head appears, the midwife or doctor will try to manually control the delivery of the baby's head. Once the head and then the shoulders emerge, the baby's airway is cleared by the midwife or doctor of all mucus and fluid and the rest of the body follows quickly.

Delivery of the placenta comes shortly after the baby is born. Usually the placenta detaches following the first or second contraction after delivery, but the doctor or midwife may help it along by massaging the abdominal area. The mother is usually asked to push one more time once the placenta has detached and a gush of blood will come out with the placenta. The doctor will examine the placenta to make sure that it is intact, and, if it is not, the remaining pieces must be removed. As soon as the placenta is delivered, the doctor may stitch any tears to the cervix or vagina, and the mother is given oxytocin to help the uterus to contract and stop any excessive bleeding from where the placenta was attached. The next 3-4 hours are a very special time where the mother and baby get to bond and the baby will nurse for the first time.

Breastfeeding

Breast milk is the ideal food for the newborn baby. The pituitary, ovarian, and placental hormones prepare the breasts for feeding. After the baby has been delivered, the breasts begin to secrete colostrum for the first five days. Colostrum is a translucent, yellow-colored liquid that contains more minerals and protein and less sugar and fat than the mother's mature milk. Over the next few days as the mother continues to breastfeed, the colostrum matures into normal human breast milk. Breast milk and colostrum both contain white blood cells and antigens that protect the baby against pathogens. It also changes the pH of the baby's stool and promotes healthy intestinal flora to prevent bacterial infections in the intestinal tract. Breast milk also contains the ideal ratio of nutrients to support proper growth and development for the new baby.

At first, milk production may seem insufficient and the process of having the newborn "latch on" to the breast may seem awkward and uncomfortable. Over time with continued feeding, milk production increases and both the mother and baby become more comfortable with the whole process. Typically, a mother breastfeeds during the first six months of the baby's life and continues to do so as the baby explores solid foods.

Ovulation is usually suppressed while the mother is breastfeeding frequently. This is because the hormone prolactin is released with suckling, thus suppressing ovulation. As the mother begins to decrease her breastfeeding sessions, she is more likely to ovulate. On average, most women who do breastfeed can expect their menses to return within 36 weeks of delivery. Even with regular and frequent breastfeeding, it is still possible for ovulation to occur. If the mother chooses to not breastfeed, ovulation typically returns 2-3 weeks after delivery.

Menopause

Menopause is the permanent cessation of menstruation caused by the failure of ovarian follicular development and estradiol production in the presence of elevated gonadotropin levels, namely FSH. Menopause literally refers to the date of the last menstrual period. The exact time of menopause is usually made in hindsight, namely one year without menses in women who are not pregnant or lactating and still have a uterus. It is a natural process where the cyclic function of the ovaries stops and the menstrual cycle ceases. A woman's ovaries become unresponsive to FSH and do not recruit and mature a dominant follicle in the ovary for ovulation. It is the follicle that is responsible for the production of estradiol and progesterone, and, in the absence of such follicles, estrogen and progesterone levels drop. This triggers the pituitary gland to release more FSH to mature a new follicle. Nevertheless, the ovaries remain unresponsive, and a woman's cycles become more erratic and unpredictable, leading eventually to menopause.

On average in the West menopause occurs at 51 years of age, but it is normal for it to occur in women as young as 40. If menopause occurs before the age of 40, this is called premature ovarian failure or premature menopause and, unlike menopause, it is a disorder. Perimenopause is the time between the onset of irregular menses and permanent cessation of menstruation. It can start anywhere from 35-50 years of age and can last from 2-10 years. The average duration is four years. The stage preceding menopause is characterized by hormonal fluctuations which lead to a whole range of typical menopausal symptoms. The follicles that are in the ovaries of a perimenopausal woman are less sensitive to the stimulation of FSH. Therefore, there will be fewer cycles where a follicle fully matures, leading to a decrease in the amount of estrogen produced. When levels of estrogen remain low, FSH levels remain high in an attempt to mature the follicle. Low estrogen levels may also fail to trigger the LH surge needed to rupture a follicle for ovulation to occur. Progesterone also declines during this period, and the decrease in both progesterone and estrogen results in a shorter time between menstrual cycles. These shortened or irregular cycles are sometimes one of the first signs that perimenopause has begun.

Typical symptoms of perimenopause and menopause include:

- Hot flashes, night sweats
- Insomnia, sleep disturbances
- Mood swings, irritability
- Memory lapses, poor concentration
- Vaginal dryness and atrophy, changes in libido
- Low bone mass and the risk of osteoporosis
- Joint pain, muscle pain, back pain
- Headaches
- Weight gain
- Changes in hair quality, aging skin
- Lack of energy
- Depression and/or anxiety
- Palpitations
- Irregular menses, anovulation

Hot flashes are the sensations of heat in the upper part of the body that are often accompanied by excessive sweating. They can last anywhere from 30 seconds to five minutes. Hot flashes usually last for more than a year and, in some women, may continue more than five years.

Osteoporosis is a big concern for women in menopause and steps need to be taken to prevent the thinning of the bones. Women who smoke, drink excessive amounts of alcohol, do not exercise, and eat a poor diet lacking in nutrients, especially calcium and magnesium, are at the highest risk of osteoporosis. Most bone loss occurs during the first five years of menopause, where a woman can lose up to three percent of her bone mass per year. Bone loss continues for the rest of a woman's life at a rate up to 1-2% per year. Drinking caffeine can also increase the rate of bone loss. Estrogen replacement therapy (ERT) may help to prevent the loss of bone, but eating well, exercising, and not smoking or drinking caffeine and alcohol excessively, go a long way in keeping bones strong and healthy.

As estrogen levels decrease, atherosclerosis can also become a health concern in menopausal women. Estrogen has a positive effect on keeping cholesterol levels in check. When the estrogen levels decrease, the "bad" cholesterol (low-density lipoprotein, LDL) tends to increase and the "good" cholesterol (high-density lipoprotein, HDL) tends to decrease. This can lead to atherosclerosis and coronary artery disease (CAD).

As of this writing, the main Western medical treatment for women going through menopause is hormone replacement therapy (HRT) using estrogen with progestin. While this therapy has the benefits of decreasing the chances of osteoporosis, it can increase the chance of endometrial cancer, breast cancer, stroke, and gallbladder disease. Giving progestin with estrogen decreases the risk of endometrial cancer. There is also a class of drugs called selective estrogen receptor modulators (SERMs) which can be used in place of estrogen/progestin HRT. Selective estrogen receptor modulators are a class of medication that acts on the estrogen receptor. A characteristic that distinguishes these substances from pure receptor agonists and antagonists is that their action is different in various tissues, thereby allowing the possibility to selectively inhibit or stimulate estrogen-like action in specific tissues. The SERM most helpful for menopausal symptoms, especially hotflashes and loss of bone density, is Fosomax®.

2

Introduction to
TCM Gynecology

Traditional Chinese Medicine (TCM) is based upon the belief that the human being is a holistic and integrated system and that disease is a manifestation of imbalance within this intricate, interrelated system. Accordingly, disease is not understood through reduction to isolated causes, such as bacteria and viruses or even specific hormones, but rather as the loss of normal interaction of certain key elements of the human system. These key elements are the channels (or channels and network vessels), the organs (literally, the "viscera and bowels"), and the body substances. Within TCM as a whole, there are 14 main channels and network vessels, five viscera and six bowels, and a number of body substances. However, in the specific study of Chinese medical gynecology, some of these channels, organs, and substances are more important than others. Those channels, organs, and body substances most germane to gynecology are those discussed below. Since gynecology is a specialty within Chinese medicine, it is assumed that the reader is already familiar with basic Chinese medical theory.

Channels

The channels most central to female reproductive physiology and pathology include the controlling (ren 任) vessel, penetrating (chong 冲) vessel, governing (du 督) vessel, and girdling (dai 带) vessel.

The controlling vessel controls the body's yin which is vital for maintaining the proper function of the female organs and shares a common source with blood. The penetrating vessel communicates directly with the uterus. The governing vessel controls the body's yang which provides the motive power and warmth to drive the functioning of the reproductive system. Without correct flow of yang, for example, infertility may result. The girdling vessel wraps around the waist. Both by virtue of its location and its action of regulating the flow of qi between the upper and lower body, the girdling vessel assists in the functioning of the female reproductive system. Blockage or damage to the girdling vessel can trap evil repletions in the lower body as well as prevent sufficient qi and blood flow to the area.

Organs

The TCM organs most central to female reproductive physiology and pathology are the kidney, liver and spleen.

The kidney is the source of the body's yin and yang. It also stores essence which is necessary for proper growth and development as well as reproductive capability. Kidney qi plays a primary role in driving the sexual and reproductive functioning of both the male and female. The genitals as well as the internal reproductive anatomy depend upon the kidney for both form and function.

The liver regulates qi and blood flow and, as such, is intimately connected with the female menstrual cycle. Regular menstruation of appropriate amount and color, without pain or premenstrual symptoms, depends upon correct functioning of the liver.

The spleen is responsible for both transforming and engendering and containing the blood in the vessels. The spleen also governs the transformation and movement of body fluids. Thus the spleen's transforming aspect is responsible for keeping dampness from accumulating in the body. As it ensures the availability of blood and prevents abnormal bleeding, the spleen is central in the establishment and maintenance of regular menstruation. Proper functioning of the spleen also guards against blockage caused by dampness which has a tendency to manifest in the lower body because of its yin (*i.e.*, heavy, downward-seeping) nature.

Body Substances

In addition to the organs and channels named above, qi and blood play important roles in gynecological physiology and pathology. Essentially, qi is function and blood is nutritive substance. Specifically, qi has five functions: to move (yun 运), transform (hua 化), defend (wei 卫), warm (wen 温), and contain (she 摄). Blood's job is to moisten (run 润) and nourish (yang 养) the physical body. In addition, the timely discharge of the menstrual blood is dependent on a sufficient amount of blood which flows freely to and from the uterus. Further, both the fetus and breast milk are largely transformed and engendered from the blood.

General Patterns of Pathology

While there are several hundred potential patterns in Chinese medicine, only certain patterns commonly manifest in gynecological complaints. The following are the most commonly seen TCM patterns presenting in gynecological conditions.

Kidney patterns

1. Kidney qi vacuity (*shen qi xu* 肾气虚)

Kidney qi supports the functional integrity of the reproductive system. This is based on the saying, "The kidney governs reproduction." If kidney qi is vacuous, there may be heavy bleeding because the kidney qi cannot hold or secure the blood within the uterus. Similarly, there may be premature labor or miscarriage because the kidney qi cannot hold the baby within the womb. There may also be uterine prolapse because the kidney qi is not holding up the uterus.

2. Kidney yin vacuity (*shen yin xu* 肾阴虚)

Kidney yin is the root of yin of the whole body, and one of the duties of yin is to hold yang in check. Therefore, lack of kidney yin can result in hyperactivity of yang and vacuity heat. In such cases, this heat may cause menstruation to come earlier or may force the blood outside the vessels, resulting in heavy bleeding. Essence (*jing* 精) is the basis of yin, and essence insufficiency may manifest as amenorrhea or congenital infertility. Heat may also cause symptoms of menopause, such as hot flashes and sweating as well as anxiety and restlessness during pregnancy.

3. Kidney yang vacuity (*shen yang xu* 肾阳虚)

Within TCM, the concept of yang includes warmth. In terms of gynecology, kidney yang is necessary to warm the uterus, and, without it, infertility and miscarriage may result from cold. Because of the interdependence of the former heaven kidney and latter heaven spleen, kidney yang also supports spleen function. Therefore, kidney yang vacuity may result in diarrhea around the time of menstruation as well as clear, copious vaginal discharge without odor. Kidney yang is also necessary for the proper elimination of excess water from the body through urination. Hence, lack of kidney yang may lead to edema or symptoms of bloating.

Liver patterns

1. Liver depression qi stagnation (*gan yu qi zhi* 肝郁气滞)

The liver regulates the qi and, as such, plays a vital role in the regularity and rhythm of the menstrual cycle. As it is said:

> The qi moves the blood. If the qi stops, the blood stops.

Thus, when qi does not flow smoothly, the timing of the menstrual cycle may be affected and menstruation may become irregular. Additionally, because of stagnant qi, symptoms such as dysmenorrhea, breast tenderness, and mood swings may develop. If qi stagnation is significant, amenorrhea or infertility may result. The liver channel also travels through the breast area. Therefore, stagnation in the liver channel may limit the flow of milk in breast-feeding mothers, resulting in insufficient lactation.

2. Liver depression transforming heat (*gan yu hua re* 肝郁化热)

Qi is yang, and one of its essential qualities is warmth. Therefore, like resistance in an electric circuit, qi stagnation can cause heat to arise in the body. This heat is called either depressive heat (*yu re*) or transformative heat (*hua re*). This heat may hurry the blood so that menstruation comes earlier, or it may force the blood outside the vessels to cause heavy bleeding. Because heat has an innate tendency to rise upward, there may also be nosebleeding during menstruation. From the point of view of five phase theory (*wu xing xue*), this is a specific effect of the relationship between the liver and the lung. Normally, metal (lung) controls wood (liver), but, as the liver qi becomes replete due to depression and creates heat, this heat scorches the lung.

3. Liver depression with dampness & heat (*gan yu shi re* 肝郁湿热)

Dampness may arise in conjunction with depressive heat due to liver depression counterflowing horizontally to attack and weaken the spleen. Dietary and lifestyle factors can also contribute to creating dampness. In this case, the dampness, although originally engendered in the middle burner, commonly seeps downward to the lower burner or body. This is once again because dampness is a yin evil. When this dampness combines with depressive heat, it transforms to become damp heat. A clinical example of this may be yellow vaginal discharge that is malodorous along with itching or burning.

4. Ascendant liver yang hyperactivity (*gan yang shang kang* 肝阳上亢) & internal stirring of liver wind (*gan feng nei dong* 肝风内动)

When there is insufficient yin to control or "anchor" liver yang, yang may become hyperactive and this may produce wind. In that case, wind tends to rise upward with yang since it is a yang evil. Characteristic symptoms include headaches before menstruation or during menopause (especially headaches that occur at the temples, vertex, or behind the eyes) and migraines. During pregnancy, such wind may manifest initially as dizziness but may then progress to hypertension, convulsions, and full eclampsia.

Spleen patterns

1. Spleen qi vacuity (*pi qi xu* 脾气虚)

The spleen qi is up-bearing, meaning it inherently has a tendency to move upward. It is this upward movement of the spleen qi that holds the abdominal organs in place. Thus, if spleen qi becomes vacuous and weak, it may fail to support these organs properly. In that case, uterine prolapse and even miscarriage may occur. Spleen qi also both transforms, engenders, and contains the blood. Therefore, when the spleen is weak, the blood cannot be contained and menstruation may be early and heavy in volume. Weakness of the spleen may also cause lack of blood which may lead to amenorrhea or insufficient lactation. Remember: "Blood and breast [milk] share a common source." As an extension of this, difficulty in containing blood can also cause milk to be uncontained and leak out, resulting in galactorrhea. Finally, if the spleen's transformative function is affected, symptoms of dampness such as vaginal discharge and morning sickness are possible.

2. Spleen yang vacuity (*pi yang xu* 脾阳虚)

When spleen yang is vacuous the spleen is unable to properly move and transform fluids. This causes the engenderment of dampness. Symptoms of this may include vaginal discharge that is white or clear and without odor, and diarrhea around the time of menstruation. The spleen is especially challenged during pregnancy when it must support and nourish the baby as well as the mother. Thus spleen yang vacuity may occur in pregnancy, causing the water swelling commonly seen during the last trimester.

3. Phlegm damp obstruction (*tan shi zu zhi* 痰湿组滞)

Phlegm damp obstruction may begin due to spleen qi vacuity or it may be the result of poor dietary or lifestyle habits. Either way, dampness may manifest as morning sickness, nausea, and vaginal discharge. When dampness begins to congeal further into phlegm, masses and tumors may develop leading to severe obstruction of the uterus, fallopian tubes, or ovaries that may result in infertility.

Qi patterns

1. Qi vacuity (*qi xu* 气虚)

In gynecological conditions, qi vacuity is usually associated with the kidney and spleen. Among other things, it affects the containment of blood and the securing of essence as well as the structural support of the body's organs. Qi vacuity may result in menstruation that comes earlier and heavier than usual as well as postpartum hemorrhage. It may also result in uterine prolapse which may occur after a series of difficult pregnancies.

2. Qi stagnation (*qi zhi* 气滞)

As stated above, qi stagnation may be thought of as "resistance in the circuit." Qi stagnation may cause menstruation to be delayed or even absent, not to mention painful. Because the qi moves the blood, lack of qi flow may also result in blood stasis. This, in turn, can create masses, such as uterine fibroids. When qi stagnates in the breast area, the milk will not descend and the breasts will feel painfully distended and hard to the touch.

Blood patterns

1. Blood vacuity (*xue xu* 血虚)

Without adequate blood to fully build the uterine lining in a timely manner, menstruation will come late or will not come at all. Additionally, the flow may be lighter, pale in color, and thin or watery in consistency. There may be soreness in the lower abdomen following menstruation because there is not enough blood to nourish the uterus. Without the nourishment of blood, there may also be infertility and miscarriage may result if there is not enough blood to nourish the baby. Because blood and milk share a common source, lack of blood may cause insufficient lactation in nursing mothers.

2. Blood stasis (*xue yu* 血瘀)

When the blood does not move through the vessels freely, blood stasis may result. As the stagnant blood blocks the channels, there is often severe pain. If the obstruction to the reproductive system is significant, menstruation may be scanty or absent. Examples of gynecological conditions involving blood stasis include tumors, and fibroids, endometriosis, heavy uterine bleeding, postpartum cramping and hemorrhage, and ectopic pregnancy.

3. Blood cold (*xue han* 血寒)

Vacuity cold (*xu han* 虚寒)

Vacuity cold is the result of insufficient kidney yang. The blood flows slowly; so menstruation may come late or possibly not at all. There may also be pain that is relieved by warmth, and copious, clear vaginal discharge without smell. When the kidney yang cannot warm the uterus, infertility may result.

Replete cold (*shi han* 实寒)

Replete cold often causes severe sharp cramping that is relieved by heat. Similar to vacuity cold, it causes the blood to flow slowly and delays menstruation.

4. Heat (*re* 热)

Vacuity heat (*xu re* 虚热)

Vacuity heat is the result of insufficient kidney yin. In this case, menstruation may arrive early, the flow may be heavier, and the color is typically bright red. In pregnancy, heat may quicken the blood, make the baby restless, and cause miscarriage or premature labor.

Replete heat (*shi re* 实热)

Replete heat also may cause early menstruation. Heat is a yang evil that rises and forces the blood from the vessels. So it may also cause nosebleeding during menstruation.

If one knows how to reliably identify these main patterns, one should be able to pattern discriminate the overwhelming majority of gynecological conditions. However, one should be aware that these patterns tend to be only building blocks of more complex, multi-pattern presentations. One should not expect to see these patterns in their pure, discrete, textbook manner.

Main Treatment Principles

In TCM methdology, one begins by diagnosing the patient's disease. Then one identifies their presenting pattern(s). Next one states the treatment principles (*zhi ze*, 治则) necessary to rebalance the imbalance implied in the name of the pattern. Thus it is said that the treatment principles are the bridge between the patterns and the treatment plan. Therefore, it is extremely important to always state the requisite treatment principles before attempting to erect a treatment plan. However, because only certain patterns present in the majority of gynecological cases, only certain treatment principles are routinely used. The main treatment principles employed in TCM gynecology are:

- Nourish kidney yin
- Warm kidney yang
- Supplement the kidney qi
- Course the liver and rectify the qi
- Calm wind and subdue yang
- Supplement the spleen qi
- Move and nourish the blood
- Warm cold
- Clear heat
- Disinhibit dampness and dispel phlegm

As one can see, these treatment principles basically correlate with the main patterns presented above. Once one states in theory what needs to be done via these treatment principles, then the practitioner should know what Chinese herbal medicinals and acupoints accomplish these goals. If the patterns, treatment principles, and treatment plan all correspond, there is a high degree of probability that the treatment will achieve its intended effect.

3

Irregular Menstruation

Western Medical View

Definition of normal menstruation:

- Onset of menarche in industrialized countries usually occurs between 12-13 years of age
- Normal menstruation is characterized by a regular cyclical pattern
- Average length between menses is 28 days; variation of up to seven days is considered normal
- Average length of bleeding is four days; variation between 2-6 days is normal
- Average blood loss is 30-80 milliliters
- Blood shed from the uterine lining normally does not coagulate into clots
- Normal menstruation is generally painless
- Oral contraceptive pills tend to keep menstruation regular, with scanty blood flow
- Intrauterine devices (IUDs) typically cause heavier bleeding and more painful menstruation

Hormones involved:

- Gonandotropin-releasing hormone (GnRH)
- Follicle-stimulating hormone (FSH)
- Luteinizing hormone (LH)
- Estrogen
- Progesterone

Menstrual problems:

1. Irregular menstruation
   a. Early menstruation

  b. Late menstruation
2. Amenorrhea
3. Menorrhagia
4. Hypomenorrhea

Types of cycle variation:

1. Irregular menstruation:

Unpredictable, irregular cycles that are sometimes early and sometimes late

Cause: Disruptions anywhere within the menstrual hormone system, caused by organic problems in the reproductive tract or as a result of other illnesses

> **A. Early menstruation (a.k.a. polymenorrhea):** Menstrual cycles shorter than 21 days
>
> > **Cause:** Low levels of progesterone and early ovulation
>
> **B. Late menstruation (a.k.a. oligomenorrhea):** Cycles over 35 days or no menstruation for less than six months
>
> > **Causes:**
> > a. Scanty, non-secretory endometrium that is difficult to slough
> > b. Hormonal imbalances due to anorexia nervosa, stress, sudden weight change, increased exercise, perimenopause or polycystic ovary syndrome (PCOS)
> > c. Elevated prolactin levels (hyperprolactinemia) often caused by a benign tumor of the pituitary gland (pituitary adenoma)
> > d. Hypothyroidism

Treatment:
- Treat underlying diseases
- Modify lifestyle choices
- Hormone therapy as needed

2. Amenorrhea:

- Late or skipped menstruation or lack of menstruation for six months or longer
- Cycles late with scanty menses (oligomenorrhea)
- Heavy bleeding or dysfunctional uterine bleeding in some cycles

Cause: Failure of ovary to release egg from the corpus luteum

Diagnosis: Measurement of basal body temperature or progesterone to determine if ovulatory cycles are present

Treatment: Anovulation due to egg release failure typically treated with a weak selective estrogen receptor modulator (SERM, *e.g.* clomiphene citrate)

3. Menorrhagia:

Large volume of flow (80 milliliters or more of blood) and/or long duration of flow (seven or more days of bleeding)

Causes:
 a. Disease in the reproductive tract – hormone-secreting tumors, fibroids, endometrial polyps
 b. Inflammation (cervicitis, endometritis, vulvovaginitis, pelvic Inflammatory disease)
 c. Trauma–abortion, IUD
 d. Systemic factors such as clotting disorders (hemophilia), leukemia, hyper- or hypothyroidism
 e. Liver cirrhosis
 f. Dysfunctional uterine bleeding (menorrhagia or metrorrhagia) without obvious organic cause
 g. Abnormal growths of endometrial glands

Diagnosis:
- Reproductive tract abnormalities are diagnosed by visualizing instrumentation
- Pelvic sonography (ultrasound)
- Hysterosalpingography
- Hysteroscopy
- Sonohysterography
- Blood tests to check for other systemic diseases
- Magnetic resonance imaging (MRI)
- Computerized tomography (CT) scan

Treatment:
- Antibiotics for inflammatory causes
- Oral estrogen for short-term treatment of acute bleeding

- Dilation and curretage (D&C) if over 35 years of age and severe anemia
- Hormonal treatment for long-term maintenance
- Surgery, chemotherapy or radiation for cancerous conditions

4. Hypomenorrhea: Scanty menstrual flow or short menstrual duration

Causes:
a. Failure of egg to release from ovary
b. Hypothyroid or hyperthyroid
c. Hypothalamic insufficiency
d. Low estrogen levels

Diagnosis: Blood tests to determine thyroid and estrogen levels

Treatment:
- Hypothyroidism is treated with thyroid hormone replacement therapy (*i.e.*, levothyroxine, Synthroid®, Euthyrax®)
- Hyperthyroidism is treated with propylthiouracil or methimasole
- Hormonal treatment for failure of egg to release from the ovary and for low hormone levels
- Lifestyle alteration as appropriate

Traditional Chinese Medical View

Irregular menstruation in TCM can refer to menstrual cycles that are shorter than 21 days, longer than 35 days, or both. There are several pathological processes that can lead to this. The main patterns leading to irregular menses are listed below.

Treatment based on pattern identification:

Early menstruation (*jing xing xian qi* 经行先期): Menstrual cycle less than 21 days

Replete heat (*shi re* 实热)

Signs & symptoms: Heavy bleeding with deep red, thick blood; nosebleed, thirst, vexation

Tongue: Red body with yellow dry fur

Pulse: Replete, rapid

Treatment principles: Clear heat and cool the blood

Formula: Qing Jing San (Clearing Menstruation Formula)

Shu Di Huang (Rehmanniae Radix Praeparata)
Di Gu Pi (Lycii Cortex)
Mu Dan Pi (Moutan Cortex)
Bai Shao (Paeoniae Radix Alba)
Qing Hao (Artemisiae Annuae Herba)
Huang Bai (Phellodendri Cortex)
Fu Ling (Poria)

This formula can also be used to clear vacuity heat.

Vacuity heat (*xu re* 虚热)

Signs & symptoms: Light bleeding with thick, bright red blood

Tongue: Red with scanty fur

Pulse: Thin, rapid

Treatment principles: Nourish yin and clear vacuity heat

Formula: Liang Di Tang (Rehmannia & Lycium Root Bark Decoction)

Sheng Di Huang (Rehmanniae Radix)
Di Gu Pi (Lycii Cortex)
Xuan Shen (Scrophulariae Radix)
Bai Shao (Paeoniae Radix Alba)
Mai Men Dong (Ophiopogonis Radix)
E Jiao (Asini Corii Colla)

Liver depression transforming heat (*gan yu hua re* 肝郁化热)

Signs & symptoms: Either heavy or light bleeding, purplish blood with clots

Tongue: Purplish red

Pulse: Bowstring, rapid

Treatment principles: Course the liver, rectify the qi, and clear heat

Formula: Jia Wei Xiao Yao San (Added Flavors Free Wanderer Powder)

Chai Hu (Bupleuri Radix)

Dang Gui (Angelicae Sinensis Radix)
Bai Shao (Paeoniae Radix Alba)
Bai Zhu (Atractylodis Macrocephalae Rhizoma)
Fu Ling (Poria)
Gan Cao (Glycyrrhizae Radix)
Sheng Jiang (Zingiberis Rhizoma Praeparatum)
Bo He (Menthae Herba)
Mu Dan Pi (Moutan Cortex)
Zhi Zi (Gardeniae Fructus)

Qi vacuity (*qi xu* 气虚)

Signs & symptoms: Light or heavy bleeding with pale, thin blood

Tongue: Pale

Pulse: Weak

Treatment principles: Supplement both the qi and blood

Formula: Gui Pi Tang (Spleen-returning Decoction)

Ren Shen (Ginseng Radix)
Bai Zhu (Atractylodis Macrocephalae Rhizoma)
Fu Ling (Poria)
Gan Cao (Glycyrrhizae Radix)
Huang Qi (Astragali Radix)
Dang Gui (Angelicae Sinensis Radix)
Long Yan Rou (Longan Arillus)
Suan Zao Ren (Ziziphi Spinosi Semen)
Yuan Zhi (Polygalae Radix)
Mu Xiang (Aucklandiae Radix)

Delayed menstruation (*jing xing hou qi* 经行后期): Menstrual cycle longer than 35 days

Replete cold (*shi han* 实寒)

Signs & symptoms: Light bleeding with dark blood, lower abdominal pain that is relieved by warmth and is worse with pressure

Tongue: Pale

Pulse: Slow, replete

Treatment principles: Warm the channels (menses) and expel stasis

Formula: Wen Jing Tang (Channel-warming [or Menses-warming] Decoction)

Ren Shen (Ginseng Radix)
Dang Gui (Angelicae Sinensis Radix)
Chuan Xiong (Chuanxiong Rhizoma)
Bai Shao (Paeoniae Radix Alba)
Niu Xi (Achyranthis Bidentatae Radix)
E Zhu (Curcumae Rhizoma)
Rou Gui (Cinnamomi Cortex)
Mu Dan Pi (Moutan Cortex)
Gan Cao (Glycyrrhizae Radix)

Vacuity cold (*xu han* 虚寒)

Signs & symptoms: Light bleeding with thin, clear blood, mild lower abdominal pain that is relieved by warmth and pressure

Tongue: Pale

Pulse: Deep, weak

Treatment principles: Warm the channels (or menses) and supplement the blood

Formula: Da Ying Jian (Major Construction Brew)

Dang Gui (Angelicae Sinensis Radix)
Shu Di Huang (Rehmanniae Radix Praeparata)
Gou Qi Zi (Lycii Fructus)
Du Zhong (Eucommiae Cortex)
Niu Xi (Achyranthis Bidentatae Radix)
Rou Gui (Cinnamomi Cortex)
Zhi Gan Cao (Glycyrrhizae Radix cum Liquido Fricta)

Blood vacuity (*xue xu* 血虚)

Signs & symptoms: Light bleeding with pale, thin blood

Tongue: Pale

Pulse: Thin

Treatment principles: Nourish the blood

Formula: Ren Shen Yang Ying Tang (Ginseng Construction-nourishing Decoction)

Ren Shen (Ginseng Radix)

Bai Zhu (Atractylodis Macrocephalae Rhizoma)
Fu Ling (Poria)
Zhi Gan Cao (Glycyrrhizae Radix)
Shu Di Huang (Rehmanniae Radix Praeparata)
Dang Gui (Angelicae Sinensis Radix)
Bai Shao (Paeoniae Radix Alba)
Huang Qi (Astragali Radix)
Rou Gui (Cinnamomi Cortex)
Wu Wei Zi (Schisandrae Fructus)
Yuan Zhi (Polygalae Radix)
Chen Pi (Citri Reticulatae Pericarpium)
Sheng Jiang (Zingiberis Rhizoma Recens)
Da Zao (Jujubae Fructus)

Qi stagnation (*qi zhi* 气滞)

Signs & symptoms: Purplish-red blood with clots

Tongue: Purple

Pulse: Bowstring

Treatment principles: Course the qi, quicken the blood, and regulate menstruation

Formula: Jia Wei Wu Yao Tang (Added Flavors Lindera Decoction)

Wu Yao (Linderae Radix)
Sha Ren (Amomi Fructus)
Mu Xiang (Aucklandiae Radix)
Yan Hu Suo (Corydalis Rhizoma)
Xiang Fu (Cyperi Rhizoma)
Bing Lang (Arecae Semen)
Gan Cao (Glycyrrhizae Radix)

Modification: For blood vacuity, add Dang Gui (Angelicae Sinensis Radix) and Chuan Xiong (Chuanxiong Rhizoma).

Irregular menstruation (*yue jing bu tiao* 月经不调): Sometimes the menses come early and sometimes they come late

N.B. Dr. Liang seems to be using irregular menstruation here for what is more accurately referred to as (sometimes) early, (sometimes) late, erratic menstruation (*jing xian hou wu ding qi* 经先后无定期). As the title of this chapter suggests, "irregular menstruation" is usually used as generic term covering a variety of menstrual diseases (*yue jing bing* 月经病).

Binding depression of the liver qi (*gan qi yu jie* 肝气郁结)

N.B. This is a synonym for liver depression qi stagnation.

Signs & symptoms: Alternating heavy and light bleeding, possibly with clots; breast tenderness, lower abdominal distention

Tongue: Purple

Pulse: Bowstring

Treatment principles: Course the liver and rectify the qi

Formula: Xiao Yao San (Free Wanderer Powder)

> Chai Hu (Bupleuri Radix)
> Dang Gui (Angelicae Sinensis Radix)
> Bai Shao (Paeoniae Radix Alba)
> Bai Zhu (Atractylodis Macrocephalae Rhizoma)
> Fu Ling (Poria)
> Gan Cao (Glycyrrhizae Radix)
> Pao Jiang (Zingiberis Rhizoma Praeparatum)
> Bo He (Menthae Herba)

Kidney vacuity (*shen xu* 肾虚)

Signs & symptoms: Light bleeding with pale-colored blood, sore lower back

Tongue: Kidney yin vacuity: red with cracks and scanty fur; kidney yang vacuity: pale, enlarged, moist fur

Pulse: Weak

Treatment principles: Supplement the kidney

Formula: Gu Yin Jian (Yin-securing Brew)

> Ren Shen (Ginseng Radix)
> Shu Di Huang (Rehmanniae Radix Praeparata)
> Shan Yao (Dioscoreae Rhizoma)
> Shan Zhu Yu (Corni Fructus)

Tu Si Zi (Cuscutae Semen)
Yuan Zhi (Polygalae Radix)
Wu Wei Zi (Schisandrae Fructus)
Zhi Gan Cao (Glycyrrhizae Radix cum Liquido Fricta)

One can add more kidney yang-supplementing medicinals if needed.

Clinical Treatment

In clinical practice, treatment of menstrual irregularities can be initially approached with one base formula, regardless of whether the patient experiences a cycle that is early, delayed or simply irregular. This formula is called Ding Jing Fang (Stabilize the Menses Formula).

Formula: Ding Jing Fang (Stabilize the Menses Formula)

Shu Di Huang (Rehmanniae Radix Praeparata)
Tu Si Zi (Cuscutae Semen)
Fu Ling (Poria)
Chai Hu (Bupleuri Radix)
Bai Shao (Paeoniae Radix Alba)
Dang Gui (Angelicae Sinensis Radix)
Dang Shen (Codonopsis Radix)
Shan Yao (Dioscoreae Rhizoma)
Ba Ji Tian (Morindae Officinalis Radix)
Zhi Gan Cao (Glycyrrhizae Radix cum Liquido Fricta)

Recall that potential pathologies of irregular menstruation include heat (both repletion and vacuity), cold (both repletion and vacuity), qi stagnation, qi vacuity and blood vacuity. With this in mind, consider the components of Ding Jing Fang.

Formula analysis

Within this formula, Shu Di Huang, Tu Si Zi, and Ba Ji Tian all supplement the kidney. Shu Di Huang and Tu Si Zi supplement the kidney in a broad sense, meaning both yin and yang, while Ba Ji Tian specifically supplements kidney yang. From a biomedical point of view, the Chinese medical "kidney" is the primary source in terms of hormone production and regulation. Therefore, in the case of early, delayed, or irregular menstruation, due to vacuity, the kidney is unable to perform this function. Thus supplementation is a fundamental component of treatment regardless of whatever other disease mechanisms are present. Fu Ling, Zhi Gan Cao,

Shan Yao, and Dang Shen fortify the spleen and supplement the qi. The spleen governs both the engendering and containing of the blood. Hence the spleen is closely connected to the regulation of the menstrual cycle. In particular, it is a main focus in the treatment of both qi and blood vacuity. However, although we need to supplement the spleen, we need to do so using medicinals that are fairly neutral in temperature. This is because heat or cold may be also involved in a patient's particular condition. Together, Chai Hu and Bai Shao course the liver and rectify the qi. Actually, Bai Shao nourishes the blood and this emoliates the liver. When these two medicinals are used together, their combined effect of coursing the liver and rectifying the qi is better than using qi-rectifying ingredients alone. It is important to include moving medicinals in this formula because we are trying to bring on menstruation. In order for this to happen, both qi and blood must be freely flowing. Dang Gui and Shu Di Huang both nourish the blood. Dang Gui also quickens the blood. This latter fact is important in the regulation of menstruation as mentioned above. Thus, taken as a whole, this formula both moves and supplements. This base formula then typically needs to be further modified to suit the patient's particular presenting patterns and type of menstrual irregularity, *i.e.*, delayed or early.

Modifications:

Through modification of the base formula, we can address an individual patient's specific disease mechanisms and their presenting patterns. For example:

- For early menstruation, Mo Han Lian (Ecliptae Herba) or Nu Zhen Zi (Ligustri Lucidi Fructus) may be added to cool the blood and stop bleeding. Nu Zhen Zi has the additional function of nourishing the liver and enriching yin. So it is an especially good choice in the case of yin vacuity.

- For delayed menstruation, more blood-moving medicinals may be added, such as Chuan Xiong (Chuanxiong Rhizoma), Niu Xi (Achyranthis Bidentatae Radix), Hong Hua (Carthami Flos), Tao Ren (Persicae Semen), Mu Dan Pi (Moutan Cortex), Chi Shao (Paeoniae Radix Rubra), and/or Dan Shen (Salviae Miltiorrhizae Radix). It is important to note that moving too strongly may cause dizziness. Also note that each of these medicinals has a slightly different character. Niu Xi moves downward as opposed to simply moving the blood in all directions, whereas Chuan Xiong moves blood and moves qi upward. Dan Shen, Chi Shao, and Mu Dan Pi also clear heat. Hong Hua relieves pain and promotes menstruation and is often used with Tao Ren which also moistens the intestines.

- For qi vacuity, Huang Qi (Astragali Radix) or Bai Zhu (Atractylodis Macrocephalae Rhizoma) may be added to fortify the spleen and boost the qi. Bai Zhu has the added characteristic of drying dampness.

- For qi stagnation, stronger qi-moving medicinals, such as Wu Yao (Linderae Radix), Yu Jin (Curcumae Radix), Xiang Fu (Cyperi Rhizoma), and/or Zhi Ke (Qiao) (Aurantii Fructus) may be added. Yu Jin also quickens the blood. Zhi Ke and Yu Jin are cooling medicinals, while Wu Yao is warming. This is an important aspect to consider since qi stagnation often causes heat. Xiang Fu especially enters (*ru* 入) or gathers (*gui* 归) in the liver channel and is a great choice if there is pain or mood issues due to qi stagnation.

- For cold in the uterus, warming medicinals such as Wu Yao, Rou Gui (Cinnamomi Cortex), Xiao Hui Xiang (Foeniculi Fructus), Wu Zhu Yu (Evodiae Fructus), and/or Gan Jiang (Zingiberis Rhizoma) may be added. Although all of these are acrid and, therefore, somewhat moving, Wu Yao has the strongest qi-moving action. Rou Gui warms the kidneys and promotes the movement of qi and blood. Xiao Hui Xiang, Wu Zhu Yu, and Gan Jiang are all effective at warming the middle burner, while Gan Jiang additionally transforms phlegm.

- To stop bleeding in the case of early menstruation, charred Jing Jie (Schizonepetae Herba) may be added.

Timing of treatment

The main difference in the treatment of early and late menstruation is timing. For early menstruation, the patient should be treated for *one week prior* to the start of the cycle. For delayed or irregular menstruation, the patient should be treated for *one week before a normal cycle would begin, i.e.,* days 21-27. The formula should be administered for one cycle and the outcome observed. Follow-up treatment is then adjusted based upon the patient's response to this initial intervention. If menstruation arrives, a new modification should be given to regulate the cycle. The contents of this new formula will depend on the specific symptoms the patient experiences, such as cramping or heavy or light bleeding. If menstruation does not arrive, the formula given will depend upon the underlying disease mechanism, such as qi stagnation or blood vacuity.

Acupuncture Protocols

The following sequence of point prescriptions is used together to regulate the menstrual cycle. Together these point prescriptions encourage hormonal balance and regular ovulation. Because of this, these basic point prescriptions are among the most important in my clinic and can be used for a variety of conditions that arise from or result in hormonal imbalance.

Before menstruation

ST36 (Zu San Li), KI3 (Tai Xi), GV20 (Bai Hui), Yin Tang (M-HN-3), and ear points Kidney, Spleen, and Shen Men

Protocol analysis

ST36 is a main point for supplementing qi and blood. The primary focus of this prescription is to supplement the blood so that the body is able to menstruate. KI3 is the source point of the kidney and nourishes yin while also supplementing kidney yang and qi. As stated above, the kidney is the main source associated with the producing hormones in general and the sex hormones in particular. Therefore, supplementation of the kidney is vital for hormonal regulation. Yin Tang quiets the spirit, and has a particularly calming effect when combined with GV20. This is important because stress often interferes with hormonal regularity by affecting the smooth flow of the liver qi and this, in turn, can cause menstruation to become irregular. From a Western medical perspective, quieting the spirit activates the parasympathetic nervous system which encourages the endocrine system to function in a smooth and regular way. The endocrine system must be in balance in order to properly regulate the hormonal cycles of the body.

The ear points of the Kidney and Spleen are chosen to supplement respectively the former and latter heaven essences. The kidney is the source of former heaven essence, and the spleen is the source of latter heaven essence. Because the functions of essence include governing development, growth, and reproduction, I believe essence can be seen as equivalent to the sex hormones. Ear Shen Men is added to further calm and relax the patient similar to GV20 and Yin Tang.

During menstruation

SP10 (Xue Hai), LI4 (He Gu), LR3 (Tai Chong), CV4 (Guan Yuan), SP6 (San Yin Jiao), Yin Tang (M-HN-3)

Protocol analysis

The emphasis in this prescription is on moving the qi and quickening the blood, although the formula does also nourish secondarily. SP10 quickens the blood and especially blood in the uterus. LI4 directs the qi downward and promotes menstruation to come in this way. LR3 moves the blood and qi in the liver channel which circulates up through and around the uterus. Additionally, this point is the source point of the liver channel. So it nourishes liver blood and yin as well. CV4 is an intersection point for the three yin channels of the leg, *i.e.*, spleen, kidney, and liver. It is a primary point for the uterus, since each of these channels has a close relationship with female reproduction. CV4 has the advantage that it can both regulate qi and nourish yin and blood. SP6 is also an intersection point for the three leg yin channels. Like CV4, it is able to both move and nourish. Yin Tang quiets the spirit and helps alleviate stress, thus promoting the free flow of qi by discouraging stress-related qi stagnation.

After menstruation

SP6 (San Yin Jiao), GV20 (Bai Hui), ST36 (Zu San Li), Yin Tang (M-HN-3), LI4 (He Gu), Zi Gong Xue (M-CA-18)

Protocol analysis

Following menstruation, the sea of blood is empty. Therefore, we wish to nourish the kidney as well as the blood and qi and to ease or soothe flow of the liver qi. From a Western medical perspective, this combination also promotes ovulation. This requires the dual approach of nourishing and gentle moving. For this reason, SP6 is a clear first choice. As described above, this point powerfully nourishes the three main viscera related to female reproduction as well as moves the qi and blood in their corresponding channels. This point is then combined with ST36, a point which is potent for supplementing the qi and blood. GV20 and Yin Tang once again are used to quiet the spirit and encourage the free flow of qi by alleviating stress. As described above, in Western medicine, this can be thought of as activation of the parasympathetic system which is important to endocrine balance. In particular, GV20 has an adaptogenic effect on the pituitary, causing either an increase or decrease in the secretion of FSH to bring the hormonal levels into normal range. LI4 descends and soothes the flow of qi, guiding the qi to the lower burner for ovulation. Finally, the two Zi Gong Xue are used as local points to directly stimulate the ovaries to release an egg and improve ovarian function.

Case Study

The patient was a 30-year-old female student whose menses usually came 7-20 days late. Once menstruation came, the bleeding was light and only lasted 2-3 days. Thus the woman also had hypomenorrhea. The patient felt very tired and lacked energy and said she felt stressed by school. She also reported lower back pain and dizziness. The woman was not thirsty and her bowel movements and urination were both normal. She usually had cold hands and feet. Her tongue was pale, enlarged with teethmarks on its edges and had thin, white fur. Her pulse was small and bowstring overall and especially weak at the cubit positions.

Pattern identification: Blood and kidney yang vacuity with liver depression qi stagnation

Blood vacuity was evidenced by the light bleeding, fatigue, dizziness, and small pulse. Kidney yang vacuity was clearly shown by her lower back pain and cold hands and feet combined with a pale, enlarged tongue, and a pulse that was weak in the cubit positions. The patient told us that she was under great stress. This and the bowstring pulse suggest an element of liver depression qi stagnation. Delayed menstruation may be due to any one of these factors: vacuity of blood, vacuity cold, and/or qi stagnation. In this case, it was probably due to a combination of all three.

Treatment principles: Nourish the blood and supplement kidney yang, course the liver and rectify the qi, quicken the blood and free the flow of menstruation

Formula: Modified Ding Jing Fang (Stabilize the Menses Formula)

Dang Gui (Angelicae Sinensis Radix)
Bai Shao (Paeoniae Radix Alba)
Shu Di Huang (Rehmanniae Radix Praeparata)
Chai Hu (Bupleuri Radix)
Shan Yao (Dioscoreae Rhizoma)
Fu Ling (Poria)
Tu Si Zi (Cuscutae Semen)
Zhi Gan Cao (Glycyrrhizae Radix cum Liquido Fricta)
Ba Ji Tian (Morindae Officinalis Radix)
Dang Shen (Codonopsis Radix)
Rou Gui (Cinnamomi Cortex)
Niu Xi (Achyranthis Bidentatae Radix)
Dan Shen (Salviae Miltiorrhizae Radix)
Chen Pi (Citri Reticulatae Pericarpium)
Bai Zhu (Atractylodis Macrocephalae Rhizoma)

Formula analysis

Ding Jing Fang is the recommended base or guiding formula in the clinical treatment section in this chapter. The main thrust of this formula is that it is both supplementing (kidney, spleen, and blood) and regulating (liver). The last five medicinals are added to modify the formula for this specific patient as follows. Rou Gui assists Ba Ji Tian by warming the kidney and invigorating yang as well as by moving qi and blood. Niu Xi guides the qi and blood downward, dispersing stagnation and encouraging menstruation in a timely manner. Dan Shen is an excellent medicinal in this case as it both quickens and nourishes the blood. It also gathers in the heart where it quiets the spirit. Chen Pi moves the qi in the chest and abdomen and supports the spleen's function of transformation. Bai Zhu supplements the spleen. Together, these two medicinals are helpful in strengthening the spleen's ability to transform and thus to engender the blood. It is important to note that, in this case, we supported the supplementation of the blood from several angles, both by nourishing it directly and by supporting the creation of blood through supplementing the spleen.

Outcome

Follow-up testing with a physician revealed a diagnosis of polycystic ovarian syndrome (PCOS), a condition of hormonal imbalance in which eggs are not released consistently from the ovarian follicles. After three months of treatment with the above formula and acupuncture, the patient established regular ovulatory cycles of 28 days with normal quantity and quality of menstrual bleeding.

4

Amenorrhea

Western Medical View

The absence of menstruation for more than three consecutive months. However, amenorrhea is a normal physiological state during pregnancy, when one is lactating, and during or after menopause.

Categories:

- Primary amenorrhea
- Secondary amenorrhea

Primary amenorrhea:

The failure to menstruate by 16 years of age with otherwise normal development of secondary sexual characteristics.

Causes:

- Anatomical abnormalities (uterine or vaginal malformations, *e.g.*, completely closed hymen)
- Hypothalamic or pituitary diseases
- Genetic factors
- Hormonal imbalances

Secondary amenorrhea:

The absence of menstruation for three months or more in women who have previously had regular cycles.

Causes:

- Pregnancy

- Breastfeeding
- Cessation of oral contraceptives, *i.e.*, birth control pills
- Menopause
- Chemotherapy
- Stress causing interruption of hormonal interactions and the feedback mechanisms of the hypothalamic-pituitary-ovarian axis
- Rapid weight change causing changes in the ratio of fat cells which, in turn, may affect hormonal regulation
- Intensive exercise, such as in ballet dancers, runners, and other athletes, which inhibits GnRH secretion from hypothalamus
- Eating disorders
- Obesity
- Diabetes
- Thyroid dysfunction (hyper- or hypothyroidism)
- Medications, including psychiatric, blood pressure, pain medications, narcotics, and tranquilizers
- Anemia
- Ovarian dysfunction:
  - Cysts or tumors
- Malfunction of ovarian feedback mechanism
- Failure to respond to hypothalamic gonadotropins
- Polycystic ovarian syndrome (PCOS)
- Hirsutism (increased body and facial hair)
- Infertility, obesity, insulin resistance (IR), excess androgens
- Pituitary abnormalities or adenomas
- Interruption of normal hypothalamic hormone feedback system

Treatment plan (as appropriate):

- Physical exam of the uterus, vagina, and ovaries
- Hormone level testing of FSH, estrogen, progesterone, TSH, T4, T3, and Prolactin
- Ultrasonography to detect anatomical problems associated with PCOS, cysts or tumors
- MRI to rule out pituitary adenoma
- Progestin challenge test to determine adequate ovarian production of estrogen
- Karyotyping to determine genetic defects, such as Turner's syndrome
- Hormonal therapy: Estrogen and/or progestin, thyroid hormones
- Surgery

• Calcium: Non-menstruating women may be more susceptible to osteoporosis

If no underlying organic cause can be determined, treatment may be unnecessary, although modern Western thinking is that hormone replacement therapy (HRT) may prevent or delay the onset of cardiovascular disease or osteoporosis.

Traditional Chinese Medical View

The absence of menstruation for more than three consecutive months in a woman with previously regular cycles or no periods at all by age 16.

Treatment based on pattern identification:
Kidney vacuity (*shen xu* 肾虚)

Signs & symptoms: Amenorrhea; history of scanty bleeding and/or irregular cycles; history of late menarche (18 years or later); menstrual blood that is thin and light colored; weakness and fatigue; low back pain; possible night sweats; dizziness

Tongue: A pale tongue if tending to yang vacuity or a red tongue with peeled coat if tending to yin vacuity

Pulse: Weak and deep in the cubit pulses

Treatment principles: Supplement both kidney yin and yang, regulate menstruation

Formula: Gui Shen Wan (Restore the Kidney Pill)
Shu Di Huang (Rehmanniae Radix Praeparata)
Shan Yao (Dioscoreae Rhizoma)
Shan Zhu Yu (Corni Fructus)
Tu Si Zi (Cuscutae Semen)
Gou Qi Zi (Lycii Fructus)
Du Zhong (Eucommiae Cortex)
Dang Gui (Angelicae Sinensis Radix)
Fu Ling (Poria)

Modification: If there is more kidney yang vacuity, one may add Ba Ji Tian (Morindae Officinalis Radix), Zi He Che (Hominis Placenta), Xian Mao (Curculiinis Rhizoma, Yin Yang Huo (Epimedium Herba).

Qi & blood dual vacuity (*qi xue liang xu* 气血两虚)

Signs & symptoms: Amenorrhea; history of slow and scanty flow, late menses, and/or hemorrhaging; pale face, lips, tongue, nails; dry skin, dry nails; possible digestive disorders; fatigue; dizziness

Tongue: A pale, small, dry or pale, swollen tongue with teethmarks on it edges

Pulse: A fine, weak, or small pulse

Treatment principles: Supplement the qi and blood, regulate menstruation

Formula: Ba Zhen Tang (Eight Pearls Decoction)

>   Shu Di Huang (Rehmanniae Radix Praeparata)
>   Dang Gui (Angelicae Sinensis Radix)
>   Bai Shao (Paeoniae Radix Alba)
>   Chuan Xiong (Chuanxiong Rhizoma)
>   Ren Shen (Ginseng Radix)
>   Bai Zhu (Atractylodis Macrocephalae Rhizoma)
>   Fu Ling (Poria)
>   Zhi Gan Cao (mixed-fried Glycyrrhizae Radix)

Modification: If there is more blood vacuity, add He Shou Wu (Polygoni Multiflori Radix), Gou Qi Zi (Lycii Fructus), and Ji Xue Teng (Spatholobi Caulis).

Qi stagnation & blood stasis (*qi zhi xue yu* 气滞血瘀)

Signs & symptoms: Amenorrhea with sudden onset; breast distention; abdominal bloating and/or pain; irritability, moodiness; migraines or headaches with menses; rib-side pain or distention

Tongue: A purplish red tongue with purple speckles

Pulse: A string-like (*i.e.*, bowstring) or replete pulse

Treatment principles: Move the qi and quicken the blood, regulate menstruation

Formula: Xue Fu Zhu Yu Tang (Blood Mansion Stasis-dispelling Decoction)

>   Dang Gui (Angelicae Sinensis Radix)

Sheng Di Huang (Rehmanniae Radix)
Chuan Xiong (Chuanxiong Rhizoma)
Chi Shao (Paeoniae Radix Rubra)
Tao Ren (Persicae Semen)
Hong Hua (Carthami Flos)
Chai Hu (Bupleuri Radix)
Zhi Ke (Qiao) (Aurantii Fructus)
Jie Geng (Platycodonis Radix)
Chuan Niu Xi (Cyathulae Radix)
Gan Cao (Glycyrrhizae Radix)

Modification: For stagnation due to cold, add Xiao Hui Xiang (Foeniculi Fructus), Gan Jiang (Zingiberis Rhizoma), Rou Gui (Cinnamomi Cortex), and Gui Zhi (Cinnamomi Ramulus).

Phlegm damp obstruction (*tan shi zu zhi* 痰湿组滞)

Signs & symptoms: Amenorrhea with sudden or gradual onset; oftentimes, overweight or prone to edema; fatigue; chest oppression; epigastric distention; abnormal vaginal discharge

Tongue: A swollen, wet tongue with thick, white, moist fur

Pulse: A slippery or soft pulse

Treatment principles: Transform phlegm and eliminate dampness, fortify the spleen, quicken the blood, regulate menstruation

Formula: Cang Fu Dao Tan Wan (Atractylodes & Cyperus Phlegm-abducting Pill)
Ban Xia (Pinelliae Rhizoma)
Chen Pi (Citri Reticulatae Pericarpium)
Fu Ling (Poria)
Gan Cao (Glycyrrhizae Radix)
Dan Nan Xing (Arisaema cum Bile)
Zhi Ke (Qiao) (Aurantii Fructus)
Cang Zhu (Atractylodis Rhizoma)
Xiang Fu (Cyperi Rhizoma)
Sheng Jiang (Zingiberis Rhizoma Recens)

Modification: If there is more phlegm, add Dan Xing (Arisaema cum Bile) and Yi Yi Ren (Coicis Semen).

Clinical Treatment

The TCM patterns presented above are the main ones seen in clinical practice which cover amenorrhea. These include kidney vacuity as well as qi and blood vacuity, qi stagnation and blood stasis, and phlegm damp obstruction.

Kidney vacuity may present as congenital problems anatomically or functionally with the reproductive system. This may manifest, in a Western medical sense, as problems with the endocrine system. There may be ovarian or pituitary dysfunction in which hormones such as FSH, estrogen, and progesterone are not produced in sufficient quantities or at appropriate times to initiate and support a menstrual cycle.

In the case of qi and blood vacuity, there may not be enough blood to menstruate in a timely manner and qi may be insufficient to engender and move the blood.

When the liver qi is stagnant, sluggish qi cannot move the blood and blood stasis may result. When the blood is severely stagnant, menstruation will not come.

Phlegm damp obstruction may occur in women who are obese. Phlegm and dampness can block the channels, especially the controlling vessel, penetrating vessel, and girdling vessel, and interfere with menstruation.

Currently the Western medical treatment for amenorrhea is to administer hormone replacement therapy, usually in the form of oral contraceptive pills (OCP). Combined estrogen and progestin are administered for three weeks to promote the building of the uterine lining, followed by seven days without hormones. (Usually the patient is given a seven-day course of inert pills, or asked to cease taking any pills altogether for seven days.) Cessation of hormonal administration during this seven-day period mimics the normal late-cycle decrease in estrogen and progesterone and promotes the shedding of the endometrial tissue as menstrual flow. When used for a few months, hormone replacement therapy is not a problem. However, there is some evidence to suggest that its use over many years may weaken ovarian function, and, subsequently, it is possible the body may become less able to produce the hormones on its own. Additionally, there may be side effects, such as cysts caused by eggs that form but are not released by the ovaries.

Traditional Chinese medicine can be used in combination with Western medical interventions to support ovarian function so that, once the hormone replacement therapy has established a physiological cycle, the ovaries can begin to work by themselves. During the three weeks of hormonal administration, Tiao Jing Fang (Regulate Menstruation Formula) is given to supplement and nourish. Upon cessation of hormones (and during the period that follows), Xing Jing Fang (Move Menstruation Formula) is given to move the qi and blood and promote menstruation as well as to supplement the qi and nourish the blood. In this way, TCM and Western medicine may be combined to treat this condition, with TCM used to support the body and reinforce the action of the hormonal treatment.

In general, whether in combination with Western medical therapy or not, the TCM approach will follow this same pattern. This method of treatment is discussed in detail below.

Treatment method:

Week 1 (no hormones; taking sugar pills or no pills)

Treatment principles: Nourish blood, move qi and quicken the blood to promote menstruation

Formula: Xing Jing Fang (Move Menstruation Formula)

Shu Di Huang (Rehmanniae Radix Praeparata)
Dang Gui (Angelicae Sinensis Radix)
Bai Shao (Paeoniae Radix Alba)
Chuan Xiong (Chuanxiong Rhizoma)
Gou Qi Zi (Lycii Fructus)
Xiang Fu (Cyperi Rhizoma)
Dan Shen (Salviae Miltiorrhizae Radix)
Niu Xi (Achyranthis Bidentatae Radix)

Formula analysis

Within this formula, Shu Di Huang, Dang Gui, Bai Shao, and Chuan Xiong are the ingredients of Si Wu Tang (Four Agents Decoction), the basic blood-supplementing formula of Chinese medicine. This formula already does contain both nourishing and moving ingredients. However, Dan Shen is added to the formula because the moving components of Si Wu Tang, Chuan Xiong and Dang Gui, are not enough by themselves. Making sure the blood is moving properly is important, especially in gynecological conditions. Along with Si Wu Tang, Gou Qi Zi is added to nourish the blood. Gou Qi Zi also supplements the kidney which makes it a natural choice for gynecological conditions (such as amenorrhea) that may involve kidney vacuity as well as blood vacuity. Moving is an important part of this formula. While Chuan Xiong and Dang Gui quicken the blood, Xiang Fu is added to move the qi. Since Xiang Fu homes to the liver, it is an especially appropriate choice as a qi-moving agent in a gynecological formula. Niu Xi is added to guide downward movement and, thereby, promote the initiation of menstrual flow.

Modifications:

- For qi vacuity, Dang Shen (Codonopsis Radix) may be added.

- For blood vacuity, Huang Jing (Polygonati Rhizoma) or extra Si Wu Tang may be added. Huang Jing supplements the qi in addition to the blood, and Si Wu Tang contains blood-moving components in addition to blood-nourishing ingredients.

- For lower abdominal cold or kidney yang vacuity, warming herbs such as Gui Zhi (Cinnamomi Ramulus) and Xiao Hui Xiang (Foeniculi Fructus) are good choices. The former helps to quicken the blood and warm the channels, while the latter moves the qi and is especially excellent for abdominal pain due to cold.

- For heat signs or kidney yin vacuity, add Sheng Di Huang (Rehmanniae Radix) and Mai Men Dong (Ophiopogonis Radix).

Weeks 2-4

Treatment principles: Supplement the kidney, fortify the spleen and supplement the qi, nourish the blood and course the liver

Formula: Tiao Jing Fang (Regulate Menstruation Formula)

Shu Di Huang (Rehmanniae Radix Praeparata)
Tu Si Zi (Cuscutae Semen)
Fu Ling (Poria)
Chai Hu (Bupleuri Radix)
Bai Shao (Paeoniae Radix Alba)
Dang Gui (Angelicae Sinensis Radix)
Dang Shen (Codonopsis Radix)
Ba Ji Tian (Morindae Officinalis Radix)
Zhi Gan Cao (Glycyrrhizae Radix cum Liquido Fricta)

Xiang Fu (Cyperi Rhizoma)
Shan Yao (Dioscoreae Rhizoma)

Formula analysis

Within this formula, Shu Di Huang and Tu Si Zi supplement the kidney in a broad sense (meaning both yin and yang), while Ba Ji Tian specifically invigorates kidney yang. From a biomedical point of view, the kidney is the primary source of hormone production and regulation. The kidney is clearly unable to perform this function in the case of amenorrhea, and kidney yang vacuity specifically may be implicated. Supplementing the kidney and warming yang is, therefore, a fundamental component of treatment regardless of what other patterns are present. Fu Ling, Zhi Gan Cao, and Dang Shen are three of the four components of Si Jun Zi Tang (Four Gentlemen Decoction), the basic formula for supplementing the spleen qi in Chinese medicine. The spleen is responsible for both engendering and containing the blood. Without sufficient spleen qi, there may not be enough qi to engender the blood or to move it, and this may result in amenorrhea. Therefore, we need to support the spleen function. However, it is best to do so with medicinals that are fairly neutral in temperature (since heat or cold may be also involved in a patient's particular condition). Bai Zhu, the fourth ingredient in Si Jun Zi Tang, is not necessary to include here unless there is also dampness as it is quite drying, and, with amenorrhea, we must protect the fluids. Chai Hu, Xiang Fu, and Bai Shao regulate the liver qi. It is important to include moving medicinals in this formula because we are trying to clear any qi stagnation in order to allow menstruation to resume. In order for this to happen, both the qi and blood must be flowing without obstruction. Dang Gui and Shu Di Huang nourish the blood. Dang Gui also quickens the blood which is important when encouraging menstruation.

Modifications:
- For kidney yin vacuity, Shan Zhu Yu (Corni Fructus), Nu Zhen Zi (Ligustri Lucidi Fructus), and Sang Shen (Mori Fructus) can be added. Each of these medicinals enters the kidney and liver and nourishes yin. Shan Zhu Yu also has a securing and astringing function and helps to contain essence. Sang Shen nourishes the blood and fluids and moistens the intestines for constipation resulting from yin vacuity. Nu Zhen Zi has a special affinity for the liver and is specifically indicated for menstrual irregularities arising from vacuity. If there is yin vacuity with heat, Mai Men Dong (Ophiopogonis Radix) and Sheng Di Huang (Rehmanniae Radix) are good additions.

- For kidney yang vacuity, warm-hot herbs, such as Rou Cong Rong (Cistanches Herba), Yin Yang Huo (Epimedii Herba), Suo Yang (Cynomorii Herba), and/or Sha Yuan Zi (Astragali Complanati Semen) are good choices. Sha Yuan Zi also has mild yin-nourishing abilities.

- For blood vacuity, Gou Qi Zi (Lycii Fructus) as well as Suo Yang and Huang Jing (Polygonati Rhizoma) may be considered. Gou Qi Zi enters both the liver and kidney and nourishes the blood and yin. Suo Yang is a warm medicinal that also supplements and invigorates kidney yang as mentioned above. Huang Jing fortifies the spleen and supplements the qi and, thereby, promotes the transformation and engenderment of blood. It also fosters kidney essence.

- For spleen qi vacuity, the spleen-fortifying and drying medicinal Bai Zhu (Atractylodis Macrocephalae Rhizoma) is a good addition since spleen qi vacuity is often accompanied by dampness.

- For qi vacuity, the supplementing and securing properties of Huang Qi (Astragali Radix) make it a top choice. In this case, securing and astringing are appropriate because this helps to secure the qi that is being built by the formula.

- For phlegm dampness, drying medicinals such as Cang Zhu (Atractylodis Rhizoma), Ban Xia (Pinelliae Rhizoma), Chen Pi (Citri Reticulatae Pericarpium), and Yi Yi Ren (Coicis Semen) are appropriate. If phlegm is more of a problem than simply dampness, Ban Xia and Yi Yi Ren are preferred.

Integrative protocol: Polycystic ovarian syndrome (PCOS)

In our clinic, we combine TCM with Western medicine to help promote ovulation in patients with amenorrhea due to PCOS. For such patients, Western treatment is usually Clomid or other gonadotropins for a period of time that is case-dependent. This encourages the development of ovarian follicles. Taking Tiao Jing Fang (Regulate Menstruation Formula) for 10 days during this time will help to build the uterine lining. Once an ultrasound exam has determined the presence of mature follicles, an injection of HCG is given to trigger the ovaries to release an egg. At this time, Wen Gong Fang (Warm the Uterus Formula) should be administered for three days. This assists with the egg's release and travel through the fallopian tubes, while still nourishing the uterus. Following this, Pai Luan Huo Fang (Promote Ovulation Formula) is given for five days, followed by five days of Tiao Jing

Qian Fang (Regulate the Premenstruum Formula). At this point, menstruation should begin. During menstruation, Tiao Jing Xing Fang (Regulate Menstrual Movement Formula) or Wen Jing Xing Fang (Warm the Menstrual Movement Formula) should be given for five days. The ingredients in each of these formulas are given below.

Summary: (See charts on page 55-56)

Days 1-10 of cycle: Tiao Jing Fang (Regulate Menstruation Formula) (10 days)

Days 11-13: Wen Gong Fang (Warm the Uterus Formula) (3 days)

Days 14-18: Pai Luan Huo Fang (Promote Ovulation Formula) (5 days)

Days 19-28: Tiao Jing Qian Fang (Regulate the Premenstruum Formula) (10 days)

Days 1-5 (menses): Tiao Jing Xing Fang (Regulate Menstrual Movement Formula) or Wen Jing Xing Fang (Warm the Menstrual Movement Formula) (5 days)

Tiao Jing Fang (Regulate Menstruation Formula)

Dang Gui (Angelicae Sinensis Radix)
Bai Shao (Paeoniae Radix Alba)
Chai Hu (Bupleuri Radix)
Fu Ling (Poria)
Shan Yao (Dioscoreae Rhizoma)
Dang Shen (Codonopsis Radix)
Ba Ji Tian (Morindae Officinalis Radix)
Tu Si Zi (Cuscutae Semen)
Shu Di Huang (Rehmanniae Radix Praeparata)
Zhi Gan Cao (Glycyrrhizae Radix cum Liquido Fricta)
Xiang Fu (Cyperi Rhizoma)

Wen Gong Fang (Warm the Uterus Formula)

Dang Gui (Angelicae Sinensis Radix)
Bai Shao (Paeoniae Radix Alba)
Chai Hu (Bupleuri Radix)
Fu Ling (Poria)

Shan Yao (Dioscoreae Rhizoma)
Dang Shen (Codonopsis Radix)
Ba Ji Tian (Morindae Officinalis Radix)
Tu Si Zi (Cuscutae Semen)
Shu Di Huang (Rehmanniae Radix Praeparata)
Zhi Gan Cao (Glycyrrhizae Radix cum Liquido Fricta)
Rou Gui (Cinnamomi Cortex)

Pai Luan Hou Fang (Promote Ovulation Formula)

Dang Gui (Angelicae Sinensis Radix)
Bai Shao (Paeoniae Radix Alba)
Shan Zhu Yu (Corni Fructus)
Shu Di Huang (Rehmanniae Radix Praeparata)
Shan Yao (Dioscoreae Rhizoma)
He Shou Wu (Polygoni Multiflori Radix)
Gou Qi Zi (Lycii Fructus)
Tu Si Zi (Cuscutae Semen)
Dang Shen (Codonopsis Radix)
Wu Wei Zi (Schisandrae Fructus)

Tiao Jing Qian Fang (Regulate the Premenstruum Formula)

Dang Gui (Angelicae Sinensis Radix)
Bai Shao (Paeoniae Radix Alba)
Chai Hu (Bupleuri Radix)
Fu Ling (Poria)
Bai Zhu (Atractylodis Macrocephalae Rhizoma)
Gan Cao (Glycyrrhizae Radix)
Shu Di Huang (Rehmanniae Radix Praeparata)
Chen Pi (Citri Reticulatae Pericarpium)
Dang Shen (Codonopsis Radix)
Suan Zao Ren (Ziziphi Spinosi Semen)

Tiao Jing Xing Fang (Regulate Menstrual Movement Formula)

Dang Gui (Angelicae Sinensis Radix)
Bai Shao (Paeoniae Radix Alba)
Shu Di Huang (Rehmanniae Radix Praeparata)
Chuan Xiong (Chuanxiong Rhizoma)
Niu Xi (Achyranthis Bidentatae Radix)

Dan Shen (Salviae Miltiorrhizae Radix)
Xiang Fu (Cyperi Rhizoma)
Gou Qi Zi (Lycii Fructus)
Xiao Hui Xiang (Feoniculi Fructus)
Yan Hu Suo (Corydalis Rhizoma)

Wen Jing Xing Fang (Warm the Menstrual Movement Formula)

Dang Gui (Angelicae Sinensis Radix)
Bai Shao (Paeoniae Radix Alba)
Shu Di Huang (Rehmanniae Radix Praeparata)
Chuan Xiong (Chuanxiong Rhizoma)
Niu Xi (Achyranthis Bidentatae Radix)
Dan Shen (Salviae Miltiorrhizae Radix)
Xiang Fu (Cyperi Rhizoma)
Gou Qi Zi (Lycii Fructus)
Xiao Hui Xiong (Feoniculi Fructus)
Gui Zhi (Cinnamomi Ramulus)

Acupuncture formulas:

Before menstruation:

ST36 (Zu San Li), KI3 (Tai Xi), GV20 (Bai Hui), Yin Tang (M-HN-3), Ear: Kidney, Spleen, Shen Men

ST36 fortifies the spleen and supplements the qi and blood, thus helping to provide the blood for menstruation as well as the qi to move the blood downward. KI3 helps to supplement the kidney to regulate the hormone levels for a normal cycle.

GV20 stimulates the pituitary gland and also helps to regulate the hormone levels so that menstruation can be triggered naturally. GV20 also quiets the spirit in conjunction with Ear Shen Men and Yin Tang, remembering that relaxation is an important part of normalizing endocrine system communication and, therefore, hormone levels. Ear Kidney and Ear Spleen support the kidney and spleen respectively, both of which must be nourished and fortified in order to promote regular menstrual periods.

During menstruation:

SP10 (Xue Hai), LI4 (He Gu), LR3 (Tai Chong), CV4 (Guan Yuan), SP6 (San Yin Jiao), Yin Tang (M-HN-3)

SP10 and SP6 both quicken the blood to promote smooth menstrual flow. LI4 and LR3, the "Four Bars," free the flow of the channels and promote the smooth flow of qi (and, therefore, blood). CV4 and SP6 supplement and nourish the kidney, liver, and spleen. Yin Tang quiets the spirit.

After menstruation:

SP6 (San Yin Jiao), GV20 (Bai Hui), ST36 (Zu San Li), Yin Tang (M-HN-3), LI4 (He Gu), Zi Gong Xue (M-CA-18)

SP6 supplements and nourishes the liver, kidney, and spleen. GV20 and Yin Tang quiet the spirit to regulate the endocrine system, and GV20 also upbears and lifts the qi. LI4 encourages the qi to flow downward so that the uterus and ovaries can be nourished. It also helps to regulate the body's qi flow overall. Zi Gong Xue stimulates the ovaries to produce and nourish an egg.

Case Study

The patient was a 35-year-old female who complained that she had not had a menstrual period for six years. Prior to that, she had only experienced approximately five periods in her life. The woman had undergone four intra-uterine insemination (IUI) procedures and tried in vitro fertilization (IVF) twice, but all failed. She reported low energy, dizziness, low backache, cold hands and feet, and feelings of depression. She did not experience thirst. Her bowel movements were unformed and urination was frequent at night. The patient's tongue was pale, swollen, and purplish with white fur. Her pulse was small and slow as well as weak in the cubit position.

Pattern identification: Kidney yang vacuity, qi & blood vacuity

The patient's swollen, white-coated tongue and small, slow pulse that was weak in the cubit position all suggest kidney yang vacuity. Additionally, her unformed bowel movements and frequent urination as well as low backache were consistent with kidney yang vacuity. Low energy and a small, weak pulse may be a sign of qi vacuity. Dizziness, a small pulse, and a pale tongue are consistent with blood vacuity. Feelings of depression in this case seem more likely to be a result of qi and blood vacuity than qi stagnation. This is based from the overall picture of the patient, especially including her pulse. It is worth noting that vacuity of the qi and blood often result in some secondary stagnation, and this was suggested by her purplish tongue and cold hands and feet. However, stagnation was not a central issue in this patient. Rather, the picture she presented was primarily one of vacuity, and thus her treatment should emphasize supplementation over dispersal.

Treatment principles: In order to promote menstruation, a two-part approach was employed.

1. **Move the qi and quicken the blood:** This should be done for one week in order to encourage menstruation to come.

2. **Warm yang, supplement the qi, and nourish the blood:** This should be done for the following three weeks to prepare for the next cycle.

Formulas:

Week 4: Modified Xing Jing Fang (Move Menstruation Formula)

Dang Gui (Angelicae Sinensis Radix)
Bai Shao (Paeoniae Radix Alba)
Chuan Xiong (Chuanxiong Rhizoma)
Gou Qi Zi (Lycii Fructus)
Xiang Fu (Cyperi Rhizoma)
Dan Shen (Salviae Miltiorrhizae Radix)
Niu Xi (Achyranthis Bidentatae Radix)
Xiao Hui Xiang (Foeniculi Fructus)

Weeks 1-3: Modified Tiao Jing Fang (Regulate Menstruation Formula)

Tu Si Zi (Cuscutae Semen)
Fu Ling (Poria)
Chai Hu (Bupleuri Radix)
Bai Shao (Paeoniae Radix Alba)
Dang Gui (Angelicae Sinensis Radix)
Dang Shen (Codonopsis Radix)
Ba Ji Tian (Morindae Officinalis Radix)
Zhi Gan Cao (Glycyrrhizae Radix cum Liquido Fricta)
Xiang Fu (Cyperi Rhizoma)
Shan Yao (Dioscoreae Rhizoma)
Bai Zhu (Atractylodis Macrocephalae Rhizoma)
Shan Zhu Yu (Corni Fructus)
Gou Qi Zi (Lycii Fructus)

Treatment analysis

Xing Jing Fang is my standard formula used to promote the movement of blood and qi to bring on menstruation. In fact, the name itself means "move menstruation." In the case of this patient, I removed Shu Di Huang (Rehmanniae Radix Praeparata) because her bowel movements were unformed. I then added Xiao Hui

Xiang because she presented a pattern of yang vacuity and needed to be warmed. More Gou Qi Zi was added to supplement the blood and kidney.

Tiao Jing Fang is Fu Qing-zhu's famous Ding Jing Fang (Stabilize Menstruation Formula) minus Shan Yao (Dioscoreae Rhizoma) but with Xiang Fu added to make it more moving. In the case of this patient, as stated above, I removed Shu Di Huang due to her unformed stool. I also replaced Shan Yao (Dioscoreae Rhizoma) with Bai Zhu. While both supplement the spleen, Shan Yao is neutral, but Bai Zhu is warm and drying. Bai Zhu is, therefore, able to address the unformed stool by drying dampness and strengthening spleen yang in addition to fortifying the spleen qi so that the spleen may create blood and produce latter heaven qi through the transformation of food and water. Shan Zhu Yu was also added to supplement the kidney. Shan Zhu Yu supplements kidney yin as well as yang. Shan Zhu Yu and Gou Qi Zi together effectively replace Shu Di Huang. In this case, Shan Zhu Yu nourishes yin, while Gou Qi Zi nourishes the blood. The combination of these two medicinals is less difficult to digest than Shu Di Huang and is, therefore, a better choice for a patient with unformed stool.

Outcome

The patient's menstruation returned within four weeks of initiating treatment. She subsequently was able to conceive naturally and carry two pregnancies to term. She now has two healthy children.

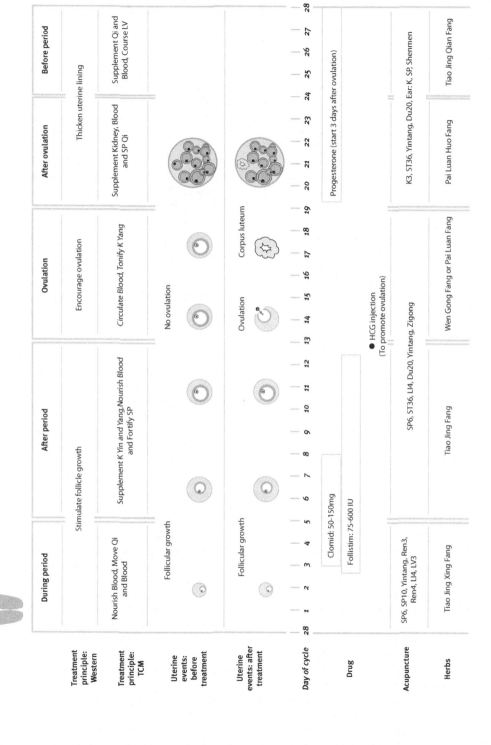

Polycystic Ovarian Syndrome: PCOS

	During period	After period	Ovulation	After ovulation	Before period
Treatment principle: Western	Stimulate follicle growth		Encourage ovulation	Thicken uterine lining	
Treatment principle: TCM	Nourish Blood, Move Qi and Blood	Supplement K Yin and Yang, Nourish Blood and Fortify SP	Circulate Blood, Tonify K Yang	Supplement Kidney, Blood and SP Qi	Supplement Qi and Blood, Course LV
Uterine events: before treatment	Follicular growth		No ovulation		
Uterine events: after treatment	Follicular growth		Ovulation	Corpus luteum	
Day of cycle	28 1 2 3 4 5	6 7 8 9 10 11 12	13 14 15 16 17 18 19	20 21 22 23 24	25 26 27 28
Drug	Clomid: 50-150mg Follistim: 75-600 IU		● HCG injection (To promote ovulation)	Progesterone (start 3 days after ovulation)	
Acupuncture	SP6, SP10, Yintang, Ren3, Ren4, LI4, LV3	SP6, ST36, LI4, Du20, Yintang, Zigong		K3, ST36, Yintang, Du20, Ear: K, SP, Shenmen	
Herbs	Tiao Jing Xing Fang	Tiao Jing Fang	Wen Gong Fang or Pai Luan Fang	Pai Luan Huo Fang	Tiao Jing Qian Fang

Missed period: Differential diagnosis

Type	Pregnancy	Amenorrhea
Missed period	(+)	(+)
Pelvic exam	Uterus: bigger and soft	Uterus: smaller
Pregnancy test	(+)	(−)
Morning sickness	(+) possible	(−)
Ultrasound fetal heartbeat	(+)	(−)
Western treatment principle	Protect miscarriage	Regulate hormones
Drug	Progesterone	Birth control pills [Estrogen +Progesterone]
TCM treatment principle	Supplement K, Blood, Qi, Quiet spirit	Supplement K, Blood, SP, Course LV qi, Regulate menses
Herbs	**K Yang vacuity:** Hu Tai Fang **K Yin and Yang vacuity:** Jing Tai Fang **K Yin vacuity:** Zi Tai Fang	**Day 1-7:** Tiao Jing Xing Fang **Day 8-28:** Tiao Jing Fang
Acupuncture	Yintang, Du20, Ear: K, SP, Shenmen	**Day 1-7:** Ren3, Ren4, SP10, LV3, SP6, LI4, Yintang **Day 8-28:** ST36, K3, SP6, LI4, Zigong, Yintang

5

Abnormal Uterine Bleeding

Western Medical View

Types of abnormal uterine bleeding:

- Dysfunctional uterine bleeding
- Menorrhagia (hypermenorrhea)
- Metrorrhagia (intermenstrual bleeding)
- Polymenorrhea
- Contact bleeding

Most types of abnormal uterine bleeding are treated with hormone therapy. If cancerous conditions are present, the appropriate surgical procedures are used.

Dysfunctional uterine bleeding

Dysfunctional uterine bleeding refers to uterine bleeding that is not due to anatomical causes or malignancy. Usually this refers to abnormal uterine bleeding that occurs between periods in regularly menstruating women. The bleeding occurs separate from ovulation and is not caused by systemic disease, pregnancy or medication use. Flow can vary from spotting to very heavy bleeding.

In menopausal women, uterine bleeding is generally caused by systemic pathology, such as thyroid imbalances, endometriosis and cancerous conditions of the uterus, ovaries or cervix.

Causes:

- Anovulation is the main cause of dysfunctional uterine bleeding during menstruating years.
- Hormonal imbalances, obesity, excessive exercise and emotional stress are contributing factors.

Diagnosis: Functional uterine bleeding is diagnosed after all other causes have been ruled out, such as infections, endometriosis, tumors, cancers, structural problems, pregnancy disorders, and medication use.

Menorrhagia (Hypermenorrhea)

Definition: Regular ovulatory cycles but with heavy or prolonged menstrual flow

Causes:

- Endometriosis
- Uterine tumors
- Polyps
- Uterine fibroids
- Intrauterine devices
- Complications of pregnancy
- Cervical cancer
- Functional uterine bleeding

Metrorrhagia

Metrorrhagia refers to uterine bleeding that occurs between periods in regularly menstruating women. It can last several weeks or even months. The bleeding may be excessive, frequent, irregular or scanty.

Causes:

- In regularly menstruating women, metrorrhagia is usually a sign of underlying hormonal disease. Other causes are anorexia, sexually transmitted diseases (STDs), endometriosis, uterine fibroids, transition into menopause (perimenopause), PCOS, yeast infections, thyroid disease, and, rarely, cancer.
- Postmenopausal uterine bleeding is not normal and indicates more pathological conditions, such as bleeding disorders, thyroid irregularities, liver disease, endometrial, cervical or ovarian cancer, hyperplasias or hormone related tumors.

Diagnosis:

- Physical exam may reveal uterine abnormalities or abdominal masses.
- Complete blood panel rules out serious blood disorders.
- Hormone levels (thyroid, prolactin, FSH, estrogen, and progesterone) are also analyzed.

- Endometrial biopsies, pap smears, hystero-sonograms and ultrasound to rule out cancers, dysplasias, fibroids, and infections

Treatment:

- Most abnormal uterine bleeding is treated with hormone replacement.
- Surgery or dilatation and curettage may be recommended if masses or cancers are present.
- If pregnancy is desired, clomiphene citrate (Clomid®) is given to stimulate ovulation.
- If excessive bleeding causes anemia, iron supplements are prescribed.

Polymenorrhea

Polymenorrhea refers to frequent menstrual bleeding (less than 24 days between periods). This has been dealt with under early menstruation in the chapter on menstrual irregularities.

Contact bleeding

Contact bleeding refers to bleeding after intercourse.

Diagnosis: Contact bleeding should be evaluated for cervical cancer, polyps, and vaginal infections.

Traditional Chinese Medical View

Flooding and spotting (or leaking) is defined as excessive or irregular uterine bleeding outside of ovulation that can last several weeks or months. The flow can vary from spotting to very heavy bleeding.

Treatment based on pattern identification:

Spleen qi vacuity (*pi qi xu* 脾气虚)

Signs & symptoms: Pale light colored, thin consistency; large amount of spotting

Tongue: Slightly pale with teethmarks on its edges

Pulse: Weak

Treatment principles: Supplement spleen and stop bleeding

Formula: Added Flavors Gu Ben Zhi Beng Tang (Root-securing Flooding-stanching Decoction)

Dang Gui (Angelicae Sinensis Radix)
Shu Di Huang (Rehmanniae Radix Praeparata)
Ren Shen (Ginseng Radix)
Huang Qi (Astragali Radix)
Bai Zhu (Atractylodis Macrocephalae Rhizoma)
Pao Jiang (Zingiberis Rhizoma Praeparatum)

Modification: For more serious spleen vacuity, one can also add Shan Yao (Dioscoreae Rhizoma) and Sheng Ma (Cimicifugae Rhizoma).

Kidney yin vacuity (shen yin xu 肾阴虚)

Signs & symptoms: Bright red, light, or heavy bleeding

Tongue: Red thin body with cracks; thin or scanty fur

Pulse: Deep, weak at the cubit; thin, weak and possibly rapid

Treatment principles: Supplement the kidney, enrich yin, and stop bleeding

Formula: Added Flavors Zuo Gui Wan (Left-restoring [Kidney Yin] Pill)

Shu Di Huang (Rehmanniae Radix Praeparata)
Shan Yao (Dioscoreae Rhizoma)
Shan Zhu Yu (Corni Fructus)
Gou Qi Zi (Lycii Fructus)
Lu Jiao Jiao (Cervi Cornus Gelatinum)
Gui Ban Jiao (Testudinis Carapacis et Plastri Gelatinum)
Tu Si Zi (Cuscutae Semen)
Niu Xi (Achyranthis Bidentatae Radix)

Modification: For more serious yin vacuity, one can add Mo Han Lian (Ecliptae Herba) and Nu Zhen Zi (Ligustri Lucidi Fructus).

Kidney yang vacuity (shen yang xu 肾阳虚)

Signs & symptoms: Pale red, heavy watery bleeding

Tongue: Pale swollen body; moist white fur

Pulse: Deep, weak at the cubit

Treatment principles: Supplement the kidney, invigorate yang, and stop bleeding

Formula: Modified You Gui Wan (Right-Restoring [Life Gate] Pill)

Shu Di Huang (Rehmanniae Radix Praeparata)
Shan Yao (Dioscoreae Rhizoma)
Shan Zhu Yu (Corni Fructus)
Rou Gui (Cinnamomi Cortex)
Fu Zi (Aconiti Carmichaeli)
Lu Jiao Jiao (Cervi Cornus Gelatinum)
Gou Qi Zi (Lycii Fructus)
Tu Si Zi (Cuscutae Semen)
Du Zhong (Eucommiae Cortex)
Dang Gui (Angelicae Sinensis Radix)

Modification: For more serious kidney yang vacuity, one can add Xu Duan (Disaci Radix) and Bu Gu Zhi (Psoraleae Fructus).

Blood stasis (*xue yu* 血瘀)

Signs & symptoms: Dark red, purple clots; heavy bleeding, pain relieved after clots

Tongue: Purplish body; thin white fur

Pulse: Rough (*i.e.*, choppy)

Treatment principles: Quicken the blood, transform stasis, and stop bleeding

Formula: Added Flavors Si Wu Tang (Four Agents Decoction) plus Shi Xiao San (Sudden Smile Powder)

Shu Di Huang (Rehmanniae Radix Praeparata)
Dang Gui (Angelicae Sinensis Radix)
Chuan Xiong (Chuanxiong Rhizoma)
Bai Shao (Paeoniae Radix Alba)
Wu Ling Zhi (Trogopteri Faeces)
Pu Huang (Typhae Pollen)

Modification: For more serious blood stasis one can add San Qi (Notoginseng Radix), Qian Cao (Rubiae Radix), Hai Piao Xiao (Sepiae Endoconcha) and E Jiao (Gelatinum).

Blood heat (*xue re* 血热)

Signs & symptoms: Bright deep red; heavy bleeding

Tongue: Red dry body; yellow dry fur

Pulse: Deep, rapid

Treatment principles: Clear heat, cool the blood, and stop bleeding

Formula: Added Flavors Qing Re Gu Jing Tang (Heat-clearing Channel-securing [or Menses-securing] Decoction)

Sheng Di Huang (Rehmanniae Radix)
Di Gu Pi (Lycii Cortex)
Huang Qin (Scutellariae Radix)
Gui Ban (Testudinis Plastrum)
Sheng Mu Li (Ostreae Concha)
E Jiao (Asini Corii Colla)
Ou Jie (Nelumbinis Rhizomatis Nodus)
Zong Lu Tan (Trachycarpi Stipulae Fibra Carbonisata)
Gan Cao (Glycyrrhizae Radix)
Mu Li (Ostreae Concha)
Zhi Zi Tan (Gardeniae Fructus Carbonisatus)
Di Yu (Sanguisorbae Radix)

Clinical Treatment

The Chinese name for metrorrhagia is beng lou (崩漏). In English, beng lou is often translated as flooding and spotting. The first Chinese character, flooding, refers to bleeding that is very severe, like an avalanche or flood. The second Chinese character, spotting, refers to spotting or a light, scanty flow. However, flooding and spotting can also refer to heavy bleeding alternating with light bleeding. This is important to remember, as it is often assumed that metrorrhagia involves only heavy bleeding.

As a young doctor in China, I treated a female patient who came to my clinic for this condition. Her bleeding was very heavy and she was in a great deal of pain. Her struggle inspired me to join a research group for uterine bleeding in China, and I subsequently spent 10 years pursuing research in this area. Sharing my experience in successfully treating metrorrhagia is, therefore, something that is especially meaningful for me.

The major Western causes associated with metrorrhagia are conditions in which ovulation is somehow impaired, such as menopause, anovulation, or PCOS. In a normal cycle, the uterine lining builds up during the estrogenic phase of the cycle. Then ovulation occurs and prompts the production of progesterone. When hormone levels then drop, the lining begins to slough off and menstruation begins. If there is no ovulation, not much progesterone is produced and the lining grows thicker over an extended time under the influence of estrogen. As hormone levels fluctuate bleeding may start and stop, but since the levels are irregular the bleeding tends to be irregular and variable in amount.

In Western medicine, several treatment methods are employed. Physicians use hormone replacement therapy to regulate the hormone levels and control the bleeding by inducing ovulation. Unfortunately, hormonal therapies have a number of side effects. Progesterone, for example, may cause depression, cramping, and fatigue. If the lining has become too thick to slough off on its own, a D & C may be performed. In this procedure, the lining is surgically removed from the uterus. If nothing else works to control the bleeding, a hysterectomy may be suggested. While a hysterectomy may be acceptable to an older patient, hysterectomy is clearly not ideal for a younger woman who wishes to retain the option to bear children.

Recall that the TCM pathologies outlined above include spleen qi vacuity, blood heat, blood stasis, and kidney yin and/or yang vacuity. From an integrative medical point of view, blood stasis should be considered when there are retained placental fragments or a history of incomplete miscarriage. Kidney vacuity is associated with endocrine system deficiencies and low hormone levels.

Here is an example of how severe blood stasis may be. While on duty at Guangzhou Hospital, I was once sent by ambulance to a small village hospital where a woman had been brought in with heavy bleeding. She was very close to death, with her blood pressure near zero. When I arrived, I found her lying on a table covered in blood. She had experienced a miscarriage, but some tissue remained inside and was blocking the cervix. In this case, surgery was the only option to save her life. I rushed her to the operating room and removed all the retained tissue. The bleeding stopped immediately and her blood pressure returned to normal.

In another example, I successfully used TCM to treat bleeding caused by blood stasis. At this time, I had been learning from a famous doctor for three years and had gained much experience. The school I attended sent me to treat the governor's wife who had been bleeding for a month without a break. I knew it was very important for me to succeed in my treatment. So I first tried to supplement the qi, blood, and kidney — all without success. I decided to change the formula and add medicinals to quicken the blood. This may at first seem counterintuitive. After all, if I wished to stop the bleeding, why would I want to move the blood more? But this case turned out to be a situation of blood stasis, and adding the blood-quickening medicinals immediately stopped the bleeding.

The point of these two stories are that, if metrorrhagia is caused by blood stasis, if one does not remove the blood stasis, the bleeding will not stop.

Treatment method: In clinic, the four TCM patterns mentioned above tend to be mixed together. This complicates the approach and means that we need a base formula that can be modified to fit the individual patient's situation. The formula I use is called **Gong Xue Fang (Uterine Bleeding Formula)**. It is composed of:

Dang Shen (Codonopsis Radix)
Bai Zhu (Atractylodis Macrocephalae Rhizoma)
Shan Zhu Yu (Corni Fructus)
Xu Duan (Dipsaci Radix)

Formula analysis

In this formula, Dang Shen supplements the qi and, along with Bai Zhu, fortifies the spleen. Shan Zhu Yu secures the kidney by supporting the yin and securing essence. Xu Duan warms and supplements kidney yang. Both Shan Zhu Yu and Xu Duan also are well-known to empirically stop uterine bleeding, although the actions by which they do so are different. Shan Zhu Yu stops bleeding by securing the kidney and liver channels, while Xu Duan promotes the movement of blood in these channels. These two medicinals complement one another very well to successfully address uterine bleeding due to a combination of kidney insecurity and blood stasis. Also, Bai Zhu and Xu Duan both "quiet the fetus" (an tai 安胎). This means that these two medicinals have a special connection with the uterus and act to reduce uterine contractility. Thus, they are first-rate choices for helping to stop uterine bleeding. Finally, the aspect of spleen qi supplementation is not to be overlooked. It is only by fortifying the spleen's function of containing the blood that a long-term resolution to abnormal uterine bleeding may be achieved. Thus this formula embodies Ye Tian-shi's three principles of stopping bleeding: 1) using empirical means to stop bleeding, 2) treating the cause of bleeding, and 3) securing the root.

Modifications:

Two main modifications of Gong Xue Fang (Uterine Blood Formula) are especially useful when treating abnormal uterine bleeding in order to more directly address the individual patient's situation.

- For significant spleen and kidney vacuity with blood stasis, use Zhi Beng Fang (Check Flooding Formula). This is Gong Xue Fang (Uterine Blood Formula) with the additions of Huang Qi (Astragali Radix) to boost the qi and supplement the middle (burner), Yi Mu Cao (Leonuri Herba) to contract the uterus and stop bleeding, and San Qi (Notoginseng Radix) to quicken the blood and stop bleeding.

- For heavy bleeding, use Da Gong Xue Fang (Major Uterine Bleeding Formula). This is Zhi Beng Fang (Check Flooding Formula) with two additional medicinals: Mo Han Lian (Ecliptae Herba) to stop heat-related bleeding, and Ai Ye (Artemisiae Argyi Folium) to stop cold-related bleeding. This is a strong formula to stop bleeding, whether the bleeding is related to heat, cold, or both.

In addition to this, individual medicinals may be added to customize the formula to the patient's needs. For example:

- For kidney yang vacuity, add Hu Jiao (Piperis Fructus) and/or Bu Gu Zhi (Psoraleae Fructus).

- For kidney yin vacuity, Nu Zhen Zi (Ligustri Lucidi Fructus) is a good choice to nourish the kidney yin without cooling the formula too much. Mo Han Lian (Ecliptae Herba) is a colder herb that can be added or increased as it stops bleeding as well as nourishing kidney yin and clearing vacuity heat.

- For spleen qi vacuity, Huang Qi (Astragali Radix) and Ren Shen (Ginseng Radix) are good choices. Both of these medicinals are warmer. Therefore, if one does not want to add warmth to the formula (as in a case of spleen yin vacuity), Shan Yao (Dioscoreae Rhizoma) may be more suitable. Shan Yao has the added benefit of nourishing the kidney.

- For vacuity heat, Sheng Di Huang (Rehmanniae Radix), Mai Men Dong

(Ophiopogonis Radix), and Zhi Zi (Gardeniae Fructus) are all appropriate. Mai Men Dong and Sheng Di Huang are more nourishing and enriching, while Zhi Zi is better for clearing vacuity fire that manifests as irritability, restlessness, and insomnia.

- For replete heat, Huang Qin (Scutellariae Radix) is a good choice. This medicinal, although typically associated with clearing heat from the upper burner, is able to quiet the fetus and stop bleeding. Thus it has a known empirical effect on uterine bleeding.

- For blood stasis, add Hong Hua (Carthami Flos), Pu Huang (Typhae Pollen), and/or Wu Ling Zhi (Trogopteri Faeces) to quicken the blood and transform stasis. Wu Ling Zhi and Pu Huang both have the additional function of stopping bleeding. In addition, Wu Ling Zhi is good for pain.

Once the root (*i.e.*, the underlying disease mechanism) has been addressed, it is important to also treat the bleeding itself (*i.e.*, the tip or branch). Many different medicinals stop bleeding. Thus one must carefully choose which ingredients are the most appropriate for the patient's condition. For example:

- For heat-related bleeding, add Di Yu (Sanguisorbae Radix) and Ce Bai Ye (Platycladi Cacumen).

- For cold-related bleeding, Ai Ye (Artemisiae Argyi Folium) and Jing Jie Tan (charred Schizonepetae Herba) are best.

- If the patient has lost a great deal of blood and is dizzy, supplement the blood and stop bleeding by adding E Jiao (Asini Corii Colla) if there is yin vacuity or Lu Jiao Jiao (Cervi Cornus Gelatinum) if there is yang vacuity.

- If the patient is passing blood clots, it is important to quicken the blood, dispel stasis, and stop bleeding by adding charred Shan Zha (Crataegi Fructus) or Xue Yu Tan (Crinis Carbonisatus).

- For heart palpitations and fright following the loss of a large quantity of blood, add Mu Li (Ostreae Concha) and Long Gu (Mastodi Ossis Fossilia). These heavy, settling medicinals both quiet the spirit as well as secure and astringe.

- Finally, in the case of continuing spotting over a long period of time, use

Xiao Gong Xue Fang (Minor Uterine Bleeding Formula). This is composed of Xiao Yao San (Free Wanderer Powder) plus Dang Shen (Codonopsis Radix) to further supplement the spleen and help it to contain the blood, Shan Zhu Yu (Corni Fructus) to supplement the kidney and nourish yin, Yi Mu Cao (Leonuri Herba) to contract the uterus and stop bleeding, and San Qi (Notoginseng Radix) to quicken the blood and stop bleeding.

Acupuncture protocols:

Basic protocol for metrorrhagia:

GV20 (Bai Hui), SP6 (San Yin Jiao), ST36 (Zu San Li), CV4 (Guan Yuan), LR3 (Tai Chong), SP1 (Yin Bai)

GV20 upbears yang. Thus it helps stop bleeding due to downward falling of the central qi (*i.e.*, spleen vacuity). SP6 is the intersection point of the three leg yin channels and is a main point for the regulation of the uterus and associated bleeding. SP6 also works in conjunction with ST36 to supplement both the qi and blood. By fortifying the spleen, we are also helping the spleen to contain the blood and stop the bleeding. CV4 is a primary local point for supplementing the qi and blood and strengthening the female gynecological system. It is also an intersection point for the three leg yin channels and acts on the uterus in a similar supportive capacity as SP6. LR3 regulates the blood as it relates to the reproductive cycle. SP1 is an empirical point used to effectively stop uterine bleeding.

Modifications:
- If kidney yin vacuity is evident due to symptoms such as night sweating, hot flashes, five-center heat, malar flushing, and/or difficulty sleeping through the night, KI6 (Zhao Hai) should be added to enrich yin.

- If there is pain, clotting, and spotting due to blood stasis, add SP10 (Xu Hai) and LR8 (Qu Quan). If the pain is severe, SP8 (Di Ji) is a better choice than SP10.

- For cases involving cold signs suggesting kidney yang vacuity, moxa should be applied to CV6 (Qi Hai), ST36, and GV20.

- If blood heat is a factor, it can be cleared by adding LI11 (Qu Chi) and SP10 (Xue Hai). If there are also signs of liver heat, such as irritability, red eyes, or burning urination, LR2 (Xing Jian) can be used.

Case Study

The patient, a 46-year-old female, came to the hospital where I worked complaining of heavy uterine bleeding for 17 days. At admissions, the woman had suddenly lost consciousness and fell to the floor, and the admitting nurse called me to help her. I immediately saw a lot of blood on the floor and knew I needed to act quickly. I first administered acupuncture at GV20 (Bai Hui), and then moxibustion. The patient regained consciousness and I gave her a piece of Ren Shen (Ginseng Radix) which she chewed and then swallowed. Ren Shen is very effective at greatly supplementing the qi and stemming desertion. Thus it helps stop bleeding in a situation like this. To be optimally effective, Ren Shen should be cooked in a double boiler for at least an hour. However, it is fine when dealing with an emergency situation such as this to give the uncooked Ren Shen first.

The patient's face was very pale and she was very fatigued. She was frightened and had heart palpitations. Her hands and feet were cold and numb, and she felt an aversion to wind. Her appetite was poor and she experienced nausea and unformed bowel movements. She felt slight pain in her lower abdomen and had heavy bleeding with some clots. Her tongue was pale and slightly purple, with teethmarks on its edges and white fur. Her pulse was slow, deep, and weak.

Pattern identification: Heart-spleen dual vacuity, kidney yang vacuity, and blood stasis

This patient was a picture of vacuity with the exception of the lower abdominal pain and bleeding with clots which, along with a slightly purple tongue, suggested an element of blood stasis. Fatigue, poor appetite, nausea, and unformed bowel movements in conjunction with a pale, teethmarked tongue and weak pulse suggested spleen qi vacuity. Additionally, she had cold signs and a slow, deep pulse which tell us that there was yang vacuity. Finally, she was frightened, experienced heart palpitations, and had a pale face. These were signs of heart blood vacuity.

Treatment principles:

Fortify the spleen and supplement the qi, warm the kidney and supplement yang, quicken the blood and stop bleeding, nourish the heart and quiet the spirit

Formula: Modified Da Gong Xue Fang (Major Uterine Bleeding Formula)

Dang Shen (Codonopsis Radix)
Bai Zhu (Atractylodis Macrocephalae Rhizoma)

Shan Zhu Yu (Corni Fructus)
Xu Duan (Dipsaci Radix)
Huang Qi (Astragali Radix)
Bu Gu Zhi (Psoraleae Fructus)
San Qi (Notoginseng Radix)
Ai Ye (Artemisiae Argyi Folium)
Mu Li (Ostreae Concha)
Long Gu (Mastodi Ossis Fossilia)

Acupuncture protocol:

Moxa was applied at LR1 (Da Dun), SP1 (Yin Bai) and GV20 (Bai Hui); needles were applied at GV20 (Bai Hui), ST36 (Zu San Li), SP6 (San Yin Jiao), LI4 (He Gu), CV6 (Qi Hai), KI3 (Tai Xi), Ear (Kidney, Spleen, Shen Men).

Treatment analysis:

Because the bleeding was heavy, I used Da Gong Xue Fang as my base formula (see above for detailed analysis). In this case, I removed Mo Han Lian (Ecliptae Herba) and Yi Mu Cao (Leonuri Herba) because the patient exhibited yang vacuity and thus cold medicinals for her would not be a good idea. To stop bleeding, the primary medicinals were San Qi and Ai Ye. San Qi is especially good to both quicken the blood and stop bleeding, while Ai Ye is good for bleeding due to cold. To help Xu Duan supplement the kidney and warm yang, I added Bu Gu Zhi. This herb is warmly astringing and also helped with the unformed stool. I added Huang Qi to help Dang Shen and Bai Zhu fortify the spleen and supplement the qi. Huang Qi also upbears the clear qi. Thus it is similar in effect to needling GV20. This helps to discourage the downward sinking of qi and, therefore, the movement of blood downward, remembering that the qi moves the blood. In this way, this medicinal helps to stop bleeding even though it is not categorized as a bleeding-staunching medicinal. To quiet the spirit and secure and astringe the fluids of the heart, I added Mu Li and Long Gu.

LR1 and SP1 were chosen because they are the Jing well points of the channels. Jing well points regulate and control blood and are empirically effective for uterine bleeding in particular. GV20 was used to upbear yang and, therefore, discourage the downward flow of blood. Because of the vacuity cold, I knew this patient would benefit from the warmth of the moxa which helped fortify the spleen qi on one hand and invigorate kidney yang on the other. SP6 is the intersection point of the three leg yin channels and was used here to regulate the uterus and stop uterine bleeding. SP6 and ST36 together were used to supplement and regulate the qi and blood. CV6 was chosen to supplement the kidney yang. LI4 was used to regulate the upbearing and downbearing of the qi dynamic or mechanism. LI4 also assists the uterus to expel any blood stasis that is contributing to the bleeding. Because LI4 promotes upbearing and downbearing, it does not simply sink the qi (which clearly, with yang and spleen qi vacuity, was already a problem). Finally, the source point KI3 was included for general supplementation of the kidney. Ear Spleen and Kidney points were chosen to supplment the spleen and kidney, while Ear Shen Men was meant to quiet the patient's spirit.

Outcome

After three packages of these medicinals, the bleeding stopped completely. The patient was kept in the hospital for another month and continued to take Tiao Jing Hou Fang (Regulate Menses After Period Formula). Readers should recall that this is Ding Jing Fang (Stabilize the Menses Formula), our basic cycle-regulating formula, with Wu Wei Zi (Schisandrae Fructus) added. This resulted in the patient's menses coming at the regular interval with a normal amount of bleeding.

6

Premenstrual Syndrome (PMS)

Western Medical View

Premenstrual syndrome (PMS) is a complicated mixture of physical and psychological conditions whose causes are still unknown. It occurs only in the second half of the menstrual cycle (the luteal phase) and is relieved by the onset of menses. Approximately 40% of women experience widely varying symptoms during the two weeks preceding menses. Approximately 2-3% of women experience such severe symptoms that their personal and professional lives are disrupted.

Causes:

The main risk factors for experiencing PMS are:
- Stressful lifestyle
- Family history of PMS
- Hypoglycemia
- Vitamin B-6 deficiency
- Prolactin excess
- Lowered levels of neurotransmitters
- Estrogen excess
- Estrogen/progesterone imbalance
- Hormone allergy

Symptoms: The main hallmark of PMS is that symptoms occur only during the second half of the menstrual cycle. These symptoms include physical, psychologcal, and behavioral changes.

Physical symptoms vary greatly among women, but the most commonly seen physical symptoms of PMS are:

- Fluid retention

- Breast tenderness
- Headaches
- Pain in the pelvic region
- Diarrhea or constipation
- Hot flashes
- Acne or other skin problems
- Food cravings, particularly for sweets

Psychological symptoms:

- Emotional lability
- Irritability, anxiety, depression, crying spells, aggression
- Changes in libido
- Fatigue
- Insomnia
- Decreased concentration

Diagnosis:

- Rule out any symptoms that occur during the first half of the menstrual cycle
- To establish history, record a diary of symptoms for at least two consecutive months
- Rule out other psychiatric disorders

Treatment:

Most cases of PMS are treated with:
- Dietary changes and regular exercise 3-4 days a week
- High protein diet
- Vitamin B-6 supplementation

More severe cases are treated with:
- Nonsteroidal anti-inflammatory drugs (NSAIDs)
- Potassium-saving diuretics
- Prolactin inhibitor (bromocriptine)
- Testosterone agonist (Danazol®)
- Antianxiety drugs
- Psychotherapy
- Progesterone
- Surgery, in extreme cases resistant to other forms of treatment

Traditional Chinese Medical View

Premenstrual syndrome (PMS) refers to the physical or emotional symptoms or changes that occur between ovulation and onset of menstruation, usually starting 7-10 days before the onset of menstruation. These symptoms may include breast distention and pain, cravings, fatigue, insomnia, headaches, diarrhea, lower abdominal distention and pain, lower back pain, dizziness, chills, and mood changes, such as irritability, tearfulness, depression, and anxiety.

Treatment based on pattern identification:

Liver qi depression & binding (*gan qi yu jie* 肝气郁结)

Signs & symptoms: Irritability, mood swings, headaches, dizziness, restlessness, breast distention, ribside distention or pain, insomnia. If the liver counterflows horizontally and assails on the spleen, there may be diarrhea or abdominal distention.

Tongue: Purplish red

Pulse: Bowstring, possibly rapid (if depression has transformed heat)

Treatment principles: Course liver and resolve depression

Formula: Xiao Yao San (Free Wanderer Powder)

> Chai Hu (Bupleuri Radix)
> Bai Shao (Paeoniae Radix Alba)
> Dang Gui (Angelicae Sinensis Radix)
> Bai Zhu (Atractylodis Macrocephalae Rhizoma)
> Fu Ling (Poria)
> Bo He (Menthae Herba)
> Sheng Jiang (Zingiberis Rhizoma Recens)
> Zhi Gan Cao (Glycyrrhizae Radix cum Liquido Fricta)

Modifications:
- For heat due to depression, add Zhi Zi (Gardeniae Fructus) and Mu Dan Pi (Moutan Cortex).

- For more severe liver depression qi stagnation, add Xiang Fu (Cyperi Rhizoma), Yu Jin (Curcumae Radix), Zhi Ke (Qiao) (Aurantii Fructus), Chuan Xiong (Chuanxiong Rhizoma), and/or Chen Pi (Citri Reticulatae Pericarpium).

- For ascendant liver yang hyperactivity, add Tian Ma (Gastrodiae Rhizoma), Gou Teng (Uncariae Ramulus cum Uncis), and/or Ci Ji Li (Tribuli Fructus).

- For breast distention and pain, add Wang Bu Liu Xing (Vaccariae Semen), Ju He (Citri Reticulatae Semen), Zhe Bei Mu (Fritillariae Thunbergii Bulbus), Ban Xia (Pinelliae Rhizoma), Qing Pi (Citri Reticulatae Pericarpium Viride), and/or Gua Lou (Trichosanthis Fructus).

- For diarrhea caused by liver qi assailing the spleen, add Chen Pi (Citri Reticulatae Pericarpium) and Fang Feng (Saposhnikoviae Radix).

- For insomnia and to quiet the spirit, add Suan Zao Ren (Ziziphi Spinosi Semen) and Wu Wei Zi (Schisandrae Fructus).

Blood vacuity (*xue xu* 血虚)

Signs & symptoms: If blood does not nourish liver yin, ascendant liver yang hyperactivity and internal stirring of liver wind signs may be seen, such as headache, migraine, dizziness, restlessness, and light-headedness. If blood does not nourish the heart, insomnia, difficulty concentrating, and poor memory may be seen. If blood does not nourish the body, it produces body aches.

Tongue: Pale and small with thin, dry fur. If there is ascendant liver yang hyperactivity or liver fire flaming upward, the tongue will be red.

Pulse: Thin, small. If there is ascendant liver yang hyperactivity or liver fire flaming upward, the pulse may be bowstring, thin, and rapid.

Treatment principles: Nourish blood, calm (or level) liver and extinguish wind. Calm the liver and subdue yang if necessary.

Formula: Qi Ju Di Huang Wan (Lycium Berry, Chrysanthemum & Rehmannia Pill)

> Shu Di Huang (Rehmanniae Radix Praeparata)
> Shan Zhu Yu (Corni Fructus)
> Shan Yao (Dioscoreae Rhizoma)
> Ze Xie (Alismatis Rhizoma)
> Mu Dan Pi (Moutan Cortex)
> Fu Ling (Poria)
> Gou Qi Zi (Lycii Fructus)
> Ju Hua (Chrysanthemi Flos)

Modifications:
- For internal stirring of liver wind, add Gou Teng (Uncariae Ramulus cum Uncis), Tian Ma (Gastrodiae Rhizoma), Mu Li (Ostreae Concha), Long Gu (Mastodi Ossis Fossilia), and/or Shi Jue Ming (Haliotidis Concha).

- For heart yin-blood vacuity, add Mai Men Dong (Ophiopogonis Radix) and Dan Shen (Salviae Miltiorrhizae Radix).

- For insomnia and to quiet the spirit, add Suan Zao Ren (Ziziphi Spinosi Semen) and Wu Wei Zi (Schisandrae Fructus).

- For wind-damp causing headache, use Wen Dan Tang (Gallbladder-warming Decoction) plus Tian Ma (Gastrodiae Rhizoma), Gou Teng (Uncariae Ramulus cum Uncis), and Bai Shao (Paeoniae Radix Alba).

Spleen-kidney yang vacuity (*pi shen yang xu* 脾肾阳虚)

Signs & symptoms: When yang (fire) of the spleen and kidney is vacuous, cold may constrict and accumulate in the body causing such symptoms as water swelling, diarrhea, and lower back pain.

Tongue: Pale and swollen with teethmarks on its edges and moist, thin, white fur

Pulse: Deep, weak

Treatment principles: Fortify the spleen and supplement the qi, supplement the kidney and warm yang

Formula: Jian Gu Tang (Fortifying & Securing Decoction)

Dang Shen (Codonopsis Radix)
Bai Zhu (Atractylodis Macrocephalae Rhizoma)
Fu Ling (Poria)
Yi Yi Ren (Coicis Semen)
Ba Ji Tian (Morindae Officinalis Radix)

Modifications:

- For abdominal distention, add Chen Pi (Citri Reticulatae Pericarpium) and Sha Ren (Amomi Fructus).

- For additional yang supplementation and warming, add Bu Gu Zhi (Psoraleae Fructus), Suo Yang (Cynomorii Herba), Rou Gui (Cinnamomi Cortex), and/or Gan Jiang (Zingiberis Rhizoma).

Clinical Treatment

As stated above, the disease mechanisms of PMS include liver depression qi stagnation, vacuities of the spleen and kidney, and vacuity of blood with ascendant liver yang hyperactivity and its evolutions of liver fire flaming upward and liver wind stirring internally. These disease mechanisms rarely occur alone in real life. Thus we often see a myriad of signs and symptoms in PMS including emotional issues, digestive problems, insomnia, fatigue, and headaches. Because the manifestations of PMS can be so varied, modifications are especially important and are detailed below.

Formulas:

Before menstruation:

Xiao Yao Fang (Relaxed Wanderer Formula) with appropriate modifications

Xiao Yao Fang (Relaxed Wanderer Formula)

> Chai Hu (Bupleuri Radix)
> Dang Gui (Angelicae Sinensis Radix)
> Bai Shao (Paeoniae Radix Alba)
> Bai Zhu (Atractylodis Macrocephalae Rhizoma)
> Fu Ling (Poria)
> Gan Cao (Glycyrrhizae Radix)

Formula analysis

Chai Hu courses the liver and rectifies the qi, while Bai Shao nourishes the blood and emoliates the liver. Together, these two medicinals harmonize the liver and get a better effect than either alone. Dang Gui and Bai Shao supplement the blood. Dang Gui also quickens the blood. Bai Zhu and Fu Ling fortify the spleen (and eliminate dampness if necessary). Gan Cao assists with supplementing the spleen as well as harmonizing the other medicinals in the formula. Bai Shao and Gan Cao together have the added benefit of helping to relieve painful cramping, as in Shao Yao Gan Cao Tang (Peony & Licorice Decoction).

Modifications:

As can be seen from this discussion, Xiao Yao Fang (Relaxed Wanderer Formula) primarily courses and harmonizes the liver and supplements the spleen. However, it also contains medicinals to nourish the blood. Of course, this formula should be modified to reflect the proportion of signs and symptoms relating to these various pathologies as well as to address kidney vacuity and ascendant liver yang hyperactivity should those elements be present. For example:

• For heat arising from qi stagnation, add Zhi Zi (Gardeniae Fructus) and Mu Dan Pi (Moutan Cortex).

• In cases of heart yin vacuity, add Mai Men Dong (Ophiopogonis Radix).

• If there is insomnia, consider including Suan Zao Ren (Ziziphi Spinosi Semen) and Wu Wei Zi (Schisandrae Fructus). The former is more nourishing and is especially appropriate in the case of heart blood vacuity, while the latter is securing and astringing and more helpful for qi and yin vacuity patterns.

• Severe liver depression qi stagnation resulting in breast pain and distention may be relieved with stronger qi-medicinals such as Zhi Ke (Qiao) (Aurantii Fructus) and Yu Jin (Curcumae Radix).

• When liver yang is rising, it may be calmed and subdued by adding Tian Ma (Gastrodiae Rhizoma) and Gou Teng (Uncariae Ramulus cum Uncis). If headache or dizziness are a problem, Ci Ji Li (Tribuli Fructus) is a good choice.

• In the event of diarrhea due to spleen-kidney yang vacuity, Dang Gui should be removed and other medicinals may be added, such as Dang Shen (Codonopsis Radix), Shan Yao (Dioscoreae Rhizoma), and Huang Qi (Astragali Radix) to supplement the spleen, and Wu Wei Zi (Schisandrae Fructus) to secure and astringe. Shan Yao also helps secure and astringe. One should be cautious with warming medicinals because there is typically a tendency toward heat due to qi stagnation in cases of PMS.

After menstruation:

Tiao Jing Hou Fang (Menstruation-regulating Later Formula) with appropriate modifications

Tiao Jing Hou Fang (Menstruation-regulating Later Formula)

Dang Gui (Angelicae Sinensis Radix)
Bai Shao (Paeoniae Radix Alba)
Wu Wei Zi (Schisandrae Fructus)
Tu Si Zi (Cuscutae Semen)
Ba Ji Tian (Morindae Officinalis Radix)
Shu Di Huang (Rehmanniae Radix Praeparata)
Fu Ling (Poria)
Shan Yao (Dioscoreae Rhizoma)
Dang Shen (Codonopsis Radix)
Zhi Gan Cao (Glycyrrhizae Radix cum Liquido Fricta)
Chai Hu (Bupleuri Radix)

Formula analysis

This formula is Ding Jing Fang (Stabilize the Menses Formula) with Wu Wei Zi added. As discussed above, within Ding Jing Fang, Shu Di Huang and Tu Si Zi supplement the kidney in a broad sense, while Ba Ji Tian specifically supplements the kidney and invigorates yang. Fu Ling, Zhi Gan Cao, Shan Yao, and Dang Shen fortify the spleen and supplement the qi. Chai Hu and Bai Shao harmonize the liver and regulate the qi. Dang Gui and Shu Di Huang nourish the blood. Dang Gui also quickens the blood. Wu Wei Zi has a securing and astringing function. Therefore, it supplments the kidney and secures the essence. It also quiets the spirit.

Modifications:

- For severe liver depression qi stagnation, the qi-moving action of the formula should be supplemented with Xiang Fu (Cyperi Rhizoma).

- If there is diarrhea, Dang Gui and Shu Di Huang should be removed and the following medicinals may be added: Chen Pi (Citri Reticulatae Pericarpium) to support the spleen and dry dampness and Shan Zhu Yu (Corni Fructus) to secure and astringe.

- When the heart is disturbed, resulting in insomnia or heart palpitations, spirit-quieting medicinals, such as Suan Zao Ren (Ziziphi Spinosi Semen), Long Yan Rou (Longan Arillus), Mu Li (Ostreae Concha), and calcined Long Gu (Mastodi Ossis Fossilia), may provide relief. Suan Zao Ren nourishes heart yin, Long Yan Rou nourishes heart blood, and Mu Li and calcined Long Gu are heavy, settling, spirit-quieting medicinals.

- For blood vacuity, supplementing agents such as Gou Qi Zi (Lycii Fructus) and Huang Qi (Astragali Radix) may be added. Gou Qi Zi supplements the kidney and blood, while Huang Qi supplements both the qi and blood and strengthens the spleen's function of engendering the blood.

- In the event of qi vacuity, Huang Qi (Astragali Radix) is recommended.

- For spleen yang vacuity, Bai Zhu is a good choice.

Acupuncture protocol:

It is important to note that PMS should not be treated only before menstruation (*i.e.*, at the time symptoms appear) but after menstruation also in order to regulate and supplement the qi, blood, yin, and yang. The symptoms of PMS are branch symptoms that are rooted in the overall imbalance of the menstrual cycle. For this reason, points in this protocol are very similar to the points used for general menstrual regulation.

Before menstruation:

ST36 (Zu San Li), SP6 (San Yin Jiao), KI3 (Tai Xi), LR3 (Tai Chong), LI4 (He Gu), Yin Tang (M-HN-3), Ear Shen Men

This protocol is for when symptoms of PMS are prevalent, and so, during this time, it is necessary to focus on moving both the qi and blood, This is because many of the symptoms at this time in the cycle, such as pain and moodiness, primarily result from stagnation. LI4 and LR3 together free the flow of the channels and regulate the qi. This helps to relieve pain, bloating, and moodiness that results from stagnant qi. When moving qi and blood, we must also be careful to supplement and nourish so that these vital substances are not dissipated. SP6 and ST36 promote the transformation and engenderment of the qi and blood as well as help to quicken the blood. KI3 supports the menstrual cycle at its foundation. The source qi of the kidney is a critical part of the engenderment of blood. Finally, we also should include points to directly quiet the spirit. Yin Tang and Ear Shen Men are excellent for this purpose.

Modifications:

- For heat arising from qi stagnation, substitute LR2 (Xing Jian) for LR3.

- In case of heart yin vacuity, HT6 (Yin Xi) may be added. However, for heart blood vacuity, use HT7 (Shen Men) instead.

- Severe liver depression qi stagnation resulting in breast pain and distention may be relieved by adding CV17 (Dan Zhong) or LR14 (Qi Men).

- GV20 (Bai Hui) can be added to help to quiet the spirit and clear the mind. If liver yang is rising, creating headache, severe anxiety, irritability, dizziness, or a sensation of heat rising to the head, KI1 (Yong Quan) may be added to move the qi downward.

- For severe lower abdominal pain, substitute SP8 (Di Ji) for SP6.

- For diarrhea due to spleen-kidney yang vacuity, warming and harmonizing moxibustion may be applied to SP6.

After menstruation:

ST36 (Zu San Li), SP6 (San Yin Jiao), KI3 (Tai Xi), Yin Tang (M-HN-3)

During this time, the underlying pattern or patterns should be addressed more directly. Because of this, point selection can be quite variable. I suggest the above point prescription as a starting place. This combination supplements the qi and blood, kidney and spleen, and quiets the spirit. SP6, the intersection point of the three leg yin channels, is also able to gently encourage the liver to move qi smoothly throughout the body. Additions can be made according to the individual patient's situation as below:

- For liver qi stagnation throughout the cycle, LR13 (Zhang Men) may be added.

- If there is diarrhea due to yang vacuity, warming and harmonizing moxibustion may be applied to SP6. If the diarrhea is due to liver assailing the spleen, LR13 should be sufficient to alleviate this.

- When the heart spirit is disturbed due to blood vacuity failing to nourish it, resulting in insomnia or heart palpitations, HT7 (Shen Men) may be added.

- For liver blood vacuity, LR3 (Tai Chong) is an appropriate addition.

Case Study

A 32-year-old patient reported symptoms of PMS beginning one week before the onset of menstruation. She felt very emotional. She cried a lot and felt easily irritated and anxious. Her breasts were sore and distended. Her sleep was poor. She felt frequently thirsty and tended towards constipation. She also experienced headaches. The patient's tongue was slightly pale with a red tip, cracks, and scanty, white fur. Her pulse was small, bowstring, slightly fast, and weak in the cubit, especially on the right side.

Pattern identification: Kidney yin vacuity, heart yin & blood vacuity, liver depression qi stagnation, spleen qi vacuity

Liver depression qi stagnation was indicated by the patient's depression and irritability. This was further supported by the presence of breast distention, headaches, constipation, and a bowstring pulse. Her cubit pulses, thirst, and cracked tongue with scanty fur support a finding of kidney yin vacuity. Anxiety, poor sleep, and the color of her tongue, body and tip, indicate heart yin and blood vacuity. Her small pulse and slightly pale tongue also suggest a possible small amount of spleen qi vacuity. Since we understand the relationship between the liver and spleen, we already know this is a likely component of the syndrome and, therefore, may include this in the diagnosis despite the lack of more prominent digestive symptoms.

Treatment principles: Nourish kidney and heart yin, course the liver and rectify the qi, fortify the spleen and supplement the qi.

Formulas:

Before menstruation:

Xiao Yao Fang (Relaxed Wanderer Formula) plus Tian Ma (Gastrodiae Rhizoma), Shu Di Huang (Rehmanniae Radix Praeparata), Zhi Ke (Qiao) (Aurantii Fructus), Suan Zao Ren (Ziziphi Spinosi Semen), Mai Men Dong (Ophiopogonis Radix)

Shu Di Huang and Zhi Ke together free the flow of the intestines, *i.e.*, promote bowel movements. In this case, Shu Di Huang moistens, while Zhi Ke regulates qi in the intestines. Suan Zao Ren and Tian Ma also have moistening properties for the intestines. Suan Zao Ren nourishes the heart and quiets the spirit. Thus it also helps with sleep. Mai Men Dong nourishes yin and clears vacuity heat. Tian Ma calms liver, subdues yang, and relieves headache.

After menstruation:

Tiao Jing Hou Fang (Menstruation-regulating Later Formula) minus Ba Ji Tian (Morindae Officinalis Radix), which is too warm for this case, but plus Suan Zao Ren (Ziziphi Spinosi Semen) and Mai Men Dong (Ophiopogonis Radix) to continue nourishing the heart blood and yin while clearing vacuity heat.

Outcome

After one month of treatment, the patient's PMS symptoms were significantly diminished. After three months of treatment, she experienced no PMS at all. She happily reported that her menstruation began so asymptomatically that she was actually surprised by its arrival.

7

Dysmenorrhea

Western Medical View

Menstrual pain in the lower abdomen.

Categories:

- Primary dysmenorrhea (functional dysmenorrhea)
- Secondary dysmenorrhea (acquired dysmenorrhea, *i.e.*, dysmenorrhea secondary to some other disease or condition)

Primary dysmenorrhea

Symptoms:

- Pain during menstruation in the lower abdominal region
- Cramping, colicky or constant dull ache
- Begins before or with menses, peaking after 24 hours and decreasing after two days
- Sometimes the pain is incapacitating, disrupting both personal and professional life
- Pain is not associated with tissue lesions or anatomical abnormalities
- May be accompanied by headache, nausea, constipation, diarrhea, frequent urination, weakness and fatigue, clots in menstrual blood
- PMS symptoms may persist during menses
- Onset usually during adolescence and often decreases with age and after pregnancy

Causes:

- Excessive uterine contractions during menstruation

- Uterine lining produces prostaglandins
- Prostaglandins cause contraction of uterine muscles to help shed lining built up during menstrual cycle
- Strong contractions can cut off oxygen flow to the uterine muscles, causing excessive prostaglandin production, contributing to a negative feedback loop
- Excess prostaglandins signal pain response in the central nervous system
- Anxiety, stress, poor diet, insufficient sleep, and lack of exercise all exacerbate the symptoms

Treatment:

- Lifestyle changes: improved nutrition, increased rest and exercise
- Use of prostaglandin synthetase inhibitors such as ibuprofen, naproxen or mefenamic acid
- Decreases prostaglandin synthesis, subjective pain sensations and may lower intrauterine pressure
- Most effective if started 24-48 hours before menses and continued for 1-2 days after onset
- Suppress ovulation if pain continues to interfere with normal activity
- Low-dose estrogen-progesterone oral contraceptives to decrease thickness of uterine lining (thinner uterine lining produces fewer prostaglandins)
- Depo-provera, 150 milligrams every 10-12 weeks may also be used. However, a side effect is calcium depletion. Therefore, care must be taken to maintain appropriate levels.
- For persistent nausea and vomiting, use antiemetics

Secondary dysmenorrhea

Symptoms:

- Pain during menstruation caused by abnormality in the pelvic region
- Lower abdominal pain, nausea, vomiting, diarrhea, headaches, weakness and fainting
- Pain similar to menstrual cramps, but often lasting longer than the menses
- Pain at any time of the month
- Usually occurs after a history of normal periods
- Onset at any time during a woman's life
- Severity varies from cycle to cycle
- Continues throughout reproductive years

Causes:

- Endometriosis (tissue from lining of uterus implants elsewhere)

- Adenomyosis (benign growths in the uterine walls)
- Cramping pain from submucosal fibroid or endometrial polyp extruding from uterus
- Pelvic inflammatory disease (PID) or other infections
- Continuous diffuse lower abdominal pain that increases with menstruation

Structural abnormalities:

- Tight cervical os (from conization, cryocautery or thermocautery) causes pain as the uterus expels tissue through a narrowed opening
- Narrow os impedes menstrual flow and results in pressure and pain
- Adhesions (scarring or adherence of two surfaces)
- Tipped or retroverted uterus makes it difficult for blood to be expelled
- Intrauterine device (IUD)
- Strong or frequent uterine contractions temporarily cut off supply of blood and oxygen to uterus

Treatment:

- Underlying cause must be diagnosed and treated
- Surgery may be required
- Medications prescribed based on the diagnosis
- Pain is treated with non-steroidal anti-inflammatory drugs (NSAIDs) or with prostaglandin synthetase inhibitors. NSAIDs should be taken with food to avoid gastric complications.

Traditional Chinese Medical View

Dysmenorrhea is pain that occurs right before the onset of or during menstruation. This is often experienced as painful cramping in the pelvic or lower abdominal region, sometimes even radiating down the thighs or to the low back, and is often accompanied by bloating and abdominal distention.

Treatment based on pattern identification:
Liver qi depression & binding (*gan qi yu jie* 肝气郁结)

Signs & symptoms: Pain before and in the first few days of menstruation, breast distention and pain, purple clots with pain that is reduced after the clots are expelled, emotional changes

Tongue: Purplish

Pulse: Bowstring

Treatment principles: Course liver and rectify the qi, quicken the blood and relieve pain

Formula: Ge Xia Zhu Yu Tang (Infradiaphragmatic Stasis-expelling Decoction)

Tao Ren (Persicae Semen)
Hong Hua (Carthami Flos)
Dang Gui (Angelicae Sinensis Radix)
Chi Shao (Paeoniae Radix Rubra)
Chuan Xiong (Chuanxiong Rhizoma)
Yan Hu Suo (Corydalis Rhizoma)
Wu Ling Zhi (Trogopteri Faeces)
Mu Dan Pi (Moutan Cortex)
Zhi Xiang Fu (mixed-fried Cyperi Rhizoma)
Zhi Ke (Qiao) (Aurantii Fructus)
Wu Yao (Linderae Radix)
Gan Cao (Glycyrrhizae Radix)

Cold damp obstruction (*han shi zu zhi* 寒湿组滞)

Signs & symptoms: Pain before and in the beginning of menstruation, prefers warmth, dark clots, a sensation of heaviness

Tongue: Pale with moist, white fur

Pulse: Slow, slippery

Treatment principles: Warm the channels and scatter cold, dispel dampness, quicken the blood, and relieve pain

Formula: Shao Fu Zhu Yu Tang (Lesser Abdomen Stasis-expelling Decoction)

Dang Gui (Angelicae Sinensis Radix)
Chi Shao (Paeoniae Radix Rubra)
Chuan Xiong (Chuanxiong Rhizoma)
Xiao Hui Xiang (Foeniculi Fructus)
Gan Jiang (Zingiberis Rhizoma)
Rou Gui (Cinnamomi Cortex)
Yan Hu Suo (Corydalis Rhizoma)
Wu Ling Zhi (Trogopteri Faeces)
Pu Huang (Typhae Pollen)
Mo Yao (Myrrha)

Modifications:

- For dampness, add Ban Xia (Pinelliae Rhizoma), Fu Ling (Poria), Yi Yi Ren (Coicis Semen), Bai Zhu (Atractylodis Macrocephalae Rhizoma), and Cang Zhu (Atractylodis Rhizoma).

- For heavy bleeding, add Yi Mu Cao (Herba Leonuri) and Wu Ling Zhi (Trogopteri Faeces).

- If pain is severe, add San Qi (Radix Pseudoginseng).

- If there is qi and blood stasis with more heat signs, use:

Xue Fu Zhu Yu Tang (House of Blood Stasis-expelling Decoction)

Tao Ren (Persicae Semen)
Hong Hua (Carthami Flos)
Chuan Xiong (Chuanxiong Rhizoma)
Dang Gui (Angelicae Sinensis Radix)
Chi Shao (Paeoniae Radix Rubra)
Sheng Di Huang (Rehmanniae Radix)
Chai Hu (Bupleuri Radix)
Chuan Niu Xi (Cyathulae Radix)
Jie Geng (Platycodonis Radix)
Zhi Ke (Qiao) (Aurantii Fructus)
Gan Cao (Glycyrrhizae Radix)

Liver-kidney vacuity (*gan shen xu* 肝肾虚)

Signs & symptoms: Pain at the end of menstruation or after menstruation, mild pain that decreases with pressure, dizziness, pale face, insomnia

Tongue: Pale

Pulse: Thin, Weak

Treatment principles: Nourish the liver and enrich the kidney

Formula: Tiao Gan Tang (Liver-regulating Decoction)

Shan Yao (Dioscoreae Rhizoma)
Dang Gui (Angelicae Sinensis Radix)
Bai Shao (Paeoniae Radix Alba)
Shan Zhu Yu (Corni Fructus)
Ba Ji Tian (Morindae Officinalis Radix)

Gan Cao (Glycyrrhizae Radix)

E Jiao (Asini Corii Colla) (For poor digestion, substitute with He Shou Wu, Polygoni Multiflori Radix, or Gou Qi Zi, Lycii Fructus.)

Qi & blood vacuity (*qi xue xu* 气血虚)

Signs & symptoms: Pain at the end of menstruation or after menstruation, mild pain, fatigue and dizziness, especially at the end of menstruation

Tongue: Pale, swollen with dry fur

Pulse: Thin

Treatment principles: Nourish blood and supplement the qi, supplement the kidney

Formula: Sheng Yu Tang (Sagacious Cure Decoction)

Huang Qi (Astragali Radix)
Dang Shen (Codonopsis Radix)
Shu Di Huang (Rehmanniae Radix Praeparata)
Dang Gui (Angelicae Sinensis Radix)
Chuan Xiong (Chuanxiong Rhizoma)
Bai Shao (Paeoniae Radix Alba)

Clinical Treatment

The three main TCM disease mechanisms associated with dysmenorrhea are qi stagnation with blood stasis, cold damp stagnation, and vacuity of qi and blood. Notice that two of these are repletion patterns and one is a vacuity pattern. In clinic, dysmenorrhea characterized by severe pain is often due directly to blockage (repletion), but this blockage may be the result of a root vacuity. The clinical presentation of dysmenorrhea is, therefore, most often a combination of repletion and vacuity, although one may predominate. However, it is possible to have a purely vacuous type of pain with dysmenorrhea. This type of pain is less severe in nature.

As with most menstrual problems, it is always important to determine when the last menstruation occurred. In this case, administration of treatment depends upon the timing of the cycle. Based on my clinical experience, dysmenorrhea is most effectively treated in three stages: the week before menstruation, the week of menstruation, and the two weeks following the end of menstruation. In order to resolve dysmenorrhea and prevent recurrence of pain, I use the following three-step approach correlated to these three periods of time.

1. Move the qi: I do this for one week before menstruation in order to prevent stagnation of qi and promote menstruation.

2. Move the qi and blood and relieve pain: I do this for one week during menstruation in order to encourage and assist the menses to flow easily and without pain.

3. Supplement qi & nourish blood: I do this for two weeks following menstruation, to support proper functioning of the system and prepare for healthy menstruation.

Treatment method

Week 4 (seven days before menstruation)

Treatment principle: Move the qi

Formula: Xiao Yao Fang (Relaxed Wanderer Formula) with appropriate modifications

Chai Hu (Bupleuri Radix)
Dang Gui (Angelicae Sinensis Radix)
Bai Shao (Paeoniae Radix Alba)
Bai Zhu (Atractylodis Macrocephalae Rhizoma)
Fu Ling (Poria)
Gan Cao (Glycyrrhizae Radix)

Formula analysis

This formula is Xiao Yao San minus Sheng Jiang (Zingiberis Rhizoma Recens) and Bo He (Menthae Herba). These two medicinals are not necessarily contraindicated here, but they are not essential to the function of the formula and other more useful ingredients may be substituted for them. Also, Bo He may cause sweating and Sheng Jiang can cause heat, neither of which we necessarily want.

Overall, Xiao Yao Fang courses the liver and moves the qi at the same time as it fortifies the spleen and supplements the qi. The medicinals in the formula work together to accomplish this as follows: Chai Hu gathers in the liver channel and moves the qi, thus addressing the liver depression qi stagnation common in PMS that can cause mood swings and physical discomfort. Dang Gui nourishes and gently quickens the blood, thus freeing the flow of menstruation. Bai Shao emolliates the liver and nourishes fluids. Along with Gan Cao, it forms Shao Yao Gan Cao Tang (Peony & Licorice Decoction), a classic formula for easing spasms and cramps. Bai Zhu and Fu Ling both fortify the spleen and help to eliminate any dampness that is either a result or a cause of spleen dysfunction. In addition, Gan Cao harmonizes all the other medicinals in the formula.

Modifications:

From the above analysis, we can see that Xiao Yao Fang is a good formula for our purposes because, prior to the onset of menstruation, we want to move the qi to prevent pain due to stagnation. However, its qi-moving function is not strong enough in this formula for the significant stagnation often seen with dysmenorrhea. Additionally, there may be other symptoms to address, such as heat. The following modifications are suggested, to be used appropriately.

- To address liver qi stagnation more strongly, add Zhi Ke (Qiao) (Aurantii Fructus), Yu Jin (Curcumae Radix), and Xiang Fu (Cyperi Rhizoma). Yu Jin is particularly good in cases of liver depression qi stagnation.

- If heat is present, add Mu Dan Pi (Moutan Cortex) and Zhi Zi (Gardeniae Fructus). This then makes Jia Wei Xiao Yao San (Added Flavors Free Wanderer Powder.

- In case of heart yin vacuity causing palpitations, add Mai Men Dong (Ophiopogonis Radix) to nourish yin and Dan Shen (Salviae Miltiorrhizae Radix) to nourish the heart.

- When headache occurs, Tian Ma (Gastrodiae Rhizoma), Shi Jue Ming (Haliotidis Concha), and Gou Teng (Uncariae Ramulus cum Uncis) are recommended to downbear counterflow and subdue yang.

- For diarrhea, various ingredients may be appropriate: Dang Shen (Codonopsis Radix) may be added to supplment the spleen, Wu Wei Zi (Schisandrae Fructus) may be added to secure the intestines, or Bu Gu Zhi (Psoraleae Fructus) may be added to both secure and warm kidney yang. Alternatively, the ingredients of Tong Xie Yao Fang (Pain & Diarrhea Formula), *i.e.*, Bai Zhu (Atractylodis Macrocephalae Rhizoma), Bai Shao (Paeoniae Radix Alba), Chen Pi (Citri Reticulatae Pericarpium), and Fang Feng (Saposhnikoviae Radix), may be added to secure and astringe, supplement the spleen and dispel dampness, and calm intestinal spasms. In the case of diarrhea, some securing and astringing may be necessary even though, typically, we would not want to strongly secure and astringe immediately prior to the onset of menstruation.

Week 1 (during menstruation when cramping is severe)

Treatment principles: Move the qi, quicken the blood, and relieve pain

Formula: Jing Tong Fang (Formula for Painful Menstruation)

Chai Hu (Bupleuri Radix)
Dang Gui (Angelicae Sinensis Radix)
Bai Shao (Paeoniae Radix Alba)
Bai Zhu (Atractylodis Macrocephalae Rhizoma)
Fu Ling (Poria)
Gan Cao (Glycyrrhizae Radix)
Xiao Hui Xiang (Foeniculi Fructus)
Gui Zhi (Cinnamomi Ramulus)
San Qi (Notoginseng Radix)
Yan Hu Suo (Corydalis Rhizoma)

Formula analysis

This formula is a modification of Xiao Yao Fang (Relaxed Wanderer Formula) discussed above. In addition to the ingredients of Xiao Yao Fang, Xiao Hui Xiang and Gui Zhi warmly move the blood. In particular, Xiao Hui Xiang gathers in the liver channel, making it especially effective for moving blood to and through the uterus. San Qi and Yan Hu Suo break stasis and relieve pain. Although both of these ingredients quicken the blood, San Qi also stops bleeding. Thus it protects against hemorrhage or excessive bleeding from the other blood-quickening medicinals.

Modifications:

- For heavy bleeding, add Shi Xiao San (Sudden Smile Powder), *i.e.*, Wu Ling Zhi (Trogopteri Faeces) and Pu Huang (Typhae Pollen). This combination has the added benefit of breaking blood stasis and, thereby, relieving pain.

- If the patient is highly emotional, consider quieting the spirit by adding Suan Zao Ren (Ziziphi Spinosi Semen) and/or Long Yan Rou (Longan Arillus). Both of these medicinals nourish the heart blood and quiet the spirit. Suan Zao Ren also enters the liver channel and has a securing and astringing function.

- In case of diarrhea, add Chen Pi (Citri Reticulatae Pericarpium) and Ban Xia (Pinelliae Rhizoma) to warmly dry dampness and regulate the qi of the digestive system, including the intestines. You may also recognize these two medicinals as central components of the formula Er Chen Tang (Two Matured Ingredients Decoction) which is very effective against dampness.

- Heart palpitations due to heart heat may be helped by the addition of Dan Shen (Salviae Miltiorrhizae Radix) and Mai Men Dong (Ophiopogonis Radix). These two medicinals work quite differently. So it is important to differentiate the pattern first. Mai Men Dong nourishes yin and clears heat while moistening. Dan Shen quickens the blood and more aggressively clears heat and relieves irritability. Unlike Mai Men Dong, it enters the liver channel, making it a good choice for heat arising from liver depression and blood stasis.

Weeks 2-3 (after menstruation)

Even if the patient's symptoms improve during her first menses following treatment, I believe it is important to ask the patient to return for treatment again after menstruation is finished. This is because the root of the condition needs to be treated in order to prevent the symptoms from returning. It should be explained to the patient that the physical structure of the uterus and cervix can contribute to cramps, for instance, if the uterus is curved or curled or if the cervix is narrow. Supplementing the kidney raises and balances hormone levels (estrogen in particular) and can help the uterus return to normal and thus help to relieve cramping. Therefore, the kidney, spleen, and blood should be supplemented and nourished. However, in doing so, we should not forget to include medicinals that support the movement of the blood and qi since we wish to prevent accumulation of stasis.

Treatment principles: Supplement the qi and nourish the blood

Formula: Jing Hou Fang (After Menstruation Formula)

Chai Hu (Bupleuri Radix)
Dang Gui (Angelicae Sinensis Radix)
Bai Shao (Paeoniae Radix Alba)
Bai Zhu (Atractylodis Macrocephalae Rhizoma)
Fu Ling (Poria)
Gan Cao (Glycyrrhizae Radix)
Dang Shen (Codonopsis Radix)
Shu Di Huang (Rehmanniae Radix Praeparata)
Rou Gui (Cinnamomi Cortex)
Gou Qi Zi (Lycii Fructus)

Formula analysis

This formula is also a modification of Xiao Yao Fang (Relaxed Wanderer Formula) discussed above. In addition to the ingredients of Xiao Yao Fang, the following medicinals are added: Dang Shen fortifies the spleen and supplements the qi. Shu Di Huang nourishes the liver and enriches the kidney. Rou Gui warms yang, guiding it into the channels. By doing so, it eases menstrual pain and promotes menstruation. Gou Qi Zi enters the liver and kidney channels and nourishes the blood.

Modifications:

- For kidney yang vacuity, Tu Si Zi (Cuscutae Semen) and Ba Ji Tian (Morindae Officinalis Radix) may be added. Tu Si Zi has the ability to supplement both yang and yin, while Ba Ji Tian focuses specifically on yang.

- For kidney yin vacuity, good choices include Nu Zhen Zi (Ligustri Lucidi Fructus) and Shan Zhu Yu (Corni Fructus). Shan Zhu Yu is a warm, securing and astringing medicinal. So it is good when there is also sweating from qi or yang vacuity. However, Nu Zhen Zi is a better choice when there is yin vacuity with heat.

- If blood vacuity is present, Huang Jing (Polygonati Rhizoma), Ji Xue Teng (Spatholobi Caulis), and He Shou Wu (Polygoni Multiflori Radix) are appropriate additions. Ji Xue Teng is helpful if there is blood stasis as well as vacuity. He Shou Wu should be used cautiously if the patient has problems with digestion, such as unformed bowel movements. Huang Jing also has a potent qi-supplementing function.

- If liver depression qi stagnation causes mood swings, move liver qi more strongly by adding Xiang Fu (Cyperi Rhizoma) and Zhi Ke (Qiao) (Aurantii Fructus).

- In cases of insomnia after menstruation, consider quieting the spirit with Suan Zao Ren (Ziziphi Spinosi Semen), Long Yan Rou (Longan Arillus), and Wu Wei Zi (Schisandrae Fructus). In this situation, the securing and astringing function of Wu Wei Zi is appropriate since menstruation has ceased and the primary treatment focus at this time is on supplementation.

The Integrated Chinese-Western Medical Treatment of Endometriosis

In Western medicine, dysmenorrhea may be due to endometriosis. This refers to an overgrowth of the uterine lining due to hormonal irregularities. Sometimes, therefore, dysmenorrhea may be addressed by regulating the hormones through the use of birth control pills. As with the case of irregular menstruation, TCM may be used in conjunction with Western hormonal treatment to support and strengthen its actions.

If the case is mild, my approach is as follows:

1. For the first two weeks of contraceptive pill administration, I prescribe Jing Hou Fang (Formula for After Menstruation).

2. For the third week of contraceptive pill administration, I prescribe Xiao Yao Fang (Relaxed Wanderer Formula).

3. For the week of no pills or placebo pills (the week of menstruation), I use Jing Tong Fang (Formula for Painful Menstruation).

If endometriosis is extensive and surgery becomes necessary:

Jing Hou Fang (Formula for After Menstruation) may be used with the addition of San Qi (Notoginseng Radix) and Dan Shen (Salviae Miltiorrhizae Radix). These two medicinals quicken the blood and help prevent scarring and adhesions. Before surgery, Xiao Yao Fang (Relaxed Wanderer Formula) may be helpful, and, since patients may be anxious and concerned, the addition of Long Yan Rou (Longan Arillus) and Suan Zao Ren (Ziziphi Spinosi Semen) are recommended to quiet the spirit. Also, the qi and blood may be further supplmented by adding Dang Shen (Codonopsis Radix) and Shu Di Huang (Rehmanniae Radix Praeparata).

If the case is more serious, stronger treatment is needed:

In that case, I use Huo Jing Zhong Zi Fang (Quicken the Channels to Plant Seeds Decoction) for the three weeks following menstruation. This formula is a modification of Xiao Yao San (Free Wanderer Powder). It moves the qi and quickens the blood, courses the liver and fortifies the spleen. Then I switch the patient to Xiao Zheng Fang (Concretion-dispersing Formula) immediately prior to and during menstruation (from day 25 to day 4 of the new cycle). This formula contains very strong blood-quickening agents. The two formulas are listed below.

Summary:

For a mild case:

Days 8-21 of cycle: Jing Hou Fang (Formula for After Menstruation) (14 days in total)

> Chai Hu (Bupleuri Radix)
> Dang Gui (Angelicae Sinensis Radix)
> Bai Shao (Paeoniae Radix Alba)
> Bai Zhu (Atractylodis Macrocephalae Rhizoma)
> Fu Ling (Poria)
> Gan Cao (Glycyrrhizae Radix)
> Dang Shen (Codonopsis Radix)
> Shu Di Huang (Rehmanniae Radix Praeparata)
> Rou Gui (Cinnamomi Cortex)
> Gou Qi Zi (Lycii Fructus)

As previously discussed, Jing Hou Fang is a modification of Xiao Yao Fang (Relaxed Wanderer Formula) with Dang Shen added to supplement the spleen, Shu Di Huang to nourish the kidney yin, Gou Qi Zi to nourish the blood, and Rou Gui to warm kidney yang.

Days 22-28: Xiao Yao Fang (Relaxed Wanderer Formula) (seven days in total)

> Chai Hu (Bupleuri Radix)
> Dang Gui (Angelicae Sinensis Radix)
> Bai Shao (Paeoniae Radix Alba)
> Bai Zhu (Atractylodis Macrocephalae Rhizoma)
> Fu Ling (Poria)
> Gan Cao (Glycyrrhizae Radix)

Xiao Yao Fang courses the qi and helps to quicken the blood very gently.

Day 1-7 (menses): Jing Tong Fang (Formula for Painful Menstruation) (seven days in total)

> Chai Hu (Bupleuri Radix)
> Dang Gui (Angelicae Sinensis Radix)
> Bai Shao (Paeoniae Radix Alba)
> Bai Zhu (Atractylodis Macrocephalae Rhizoma)
> Fu Ling (Poria)

Gan Cao (Glycyrrhizae Radix)
Xiao Hui Xiang (Foeniculi Fructus)
Gui Zhi (Cinnamomi Ramulus)
San Qi (Notoginseng Radix)
Yan Hu Suo (Corydalis Rhizoma)

Jing Tong Fang is another modification of Xiao Yao Fang (Relaxed Wanderer Formula), this time with stronger ingredients, namely San Qi and Yan Hu Suo, to quicken the blood. These medicinals also are empirically well-known for relieving pain. Also, Gui Zhi helps to move the blood. Both Gui Zhi and Xiao Hui Xiang are warm and acrid, thus encouraging the qi to move.

For a severe case:

Days 5-24: Huo Jing Zhong Zi Fang (Quicken the Channels to Plant Seeds Decoction)

Dang Gui (Angelicae Sinensis Radix)
Chai Hu (Bupleuri Radix)
Dan Shen (Salviae Miltiorrhizae Radix)
Bai Shao (Paeoniae Radix Alba)
Fu Ling (Poria)
Bai Zhu (Atractylodis Macrocephalae Rhizoma)
Zhi Ke (Qiao) (Aurantii Fructus)
Gan Cao (Glycyrrhizae Radix)

This formula is a modification of Xiao Yao Fang (Relaxed Wanderer Formula) with Zhi Ke added to strongly move qi in the middle burner.

Days 25-4 of new cycle: Xiao Zheng Fang (Concretion-dispersing Formula)

Ji Xue Teng (Spatholobi Caulis)
San Leng (Sparganii Rhizoma)
E Zhu (Curcumae Rhizoma)
Mu Dan Pi (Moutan Cortex)
Dan Shen (Salviae Miltiorrhizae Radix)
Chi Shao (Paeoniae Radix Rubra)
Tao Ren (Persicae Semen)
Zhi Ke (Qiao) (Aurantii Fructus)
Fu Ling (Poria)
Bai Zhu (Atractylodis Macrocephalae Rhizoma)

This formula contains many blood-quickening medicinals and is focused on breaking stasis and quickening the blood. This will help with any pain as well. In particular, San Leng and E Zhu form a potent combination for treating blood stasis and pain. Mu Dan Pi also clears any heat in the blood aspect that has resulted from the stagnation of blood and qi. Tao Ren and Zhi Ke together move downward, promoting the elimination of stagnation. Fu Ling and Bai Zhu fortify the spleen and dry dampness, and dampness may contribute to stagnation in the middle and lower burners.

Acupuncture formulas:

Before menstruation:

ST36 (Zu San Li), LI4 (He Gu), GV20 (Bai Hui), Yin Tang (M-HN-3), SP6 (San Yin Jiao)

Formula analysis

During this time, we primarily want to supplement the qi, nourish the blood, supplement the kidney, and quiet the spirit. We also want to prepare the body to menstruate by beginning to gently direct qi and blood downward. ST36 strongly supplements the qi and mildly supports the downward flow of qi and blood. SP6 is the intersection point for the three yin channels of the leg (liver, kidney, and spleen) and, as such, is used to nourish the kidney and blood. This point also moves the blood and qi to the uterus, thus preparing the body for menstruation by coursing stagnation in the lower abdomen. LI4 promotes the downward movement of qi and Yin Tang together quiet the spirit.

During menstruation:

SP10 (Xue Hai), LI4 (He Gu), LR3 (Tai Chong), CV4 (Guan Yuan), SP6 (San Yin Jiao), Yin Tang (M-HN-3)

Formula analysis:

At this time, our primary intent of treatment is to quicken the blood and break any stasis that is occurring and causing pain. Together LI4 and LR3 are known as "the four gates," and this point combination frees the flow of the channels and courses the qi throughout the body. As described above, SP6 quickens the blood while still nourishing. CV4 is an intersection point of the three leg yin channels. Therefore, like SP6, it regulates the flow of qi and blood in the uterus as well as nourishing the blood and yin. SP10 quickens the blood more strongly than does SP6. Finally,

Yin Tang quiets the spirit. GV20 is not used during menstruation because its action is upbearing and we wish to promote the downward flow of the blood at this time.

Modification: If there is endometriosis, Zi Gong Xue (M-CA-18) and LR8 (Qu Quan) may be added to more powerfully quicken the blood and break stasis. If pain is severe, SP8 (Di Ji) is an appropriate addition since it is the cleft point of the spleen channel and, as such, is especially indicated for pain.

After menstruation:

KI3 (Tai Xi), GV20 (Bai Hui), ST36 (Zu San Li), SP6 (San Yin Jiao), Yin Tang (M-HN-3), Zi Gong Xue (M-CA-18)

Formula analysis

Following menstruation, it is important to nourish the kidney as well as to supplement the spleen and blood. The kidney is especially important because it is the hormonal foundation of the body. To supplement the kidney, we can choose its source point, KI3. We also include Zi Gong Xue which directly stimulates the ovaries and, therefore, hormonal production. This point also encourages the movement of blood to the uterus in order to provide nourishment. SP6 is an intersection point for the three leg yin channels which include the kidney. Therefore, it nourishes kidney yin as well as the spleen and blood. ST36 is used to supplement the qi of the entire body. GV20 and Yin Tang again pair up to quiet the spirit. GV20 also stimulates the pituitary and helps to down-regulate the production of FSH, thereby improving ovarian function.

Case Study

The patient was a 28-year-old female complaining of menstrual cramps. She had suffered from painful menstruation for three years. Her symptoms were most severe on the first day of menstruation. Typically, she experienced heavy bleeding for seven days with many clots. She was fatigued and did not have much energy. She also described feeling cold in her lower abdomen and expressed a preference for warmth. She has breast distention, dizziness, low back pain, poor appetite, and nausea with her menstruation. Her urination was frequent and her bowel movements were changeable, from unformed stool to constipation. About one week prior to menstruation, she felt very sad and cried a lot. Her pulse was slow, bowstring, thin, and weak in both cubit positions. Her tongue was pale and purplish, enlarged with teethmarks, and had a white coating.

Pattern identification: Qi & blood stasis and stagnation with spleen-kidney yang vacuity

Symptom analysis

From the patient's pain presentation and quality of menses, there is evidence of blood stasis, e.g., her pain was worse on the first day of bleeding and she had many clots. Breast distention is a common symptom of liver depression qi stagnation since the liver channel passes through the area of the breasts. Changeable stools are a common result of liver depression overacting on the spleen. Mood swings the week prior to menstruation also suggest liver depression qi stagnation. Stasis and stagnation of the qi and blood was confirmed by the bowstring quality of her pulse and the purplish tongue. The patient also showed cold signs and reported low back pain and frequent urination. This, along with her slow pulse and enlarged, pale tongue, suggests an element of kidney yang vacuity. Her pulses were also weak in the cubit positions, thus confirming that the kidney is generally weak. Finally, the patient reported nausea, lack of appetite, and dizziness with her menstruation. She also described excessively profuse menstruation and general fatigue. Her tongue also had teethmarks. These all suggest spleen qi vacuity. The fact that these symptoms were worse around the time of her menses reflects the relationship between the spleen and the liver and the tendency of the liver to overact on the spleen due to increased liver depression qi stagnation prior to menstruation.

Treatment

One week before menstruation, I prescribed Xiao Yao Fang (Relaxed Wanderer Formula) plus Xiang Fu (Cyperi Rhizoma), Suan Zao Ren (Ziziphi Spinosi Semen), Dang Shen (Codonopsis Radix) and Gou Qi Zi (Lycii Fructus).

At this time, I primarily wished to course the liver and rectify the qi. This seemed to be the time when the patient reported the majority of symptoms that result directly from liver depression qi stagnation, such as her emotional and digestive problems. Of course, I also needed to nourish the blood in order to support the substance of the impending menses. Consequently, I choose Xiao Yao Fang which courses the liver, moves the qi, and supplements the blood. With this as a base, I added Xiang Fu to strengthen the formula's ability to course the liver and move the qi. I also added Suan Zao Ren to help quiet the patient's spirit during this emotionally turbulent time. Dang Shen fortifies the spleen and, therefore, helped address the fatigue and dizziness which, in this case, was due to downward falling of the central qi, not blood vacuity (which would come after menstruation). Gou Qi Zi directly nourishes liver blood but is not too enriching and stagnating for her to digest with a weakened spleen.

During menstruation, I prescribed Jing Tong Fang (Formula for Painful Menstruation) minus Yan Hu Suo (Corydalis Rhizoma) but plus Yi Mu Cao (Leonuri Herba), Huang Qi (Astragali Radix), Pu Huang (Typhae Pollen), and Wu Ling Zhi (Trogopteri Faeces).

This is the time when the patient experienced pain due to blood stasis. Therefore, it was vital to quicken the blood at this time. However, I had to be cautious not to quicken too violently because she already had heavy menstruation due to spleen qi vacuity not containing the blood. Because of this, I removed Yan Hu Suo which moves too powerfully. Instead, I added Yi Mu Cao which also is good for pain and helps to decrease bleeding. I added Huang Qi to help the spleen qi to contain the blood within its vessels and regulate its flow. Pu Huang and Wu Ling Zhi together form the formula Shi Xiao San (Sudden Smile Powder) which is very effective for the treatment of pain.

After menstruation, I prescribed Jing Hou Fang (Formula for After Menstruation) minus Shu Di Huang (Rehmanniae Radix Praeparata) and plus Shan Zhu Yu (Corni Fructus), Tu Si Zi (Cuscutae Semen), and Chen Pi (Citri Reticulatae Pericarpium).

During this time, I felt it was important to address the root vacuity issues that this patient faced, *i.e.*, spleen qi and kidney yang vacuity. Readers should recall that Jing Hou Fang is a modification of Xiao Yao San (Free Wanderer Powder) with Dang Shen (Codonopsis Radix) added to supplement the spleen, Shu Di Huang (Rehmanniae Radix Praeparata) to nourish the kidney yin, Gou Qi Zi (Lycii Fructus) to nourish the blood, and Rou Gui (Cinnamomi Cortex) to warm the kidney yang. I felt that was basically a perfect formula for this patient. However, I removed Shu Di Huang because it is difficult to digest, and I replaced it with Shan Zhu Yu (Corni Fructus). This is also a wonderful medicinal to nourish kidney and liver yin, but it is much more easily digested than Shu Di Huang. To strengthen the kidney yang-warming aspect of the formula, I also added Tu Si Zi. Finally, I added a little Chen Pi to regulate the middle burner and assist the spleen in digesting the nourishing and enriching medicinals in the formula.

Acupuncture formulas:

Before menstruation:

ST36 (Zu San Li), LI4 (He Gu), LR3 (Tai Chong), GV20 (Bai Hui), Yin Tang (M-HN-3), SP6 (San Yin Jiao), LR14 (Qi Men), PC6 (Nei Guan)

In this case, I added LR3 to my usual protocol before the patient's menses to course the liver and rectify the qi. LR14 is an interesection point for the spleen and liver channels as well as the front mu point of the liver. Thus it is an excellent point to use when there is liver depression qi stagnation overacting on the spleen. Also, LR14 and PC6 together free the flow of the breast area to alleviate distention. PC6 also helps quiet the spirit and soothe the emotions.

During menstruation:

LR8 (Qu Quan), SP8 (Di Ji), LI4 (He Gu), LR3 (Tai Chong), CV4 (Guan Yuan), SP6 (San Yin Jiao), Yin Tang (M-HN-3)

Because this patient had severe pain, I added SP8 (Di Ji). Instead of then having three spleen points, I substituted LR8 for SP10 in order to quicken the blood in the uterus.

After menstruation:

KI7 (Fu Liu), CV4 (Guan Yuan), GV20 (Bai Hui), ST36 (Zu San Li), SP6 (San Yin Jiao), Yin Tang (M-HN-3), Zi Gong Xue (M-CA-18)

Instead of needling KI3, I moxaed KI7. This is the spring point of the kidney channel and is the best distal kidney point to supplement kidney yang. I also used moxibustion on CV4 which has the ability to supplement yang in addition to yin and blood.

Outcome

After one month of treatment, the patient happily reported she experienced neither cramping nor heavy bleeding with menstruation.

8

Menopausal Syndrome

Western Medical View

Menopause refers to the absence of menstruation for a period of one year. The average age of menopause in developed countries is 41-55 years of age. The median age is 51.

Perimenopause is the time preceding the end of menstruation and usually occurs 2-5 years before true cessation of menstruation. During this time, ovulation may still occur. However, hormone production begins to decrease and menstruation becomes increasingly irregular, heavy, or scanty. Follicle stimulating hormone levels (FSH) start to rise, and some of the symptoms associated with menopause begin to appear.

Postmenopause refers to the time 12 months after the last menses when eggs are no longer released and estrogen and progesterone levels have dropped significantly.

Menopause before the age of 40 is referred to as premature ovarian failure.

Artificial menopause can be induced by removal of the ovaries, cancer, chemotherapy, and radiation or surgical damage.

Menopausal syndrome refers to recurring symptoms experienced by some women during the climacteric period. These include hot flashes, chills, headache, irritability, and depression.

"Climacteric" refers to the normal changes that occur during the transition from reproduction to nonreproduction.

N.B. It is important to remember that, in this chapter we are talking about the treatment of menopausal syndrome and not menopause *per se*.

Causes:

Aging causes natural changes in a woman's reproductive system. As the follicles diminish in number, the ovaries shrink. They no longer respond to gonadotropin releasing hormone (GnRH) and stop producing estrogen. Progesterone levels also drop and other hormonal changes associated with normal menstruation cease.

Symptoms:

Physical changes:

- Hot flashes, night sweats, sweating
- Vaginal dryness
- Frequent urination or urinary incontinence
- Digestive changes, *i.e.*, constipation, unformed bowel movements, bloating, gas
- Heart palpitations
- Headaches
- Fatigue
- Thinning of the skin
- Weight gain
- Osteoporosis

Mental changes:

- Irritability, anxiety, depression
- Poor memory, inability to concentrate
- Insomnia

Some women experience no symptoms.

Complications:

- Increased risk of cardiovascular disease
- Osteoporosis

Treatment: Hormone replacement therapy (HRT) is the treatment of choice. Estrogen or estrogen/progesterone combinations are most commonly used to relieve the discomforts of menopause. However, HRT has been associated with an increased risk of heart disease, stroke, breast cancer and endometrial hyperplasia.

Other medications (antidepressants, seizure medications, hypertension medications, or drugs that mimic estrogen) are sometimes used to relieve hot flashes or guard against osteoporosis, but each has its own set of side effects and contraindications. Vaginal estrogens are often used locally to relieve vaginal discomfort.

Self-care: Women are advised to eat a balanced diet that includes fruits, vegetables, and whole grains, and limits saturated fats, oils, and sugars. Adequate calcium (1,500 mg/day) and Vitamin D (400-800 IU per day) intake through diet or supplements is recommended. Moderate weight-bearing exercise is advised to prevent osteoporosis and reduce the risk of fractures. Regular physical activity also protects against cardiovascular disease.

Traditional Chinese Medical View

Menopause is the cessation of menstruation at approximately the age of 50, although women can experience it between the ages of 40-60.

Symptoms: One-third of women do not experience any symptoms when going through menopause. However, for the rest, the signs and symptoms can vary. These include hot flashes, night sweats or spontaneous sweating, insomnia, emotional changes, poor memory, anxiousness, depression, nervousness, palpitations, hypertension, and/or sore lower back.

Treatment based on pattern identification:
Kidney yin vacuity (*shen yin xu* 肾阴虚)

Signs & symptoms: Hot flashes, night sweating, insomnia, emotional changes, poor memory, anxiety, depression, nervousness, palpitations, hypertension, and sore lower back

Tongue: Red, cracks, scanty fur

Pulse: Thin, weak, rapid

Treatment principles: Supplement the kidney and enrich yin

Formula: Zuo Gui Yin (Left-restoring [Kidney Yin] Pill)

Shu Di Huang (Rehmanniae Radix Praeparata)
Shan Zhu Yu (Corni Fructus)
Shan Yao (Dioscoreae Rhizoma)
Gou Qi Zi (Lycii Fructus)

Fu Ling (Poria)

Zhi Gan Cao (Glycyrrhizae Radix cum Liquido Fricta)

Modifications:

- If there is more heat, add Mu Dan Pi (Moutan Cortex), Huang Bai (Phellodendri Cortex), and Zhi Mu (Anemarrhenae Rhizoma).

- For heart palpitations, add Suan Zao Ren (Ziziphi Spinosi Semen), Long Yan Rou (Longan Arillus), and Mu Li (Ostreae Concha).

- For dizziness, add Gou Teng (Uncariae Ramulus cum Uncis), Tian Ma (Gastrodiae Rhizoma), and Mu Li (Ostreae Concha).

- For hot flashes, add Gui Ban (Testudinis Plastrum) and Niu Xi (Achyranthis Bidentatae Radix).

- If easily angered, add Bai Shao (Paeoniae Radix Alba), He Huan Pi (Albizziae Cortex), Xiang Fu (Cyperi Rhizoma), Yu Jin (Curcumae Radix), Dan Shen (Salviae Miltiorrhizae Radix), and Zhi Ke (Qiao) (Aurantii Fructus).

- To quiet the spirit, add Suan Zao Ren (Ziziphi Spinosi Semen), Wu Wei Zi (Schisandrae Fructus), Long Yan Rou (Longan Arillus), Yuan Zhi (Polygalae Radix), and Bai Zi Ren (Platycladi Semen).

Kidney yang vacuity (*shen yang xu* 肾阳虚)

Signs & symptoms: Body aches, cold extremities, diarrhea or unformed bowel movements, fatigue, frequent nighttime urination, incontinence, edema

Tongue: Pale, swollen, moist fur

Pulse: Deep, weak

Treatment principles: Supplement the kidney and invigorate yang

Formula: You Gui Wan (Right-restoring [Life Gate] Pill)

Shu Di Huang (Rehmanniae Radix Praeparata)

Shan Zhu Yu (Corni Fructus)

Shan Yao (Dioscoreae Rhizoma)

Lu Jiao Jiao (Cervi Cornus Gelatinum)

Tu Si Zi (Cuscutae Semen)

Gou Qi Zi (Lycii Fructus)

Du Zhong (Eucommiae Cortex)

Dang Gui (Angelicae Sinensis Radix)
Zhi Fu Zi (mix-fried Aconiti Radix Lateralis Praeparata)
Rou Gui (Cinnamomi Cortex)

Modifications:

- If diarrhea is present, remove Shu Di Huang and/or Lu Jiao Jiao and add the ingredients of Si Shen Wan (Four Spirits Pill), *i.e.*, Wu Zhu Yu (Evodiae Fructus), Wu Wei Zi (Schisandrae Fructus), Rou Dou Kou (Myristicae Semen), and Bu Gu Zhi (Psoraleae Fructus).

- If water swelling is present, add Che Qian Zi (Plantaginis Semen) and Chen Pi (Citri Reticulatae Pericarpium). The ingredients of Wu Pi San (Five-peel Powder) can be used as well: Fu Ling Pi (Poriae Cutis), Sheng Jiang Pi (Zingiberis Rhizomatis Cortex), Da Fu Pi (Arecae Pericarpium), Chen Pi (Citri Reticulatae Pericarpium), and Sang Bai Pi (Mori Cortex).

Kidney yin & yang dual vacuity (*shen yin yang liang xu* 肾阴阳两虚)

Signs & symptoms: A combination of the signs and symptoms of the two preceding patterns

Tongue: A combination of the signs of the two preceding patterns

Pulse: A combination of the signs of the two preceding patterns

Treatment principles: Nourish kidney yin and supplement kidney yang

Formula: Er Xian Tang (Two Immortals Decoction)

Xian Mao (Curculiginis Rhizoma)
Yin Yang Huo (Epimedii Herba)
Dang Gui (Angelicae Sinensis Radix)
Ba Ji Tian (Morindae Officinalis Radix)
Huang Bai (Phellodendri Cortex)
Zhi Mu (Anemarrhenae Rhizoma)

Modification: If kidney yin vacuity is predominant, add Nu Zhen Zi (Ligustri Lucidi Fructus), Mo Han Lian (Ecliptae Herba), Gou Qi Zi (Lycii Fructus), Mai Men Dong (Ophiopogonis Radix), Shu Di Huang (Rehmanniae Radix Praeparata), and Shan Zhu Yu (Corni Fructus).

Clinical Treatment

In Chinese medicine, we describe women's reproductive lives in terms of seven-year cycles. Thus, at age 14, the *tian kui* is said to arrive. The tian kui refers to the maturation of kidney water and essence, and its arrival marks the commencement of menstruation, the ability to conceive, and thus of womanhood. The seventh cycle, starting at age 49, marks the cessation of menstruation. At this point, the essence is so diminished that menstruation is no longer supported. This is what is referred to in Western medicine as menopause.

According to Chinese medicine, because the kidney governs reproduction, the fundamental cause of menopause is kidney vacuity, remembering that menopause per *se* is a natural physiological event in the life-cycle of a female. Thus, symptoms of menopausal syndrome, meaning the constellation of pathological signs and symptoms which are commonly associated with menopause, may be due to kidney yin vacuity, kidney yang vacuity, or both. In clinic, however, experience has shown that it is also sometimes effective to treat menopause syndrome as a case of modified liver depression qi stagnation. This is not to imply that there is not fundamental kidney involvement. Simply, this approach is appropriate in certain cases in which the predominate manifestation of menopause includes a range of liver depression qi stagnation signs and symptoms, such as mood disorders, insomnia, headache, and dizziness.

In clinic, patients may usually be divided into three groups. For those who are very emotional, we may think that liver qi depression and binding is the central factor. Alternatively, if we see more kidney signs, we may categorize patients as predominantly kidney yin vacuity type or kidney yang vacuity type.

Liver qi depression & binding (*gan qi yu jie* 肝气郁结)

Signs & symptoms: Emotional depression, emotional lability, irritability, headaches, chest oppression, sighing

Tongue: Purplish

Pulse: Bowstring

Treatment principles: Course the liver and rectify the qi

Formula: Modified Xiao Yao Fang (Relaxed Wanderer Formula)

Xiao Yao Fang (Relaxed Wanderer Formula)

Dang Gui (Angelicae Sinensis Radix)
Bai Zhu (Atractylodis Macrocephalae Rhizoma)
Bai Shao (Paeoniae Radix Alba)
Chai Hu (Bupleuri Radix)
Fu Ling (Poria)
Gan Cao (Glycyrrhizae Radix)

Bo He (Menthae Haplocalycis Herba) and Sheng Jiang (Zingiberis Rhizoma Recens) have been removed from the standard version of Xiao Yao San (Free Wanderer Powder) because they tend to damage yin fluids and yin fluids tend to be vacuous in menopausal women.

Modifications:

• If there is insomnia, add Suan Zao Ren (Ziziphi Spinosi Semen), Wu Wei Zi (Schisandrae Fructus), Mu Li (Ostreae Concha), Long Gu (Mastodi Ossis Fossilia), Long Yan Rou (Longan Arillus), Bai Zi Ren (Platycladi Semen), and/or Zhen Zhu Mu (Concha Margaritifera). The specific choices of modifying medicinals rely on a correct assessment of the nature of the insomnia. Thus Suan Zao Ren and Long Yan Rou, for example, nourish the heart blood, whereas Mu Li and Long Gu are securing and astringing, heavy and settling.

• When a patient exhibits no appetite in addition to insomnia, Wu Wei Zi (Schisandrae Fructus) is especially good. The combination of sour and sweet flavors promotes the engenderment of yin while stimulating the appetite.

• For insomnia with heart palpitations, Suan Zao Ren (Ziziphi Spinosi Semen), Long Yan Rou (Longan Arillus), Mu Li (Ostreae Concha), Long Gu (Mastodi Ossis Fossilia), and Zhen Zhu Mu (Concha Margaritifera) are all effective. Other medicinals that are useful for heart palpitations include Bai Zi Ren (Platycladi Semen), Mai Men Dong (Ophiopogonis Radix), Wu Wei Zi (Schisandrae Fructus), Dan Shen (Salviae Miltiorrhizae Radix), and Gou Qi Zi (Lycii Fructus). Again, appropriate choice of modifying medicinals depends on a correct assessment of the nature of the palpitations. These may include, for example, heat harassing the heart, thus indicating Mai Men Dong or heart blood vacuity, indicating Gou Qi Zi and Dan Shen.

• In case of constipation, crushed Bai Zi Ren (Platycladi Semen) or Suan Zao Ren (Ziziphi Spinosi Semen) may be added. These two medicinals treat constipation by moistening rather than precipitating. This is important in this case because of the underlying vacuity associated with menopause.

- When there is headache due to ascendant liver yang hyperactivity or liver wind stirring internally, Tian Ma (Gastrodiae Rhizoma) and Gou Teng (Uncariae Ramulus cum Uncis) may be added to extringuish wind and downbear yang.

- If there is dizziness due to qi not ascending to the head, Gou Qi Zi (Lycii Fructus) and He Shou Wu (Polygoni Multiflori Radix) are good additions.

Kidney yin vacuity (*shen yin xu* 肾阴虚)

Signs & symptoms: Hot flashes, night sweats, low back soreness, nighttime polyuria with scanty flow

Tongue: Red, peeled fur or scanty, dry fur

Pulse: Thin, rapid

Treatment principles: Supplement the kidney and enrich yin

Formula: Zhi Ru Fang (Conception Decoction)

N.B. The name Zhi Ru Tang means "Conception Decoction." This may seem unusual since here we are treating menopause and not promoting pregnancy. However, the reader should remember that, in both cases, the primary focus is to nourish the reproductive organs in order to bring them into functional balance.

Zhi Ru Fang (Conception Decoction)

Shu Di Huang (Rehmanniae Radix Praeparata)
Shan Zhu Yu (Corni Fructus)
Shan Yao (Dioscoreae Rhizoma)
Mu Dan Pi (Moutan Cortex)
Fu Ling (Poria)
Ze Xie (Alismatis Rhizoma)
Bai Shao (Paeoniae Radix Alba)
Suan Zao Ren (Ziziphi Spinosi Semen)
Tu Si Zi (Cuscutae Semen)
Gan Cao (Glycyrrhizae Radix)

Formula analysis

This formula is simply a modification of Liu Wei Di Huang Wan (Six-ingredient Rehmannia Pill). Liu Wei Di Huang Wan is a basic and balanced formula for enriching yin. To this we have added Suan Zao Ren, Tu Si Zi, Gan Cao, and Bai Shao. Suan Zao Ren nourishes the heart and quiets the spirit, thus helping to address the insomnia that is so often present in menopause cases with predominant kidney yin vacuity. Bai Shao assists in nourishing the yin and also soothes the liver. This is helpful because the liver often becomes depressed and the qi stagnant in these patients. In such cases, Bai Shao is used to emolliate the liver and protects yin, whereas, if we used Chai Hu (Bupleuri Radix), that medicinal typically hinders the yin. Tu Si Zi supplements both kidney yin and kidney yang. Even though this is a kidney yin vacuity pattern, it is advisable nonetheless to supplement kidney yang a little. Otherwise the yin-enriching medicinals may be too cold and enriching, thus creating dampness and stagnation. Finally, Gan Cao both harmonizes all the other ingredients in the formula and fortifies the spleen. The latter is important because the spleen must be strong in order to digest the cloying, yin-enriching medicinals. Gan Cao also teams with Bai Shao to help relax the muscles and sinews. Yin vacuity includes an element of fluid dryness and, therefore, can dry the tissues and lead to body pain, tension, and spasm.

Kidney yang vacuity (*shen yang xu* 肾阳虚)

Signs & symptoms: Polyuria with long, clear stream, nocturia, cold hands and feet, aversion to cold, low back pain, decreased libido

Tongue: Pale, moist

Pulse: Deep, slow

Treatment principles: Supplement the kidney and invigorate yang

Formula: Wen Gong Fang (Warm the Uterus Formula)

Dang Gui (Anelicae Sinensis Radix)
Bai Shao (Paeoniae Radix Alba)
Shu Di Huang (Rehmanniae Radix Praeparata)
Chai Hu (Bupleuri Radix)
Shan Yao (Dioscoreae Rhizoma)
Fu Ling (Poria)
Tu Si Zi (Cuscutae Semen)
Ba Ji Tian (Morindae Officinalis Radix)
Dang Shen (Codonopsis Radix)
Rou Gui (Cinnamomi Cortex)
Zhi Gan Cao (Glycyrrhizae Radix cum Liquido Fricta)

Formula analysis

This formula is a modification of Ding Jing Fang (Stabilize the Menses Formula) with the addition of Rou Gui to warm the kidney and supplement yang. Ding Jing Fang, you will recall, is a basic formula for regulating the female hormonal system. Dang Gui and Shu Di Huang nourish the blood. Chai Hu and Bai Shao soothe the liver qi. Fu Ling and Shan Yao fortify the spleen, respectively disinhibiting and se-curing in order to maintain the correct balance of fluids. Tu Si Zi, Ba Ji Tian, and Rou Gui together supplement and warm kidney yang. It is important to notice that, although the focus of this formula is on kidney yang, there are a mixture of both yin and yang supplements in this formula. This is because yin and yang rely on each other for their engenderment and balance. If only yang medicinals were in-cluded, yin would be damaged. On the other hand, without the yin, yang would be unsupported and subsequently would also suffer. Finally, Zhi Gan Cao is used to harmonize all the other ingredients in the formula and to fortify the spleen to sup-port digestion of the rich, cloying, yin-supplementing medicinals.

Modifications:

- For yang vacuity diarrhea, add Bu Gu Zhi (Psoraleae Fructus) and Gan Jiang (Zingiberis Rhizoma). Both of these medicinals are warming and Bu Gu Zhi also secures and astringes.

- In case of frequent urination, Fu Pen Zi (Rubi Fructus) or Yi Zhi Ren (Alpiniae Oxyphyllae Fructus) may be added. Although both strengthen the kidney and assist the kidney's function of holding the urine, Fu Pen Zi is more securing and astringing, while Yi Zhi Ren is more warming. Yi Zhi Ren additionally supplements the spleen and may be a better addition if there are signs of spleen-kidney dual vacuity, such as early morning diarrhea.

- For lower back pain due to yang vacuity, Du Zhong (Eucommiae Cortex), Xu Duan (Dipsaci Radix) and Gu Sui Bu (Drynariae Rhizoma) are helpful. Each of these herbs strengthens the bones and sinews, but each also has a special aspect. Gu Sui Bu is excellent in cases where there is damage or ex-treme weakness, including traumatic injuries or fractures (such as may occur with the elderly or in cases of osteoporosis). Xu Duan and Du Zhong both move the blood and therefore are helpful analgesics. Du Zhong is especially warming, and therefore helps to open the channels that are constricted by cold.

• Water swelling may be treated with the addition of Yi Yi Ren (Coicis Semen), Bai Zhu (Atractylodis Macrocephalae Rhizoma), Chen Pi (Citri Reticulatae Pericarpium), and/or Gui Zhi (Cinnamomi Ramulus) or the ingredients of Wu Pi Yin (Five-peel Beverage). Attention should be paid to the underlying cause of the water swelling. This is most frequently a dysfunction of the spleen or kidney. Wu Pi Yin focuses on the kidney and is best in cases of pitting edema in the lower body. Gui Zhi and Bai Zhu are a combination that may be appropriately applied to water swelling resulting from spleen vacuity. Chen Pi moves the qi and warms the middle burner and, therefore, is a good addition when there are digestive signs, such as bloating, lack of appetite, and a heavy sensation in the epigastrium. Yi Yi Ren is especially effective for water swelling that occurs with urinary retention or difficulty.

An Integrated Chinese-Western Medical Treatment of Menopausal Syndrome

Since most menopausal symptoms are the direct result of changing hormone levels and, in particular, diminishing estrogen, Western medicine often addresses menopause by giving hormone replacement therapy (HRT). My experience in China suggests that one risk of long-term HRT, especially unopposed estrogen HRT, may be breast and uterine cancers. My experience has also shown that acupuncture and Chinese medicinals can help support the patient during HRT and allow a gradual decrease in dosage over time. I have found that the patient is often able to eventually cease HRT completely with such support. Usually, acute symptoms of menopause do not last longer than three years, and, therefore, treatment will not need to be continued indefinitely. In cases where women develop osteoporosis, continued treatment with acupuncture and Chinese medicinals is highly recommended.

Acupuncture formulas:

A good basic point prescription for menopausal syndrome is: Yin Tang (M-HN-3), KI6 (Zhao Hai), HT7 (Shen Men), SP6 (San Yin Jiao), ST36 (Zu San Li)

Formula analysis

Yin Tang quiets the spirit. This is very important for menopausal women because they tend to feel emotional. Strong emotions can create further problems in the body by deregulating the normal flow of qi in the channels and impacting the normal functioning of the organs. KI6 is an important kidney-supplementing point because it supplements both yin and yang. HT7 helps to quiet the spirit also, especially for women who are having heart palpitations which are not uncommon. SP6 is an intersection point for the three leg yin channels (kidney, liver, and spleen) and is a powerful point for nourishing the yin and blood. ST36 is an overall supplementation point for the qi and blood. It also has a regulatory effect on the digestive functions which are often disrupted in menopause.

Modifications:

- In cases where there is a clear element of liver depression qi stagnation, LR3 (Tai Chong) and LI4 (He Gu) can be added to course the qi in the channels. If heat due to depression is also present, LR2 (Xing Jian) may be substituted for LR3.

- Insomnia and night sweats are common problems for menopausal women. For insomnia, ear points such as Kidney, Spleen, and Shen Men are very useful, while the combination of KI7 (Fu Liu) and HT6 (Yin Xi) is a classical pairing for night sweats.

- Body soreness, particularly backache, is also commonly seen in menopausal women. In such cases, a back treatment may be indicated. The back transport points of the heart, liver, spleen, and kidney make an appropriate combination for such situations. These are BL15 (Xin Shu), BL18 (Gan Shu), BL20 (Pi Shu), and BL23 (Shen Shu). If the back soreness and coldness are due to kidney yang vacuity, moxa may be used at BL23 and GV4 (Ming Men) to warm the yang.

- If there is whole body soreness and stiffness, GB34 (Yang Ling Quan) and GB40 (Qiu Xu) are useful points. Palpate and discover where the maximum sensitivity lies or consider the quality of the area around each of the points to determine which to needle.

- For headache, consider adding Tai Yang (M-HN-7), GB20 (Feng Chi) or GB40 (Qiu Xu). In my clinical experience, most menopausal headaches are related to ascending yang in the liver and/or gallbladder channels due to vacuity of kidney yin not nourishing the liver.

- If heart palpitations are significant, CV17 (Dan Zhong) should be added.

Case Study

The patient was a 50-year-old woman who came to the clinic complaining of hot flashes, anxiety, heart palpitations, and insomnia (onset and waking throughout the night). She had not menstruated for six months. She felt irritable and stressed out and sweated more than usual. Her bowel movements and urination were both normal. Her tongue was pink with a red tip, was cracked, and had thin, white fur. Her pulse was small, rapid, and irregular. It was also bowstring and weak in the cubit positions.

Pattern identification: Kidney yin and heart blood vacuity with vacuity heat and liver depression qi stagnation

Symptom analysis

The combination of hot flashes, sweating, anxiety, heart palpitations, and insomnia are strongly suggestive of a pattern involving both the kidney and heart. In classic theory, this is often described as kidney yin not nourishing the heart possibly leading to the engenderment of vacuity heat or fire. In this case, there was both onset insomnia and waking throughout the night. This suggests that the pattern was a combination of kidney yin vacuity and heart blood vacuity. The feelings of stress and the bowstring pulse point to an element of liver depression qi stagnation.

Treatment principles: Enrich kidney yin and nourish heart blood, clear vacuity heat, course the liver and rectify the qi

Formula: Modified Zi Ru Fang (Conception Decoction)

> Shu Di Huang (Rehmanniae Radix Praeparata)
> Shan Zhu Yu (Corni Fructus)
> Shan Yao (Dioscoreae Rhizoma)
> Ze Xie (Alismatis Rhizoma)
> Fu Ling (Poria)
> Tu Si Zi (Cuscutae Semen)
> Suan Zao Ren (Ziziphi Spinosi Semen)
> Mu Dan Pi (Moutan Cortex)
> Gan Cao (Glycyrrhizae Radix)

Modifications: For fluid dryness/yin vacuity, add Wu Wei Zi (Schisandrae Fructus) and Mai Men Dong (Ophiopogonis Radix). For blood vacuity and/or stasis add Dan Shen (Salviae Miltiorrhizae Radix) and Bai Shao (Paeoniae Radix Alba).

Formula analysis

As discussed above, Zhi Ru Tang is a modification of Liu Wei Di Huang Wan (Six-ingredient Rehmannia Pill). Shu Di Huang, Shan Zhu Yu, and Shan Yao nourish yin, each focusing on a different viscus (kidney, liver, and spleen respectively). Ze Xie drains vacuity fire from the kidney. Fu Ling promotes urination to disinhibit dampness and fortifies the spleen's ability to transform fluids. It also enters the heart and quiets the spirit. Tu Si Zi is a good addition here because it can strengthen the kidney overall (yin and yang). It is also neutral in temperature and so will not aggravate vacuity heat. Wu Wei Zi addresses the insomnia and combines with the sweet Shu Di Huang and Shan Yao to engender yin. Mu Dan Pi (Moutan Cortex) is replaced by Mai Men Dong. In this case, the heat was not strong enough to warrant the use of Mu Dan Pi. Instead, Mai Men Dong engenders fluids and gently clears vacuity heat. Dan Shen clears heat from the heart and quiets the spirit to relieve irritability. Also, Shu Di Huang and Dan Shen together enter the heart and supplement the heart blood. Bai Shao assists in nourishing yin and also soothes the liver qi to relieve tension. In addition, readers should notice that the heat-clearing aspects of the formula come from both below (Ze Xie) and above (Mai Men Dong and Dan Shen). This is because part of the heat comes from kidney yin vacuity and part arises because the heart is deprived of nourishment.

Outcome

After one month of treatment, the patient reported that she was no longer experiencing hot flashes, sweating, or palpatations. Her sleep was better and she felt calmer. She said she was happy to feel like herself again. Her period returned and continued to be regular for another six years.

9

Vomiting in Pregnancy

Western Medical View

Vomiting in pregnancy (often called morning sickness) refers to moderate to intense nausea and vomiting during the first 2-3 months of pregnancy. Symptoms may be more severe in the morning but can occur any time throughout the day or night. Approximately 60-80% of pregnant women experience vomiting during pregnancy for an average of 35 days. Usually, symptoms disappear by the end of the first trimester.

Hyperemesis gravidarum is severe vomiting during pregnancy. It affects approximately one percent of pregnant women. Vomiting is prolonged and frequent, causing weight loss, dehydration, and vitamin, acid-base, and electrolyte imbalances. It is associated with potassium deficiency and, if untreated, can lead to severe mental and physical conditions.

Causes:

Although the exact cause of vomiting during pregnancy is still unknown, it is most likely due to hormonal changes, especially elevated serum levels of human chorionic gonadotropin levels (HCG). Other causes may include the lower blood sugar levels of early pregnancy, slowed stomach emptying, stress, travel, and particular foods.

Hyperemesis gravidarum is associated with potassium deficiency as well as high levels of serum HCG and/or estrogen. It can lead to deficiencies of thiamin and vitamin K. Some conditions that underlie hyperemesis gravidarum include:

- Pancreatitis
- Hyperparathyroidism

- Hyperthyroidism
- Diabetes
- Liver disease (especially fatty liver disease)
- Pheochromocytoma (a rare, usually noncancerous tumor of the adrenal medulla)

Treatment:

Treatment consists of patient counseling. Suggestions include:

- Small frequent meals
- High protein and complex carbohydrate foods
- Adequate fluid intake
- Dry crackers before rising
- Avoidance of spicy greasy foods and late meals
- Antiemetics or high doses of vitamin B6 may be prescribed
- Severe cases of hyperemesis gravidarum are treated by hospitalization to administer intravenous fluids, electrolytes, vitamins, and antiemetics. A urinalysis can reveal ketone levels and the severity of dehydration.

Traditional Chinese Medical View

Vomiting during pregnancy does not necessarily occur in the morning and is most commonly experienced between the fourth and sixth weeks of pregnancy.

Treatment based on pattern differentiation:

Spleen & stomach vacuity (*pi wei xu* 脾胃虚)

Signs & symptoms: Nausea, vomiting, decreased appetite, fatigue, possibly unformed bowel movements

Tongue: Pale with teethmarks on its edges

Pulse: Weak, thin

Treatment principles: Supplement the spleen, harmonize the stomach, and rectify the qi

Formula: Xiang Sha Liu Jun Zi Tang (Auklandia & Amomum Six Gentlemen Decoction)

Mu Xiang (Aucklandiae Radix)
Sha Ren (Amomi Fructus)
Chen Pi (Citri Reticulatae Pericarpium)

Ban Xia (Pinelliae Rhizoma)
Ren Shen (Ginseng Radix)
Bai Zhu (Atractylodis Macrocephalae Rhizoma)
Fu Ling (Poria)
Gan Cao (Glycyrrhizae Radix)

Modifications:

- To harmonize the spleen and stomach, add Sheng Jiang (Zingiberis Rhizoma Recens).

- For more qi supplementation, add Da Zao (Jujubae Fructus).

Liver-stomach disharmony (*gan wei bu he* 肝胃不和)

Signs & symptoms: Nausea, vomiting, emotional tension such as irritability or anger, hypochondriac pain, bitter taste in the mouth, high stress

Tongue: Purplish

Pulse: Bowstring

Treatment principles: Harmonize the liver and stomach

Formula: Modified Su Ye Huang Lian Tang (Perilla Leaf & Coptis Decoction)

Zi Su Geng (Perillae Caulis)
Huang Lian (Coptidis Rhizoma)
Sheng Jiang (Zingiberis Rhizoma Recens)
Ban Xia (Pinelliae Rhizoma)
Chen Pi (Citri Reticulatae Pericarpium)
Zhu Ru (Bumbusae Caulis in Taenia)
Bai Shao (Paeoniae Radix Alba)

Modifications:

- If there is more heat, add Huang Qin (Scutellariae Radix).

- For yin vacuity due to loss of fluid through vomiting, add Mai Men Dong (Ophiopogonis Radix), Tian Dong (Asparagi Radix), Sha Shen (Adenophorae seu Glehniae Radix), and/or Shi Hu (Dendrobii Herba).

- Also consider Zeng Ye Tang (Humor-increasing Decoction) to increase the function of nourishing yin and fluids: Xuan Shen (Scrophulariae Radix), Mai Men Dong (Ophiopogonis Radix), and Sheng Di Huang (Rehmanniae Radix Exsiccata seu Recens)

- To nourish both qi and yin, add Sheng Mai San (Pulse-engendering Powder): Ren Shen (Ginseng Radix), Mai Men Dong (Ophiopogonis Radix), and Wu Wei Zi (Schisandrae Fructus).

Clinical Treatment

Digestion relates to the spleen and stomach. Emotions relate to the liver which, in turn, affects the stomach's function. The standard textbook patterns of vomiting during pregnancy, therefore, include spleen-stomach vacuity, in which the normal upbearing and downbearing are disturbed, and disharmony of the liver and stomach. The presentations of these two patterns are similar and often include loss of appetite, nausea, and possibly vomiting. There may also be abdominal distention, flatulence, and diarrhea. Liver involvement is differentiated by the presence of additional symptoms such as moodiness and strong emotions. If there is significant liver depression, the resulting heat may produce a bitter taste in the mouth.

The clinical presentation is usually very simple and follows the standard patterns outlined above. My experience suggests that the best base formula to use for treating vomiting during pregnancy is Liu Jun Zi Tang (Six Gentlemen Decoction):

> Chen Pi (Citri Reticulatae Pericarpium)
> Ban Xia (Pinelliae Rhizoma)
> Ren Shen (Ginseng Radix)
> Bai Zhu (Atractylodis Macrocephalae Rhizoma)
> Fu Ling (Poria)
> Gan Cao (Glycyrrhizae Radix)

Formula analysis

This formula moves the qi and disperses stagnation, dries dampness and supports the middle burner. Within it, Ren Shen, Bai Zhu, Fu Ling, and Gan Cao form Si Jun Zi Tang (Four Gentlemen Decoction) which is the basis of the formula. These four ingredients fortify the spleen and supplement the qi. In addition, Fu Ling and Bai Zhu eliminate dampness which is both a cause and result of impaired spleen function. To this base, Ban Xia is added to dry dampness, transforms phlegm, and downbear the qi. It harmonizes the stomach to relieve vomiting. Chen Pi moves the qi and helps support spleen function while drying dampness. It is important to note that medicinals that move and disperse must be used with caution in pregnancy. For example, Zhi Shi (Aurantii Fructus Immaturus) and Hou Po (Magnoliae Offici-nalis Cortex) would normally be good for moving the qi in the middle burner, but, because they move qi downward, they can cause miscarriage and, therefore, are not advised in pregnancy.

Modifications:

- If there is evidence of liver qi depression and binding, such as moodiness, Bai Shao (Paeoniae Radix Alba) may be added to emolliate the liver.

- If liver-related symptoms are accompanied by evidence of heat, such as irri-tability or a bitter taste in the mouth, Zhu Ru (Bumbusae Caulis in Taenia) is a good addition.

- If there is flatulence and abdominal distention, Sha Ren (Amomi Fructus) can be added. This ingredient aromatically transforms dampness and checks vom-iting. Additionally, it has a gentle qi-moving action and helps to quiet the fetus.

- If there is poor appetite or poor sleep, add Wu Wei Zi (Schisandrae Fructus). Its sour flavor tends to stimulate the appetite, and it also quiets the spirit. Wu Wei Zi is also able to secure and astringe to protect yin fluids.

As mentioned above, vomiting in pregnancy can become severe enough to cause dehydration and lack of nourishment. When this occurs, qi and yin can be dam-aged. Western medical treatment for this will often include IV fluids. The formula Zeng Ye Tang (Humor-increasing Decoction) supports this Western medical treat-ment by nourishing yin. To nourish yin and supplement qi, Sheng Mai San (Pulse-engendering Powder) may be added.

Zeng Ye Tang (Humor-increasing Decoction)

Mai Men Dong (Ophiopogonis Radix)
Xuan Shen (Scrophulariae Radix)
Sheng Di Huang (Rehmanniae Radix Exsiccata seu Recens)

Formula analysis

Mai Men Dong specifically engenders stomach yin. Xuan Shen and Sheng Di Huang nourish yin in general.

Sheng Mai San (Pulse-engendering Powder)

Ren Shen (Ginseng Radix)
Mai Men Dong (Ophiopogonis Radix)
Wu Wei Zi (Schisandrae Fructus)

Ren Shen supplements the qi and engenders fluids. Mai Men Dong engenders stomach yin. Wu Wei Zi engenders fluids as well but also secures and astringes to prevent the dissipation of qi and yin. The sour and sweet flavors together engender yin.

These herbal treatments for vomiting during pregnancy will not conflict with Western medical treatments such as antiemetic drugs and B6 vitamin supplements. In fact, they work well as a combined approach. The best way to gain the most from each treatment is to take the Chinese medicinals two hours before or after any other drugs or supplements.

Acupuncture formula:

GV20 (Bai Hui), Yin Tang (M-HN-3), and Ear points Spleen, Kidney, and Shen Men.

Moxa may be used on CV12 (Zhong Wan), CV8 (Shen Que), ST36 (Zu San Li), or ST25 (Tian Shu).

Formula analysis

The main thrust of this acupuncture treatment is to calm the patient. I find that the nervous system is typically overstimulated in these patients, and this perpetuates the nausea and vomiting. GV20, Yin Tang, and Ear Shen Men therefore make an appropriate combination for these situations since these three points are very effective at quieting the spirit.

I am very conservative in my approach to needling during pregnancy and prefer not to needle body points on pregnant patients. Instead, I use Ear Kidney and Spleen to regulate these two important organs of pregnancy. The kidney is in charge of hormonal regulation as well as holding and nourishing the fetus in the uterus. The spleen is in charge of engendering the blood, making it an important adjunct for holding and nourishing the fetus. In the case of vomiting during pregnancy, the spleen needs extra support to facilitate the digestive system.

I use moxibustion instead of needles on CV8, CV12, ST36, or ST25 to downbear the qi. It is not necessary that cold be present for the use of moxibustion in this case. The stimulation should be very gentle and should not be too hot or too long in duration. CV12 and ST36 are especially good for downbearing the qi of the stomach in case of vomiting. CV8 and ST25 are better for treating unformed bowel movements, although these points will help with vomiting also by promoting the proper flow of stomach qi downward.

I recommend that practitioners be very cautious when moving or downbearing the qi in pregnant patients. The minimum possible number of points should be used and needling technique should be extremely gentle.

Case Study

The patient was a 36-year-old woman who was six weeks pregnant, vomited 3-4 times daily, and was constantly nauseous. She had difficulty bringing herself to eat and had a tendency toward gas and bloating after meals. She also reported feeling dizzy, weak, and fatigued. She was not experiencing vaginal bleeding or lower abdominal cramping. Her bowel movements were unformed and her urination was normal. She worried a lot and had a history of two miscarriages. Her pulse was slippery, bowstring, and weak at the cubit positions. Her tongue was pale with teethmarks on its edges and wet, white fur.

Diagnosis: Spleen-kidney dual vacuity with liver qi depression and binding

The digestive symptoms as well as her fatigue and weakness suggested spleen qi vacuity. This was further supported by her pale tongue with teethmarks. Her pulse was weak at the cubit positions, signifying kidney vacuity. She had a history of multiple miscarriages which further suggested kidney vacuity. The dizziness she experienced may have been the result of the spleen and kidney not upbearing the clear qi to the head. She also worried and had a bowstring pulse, leading me to the conclusion that there was also an element of liver depression.

Treatment principles: Supplement the spleen and kidney, course the liver and rectify the qi

Formula: Modified Liu Jun Zi Tang (Six Gentlemen Decoction)

Chen Pi (Citri Reticulatae Pericarpium)
Ban Xia (Pinelliae Rhizoma)
Dang Shen (Codonopsis Radix)

Fu Ling (Poria)
Bai Zhu (Atractylodis Macrocephalae Rhizoma)
Gan Cao (Glycyrrhizae Radix)
Bai Shao (Paeoniae Radix Alba)
Sha Ren (Amomi Fructus)
Sheng Jiang (Zingiberis Rhizoma Recens)
Wu Wei Zi (Schisandrae Fructus)

Acupuncture points:

Yin Tang (M-HN-3), GV20 (Bai Hui), Ear Kidney, Spleen, and Shen Men; moxibustion on CV12 (Zhong Wan) and ST25 (Tian Shu)

Treatment analysis

As discussed above, Liu Jun Zi Tang supplements the spleen qi, dries dampness, and moves the qi. In this case, Bai Shao was added to relax the uterus, prevent uterine contractions, and soothe the liver. Sha Ren was added to address the gas and bloating and, together with Sheng Jiang, helped harmonize the middle burner to stop the vomiting. Wu Wei Zi was used here to help promote the patient's appetite while also quieting her spirit. No additional medicinals were added to directly address the kidney because such medicinals would be too difficult to digest for this patient. Also, the kidney vacuity was not very acute at this point.

Yin Tang, Ear Shen Men, and GV20 quiet the spirit and help to soothe the patient. Her worrying was only contributing to the problem. This is because, when the liver is depressed, a replete liver counterflows to assail the spleen, making it vacuous and weak.

Ear Kidney and Spleen support their respective organs, addressing the patient's kidney and spleen vacuity.

Moxibustion was applied to CV12 to check vomiting by downbearing the qi. Moxibustion was also applied to ST25 to help regulate the intestines and address the patient's unformed bowel movements.

Outcome

After three treatments, the patient experienced only very slight nausea and no vomiting. She carried her pregnancy successfully to term and gave birth to a healthy baby boy.

10

Prevention of Miscarriage

Western Medical View

Miscarriage (spontaneous abortion) is the natural loss of the fetus before 20 weeks of gestation. In approximately 20% of known pregnancies, there are warning signs that a miscarriage may occur. About half of these patients (10%) actually miscarry. Some women miscarry before they even know they are pregnant. Most miscarriages happen within the first 12 weeks and are due to chromosomal abnormalities. Women who have one miscarriage usually are able to have successful pregnancies.

Types of miscarriage:

- **Threatened miscarriage (premiscarriage):** In this case, there are warning signs and half of such patients do miscarry.
- **Incomplete miscarriage (incomplete abortion):** In this case, some fetal tissue is expelled and some remains in the uterus.
- **Complete miscarriage (spontaneous abortion):** This refers to the complete expulsion of the fetus.
- **Missed abortion:** This refers to loss of pregnancy but failure to expel the fetus.
- **Inevitable miscarriage (inevitable abortion):** This refers to a miscarriage in progress that cannot be stopped.

Symptoms:

- Vaginal spotting or bleeding during the first weeks of pregnancy, sometimes accompanied by discharge of fluid or tissue
- Cramping or pain in the abdomen, lower back or pelvic area
- Rhythmic cramping or constant midline dull ache
- Membrane rupture or leaking of amniotic fluid

Diagnosis:

- Pelvic exam to check cervical dilation, size and quality of uterus (soft indicates pregnancy, hard indicates fibroids)
- Ultrasound to check for fetal heartbeat and normal embryo development
- Blood or urine pregnancy tests (measures HCG levels)

Causes (& risk factors):

- Chromosomal abnormalities in the fetus
- Advanced maternal age (over 35)
- Progesterone deficiency
- Poor egg quality
- Difficult for the uterus to support growing fetus due to decreased sensitivity to progesterone
- Increased chance of chromosomal abnormalities
- Lifestyle (cigarette smoking, caffeine, alcohol, drugs)
- Abnormalities in the uterus or cervix
- Scar tissue, uterine fibroids and adhesions within the uterus
- Weak cervical muscles unable to hold fetus within the uterus
- Blighted ovum
  Defined: Fertilized egg produces hormones of pregnancy, placenta and amniotic sac, but embryo fails to develop, often due to chromosomal abnormalities
- Molar pregnancy (Hydatidiform Mole)
  Defined: Benign mass of cysts growing within the placental tissues does not allow embryo to implant
- Vaginal infection
- Chronic maternal health conditions (diabetes, thyroid disease, infections, blood clotting disorders, autoimmune conditions)
- Environmental toxins
- Invasive prenatal tests (villus sampling, amniocentesis)

Prevention:

- Counseling and education
- Regular prenatal care
- Healthy maternal lifestyle
- Avoid known risk factors
- Keep chronic conditions under control

Treatment:

The main protocol for decreasing miscarriage risk is adequate bed rest and abstinence from sex and heavy exercise. If there is a history of recurrent miscarriages, treatment with aspirin or other blood-thinners may be suggested.

Specific treatment for actual miscarriage:

- Allow the miscarriage to progress naturally
- If necessary use medication or surgical treatment (D&C) to aid body in expelling products of conception
- Stop bleeding and prevent infection
- In case of infection (signaled by bleeding, fever, chills or severe pain), treat with antibiotics

Recovery:

- Physical recovery from miscarriage may take only a few hours
- Menstruation normally returns within four to six weeks
- Emotional pain may persist, but is eased by time

Discussion of Specific Types of Miscarriage

Threatened miscarriage (premiscarriage)

Vaginal bleeding during the first 20 weeks of pregnancy with no signs of ruptured membranes or passage of tissue. The embryo separates from the uterine wall, but the cervical os remains closed. Threatened miscarriage often has a good outcome.

Symptoms:

- Vaginal spotting, bleeding or discharge
- Pain in abdomen, pelvic area, or lower back
- Dull midline ache, constant or variable
- Rhythmic cramping

Diagnosis:

- Pelvic exam to check for dilation of the cervix
- Cervical os remains closed
- Ultrasound to test for fetal heartbeat
- If there is a fetal heartbeat, it is still possible to save the pregnancy
- Possible amniocentesis to test for chromosomal abnormalities

- Rule out ectopic pregnancy and ovarian torsion

Treatment:

- Adequate bed rest
- Avoid intercourse, heavy exercise, and traveling
- Report any increase in bleeding, cramping, passage of tissue or fever
- Minimize risk factors

Incomplete miscarriage/missed abortion/septic abortion

Loss of pregnancy with partial or complete failure to expel the dead fetus from the uterus. The cervical os is dilated or membranes have ruptured. Failure to fully expel a dead fetus can result in septic abortion, a potentially life-threatening condition.

Symptoms:

- Severe cramping, heavy bleeding
- Dizziness
- Changes in blood pressure and pulse
- Dilated cervical os

Missed abortion:

- Lack of symptoms except for amenorrhea
- Uterus does not grow as in normal pregnancy

Diagnosis:

- Check for dilated cervical os
- Ultrasound shows absence of fetal heartbeat (absence of heartbeat after week seven indicates death of the fetus)

Low levels of pregnancy hormones

Treatment:

- Allow the miscarriage to happen naturally
- Speed inevitable miscarriage with oral or vaginal medication (oxytocin used to induce uterine contractions)
- Dilation and curettage (D & C) to clean uterine lining of any remaining products of conception

Complete miscarriage (spontaneous abortion)

Approximately 15% of known pregnancies result in complete miscarriage. The embryo separates from the uterine wall and is completely expelled, along with all products of conception. After the embryo is expelled, the cervix closes on its own.

Symptoms:

- Severe cramping, bleeding and/or discharge
- Bleeding continues for 7-10 days, decreases, and then stops

Diagnosis: Ultrasound to test for embryonic/fetal and placental tissue in uterus

Treatment:

- Wait at least three months to allow the uterus to recover from the trauma
- Then attempt to conceive again

Inevitable miscarriage (inevitable abortion)

An inevitable miscarriage cannot be stopped. The cervical os is dilated and the uterus is contracting. There is vaginal bleeding, usually accompanied by cramps similar to menstrual cramps.

Symptoms:

- Membrane rupture and leaking amniotic fluid
- Vaginal bleeding, often with menstrual-like cramps

Diagnosis:

- Amniocentesis to check for chromosomal abnormalities
- Rule out ectopic pregnancy or ovarian torsion

Treatment:

- Allow the miscarriage to happen naturally
- Speed inevitable miscarriage with oral or vaginal medication
- Dilation and curettage (D & C), as necessary, to clean uterine lining of remaining fetal or placental tissue

Traditional Chinese Medical View

Miscarriage is the natural loss of the fetus before 20 weeks of gestation. If the loss occurs after 20 weeks, it is called a stillbirth or premature delivery. This is true for Western medicine too. There are four types of a miscarriage: premiscarriage, complete miscarriage, incomplete miscarriage, or inevitable abortion. In a premiscarriage, there is still a chance to be able to save the pregnancy with Chinese medicine as described below. Some of the signs of a premiscarriage are slight bleeding, slight cramping, and a closed cervix upon examination.

Treatment based on pattern identification:

Qi & blood vacuity (*qi xue xu* 气血虚)

Signs & symptoms: Bleeding with dropping or sinking sensation

Tongue: Pale

Pulse: Thin, weak

Treatment principles: Supplement the qi and blood

Formula: Tai Yuan Yin (Fetal Origin Beverage)

> Ren Shen (Ginseng Radix)
> Bai Zhu (Atractylodis Macrocephalae Rhizoma)
> Zhi Gan Cao (Glycyrrhizae Radix cum Liquido Fricta)
> Dang Gui (Angelicae Sinensis Radix)
> Shu Di Huang (Rehmanniae Radix Praeparata)
> Bai Shao (Paeoniae Radix Alba)
> Chen Pi (Citri Reticulatae Pericarpium)
> Du Zhong (Eucommiae Cortex)

Modifications:

- For more qi vacuity, add Huang Qi (Astragali Radix) and Shan Yao (Dioscoreae Rhizoma).

- For more blood vacuity, add Gou Qi Zi (Lycii Fructus) and He Shou Wu (Polygoni Multiflori Radix).

- If kidney yin vacuity is also present, add Shan Zhu Yu (Corni Fructus) and Sang Shen (Mori Fructus).

- If kidney yang vacuity is also present, add Xu Duan (Dipsaci Radix) and Bu Gu Zhi (Psoraleae Fructus).

- For kidney yin and yang dual vacuity, add Tu Si Zi (Cuscutae Semen) and Sha Yuan Zi (Astragali Complanati Semen).

- For nausea, add Sha Ren (Amomi Fructus).

- For vomiting, add Ban Xia (Pinelliae Rhizoma) and Sheng Jiang (Zingiberis Rhizoma Recens).

- For bleeding due to heat, add Mo Han Lian (Ecliptae Herba).

- For bleeding due to cold, add Ai Ye (Artemisiae Argyi Folium).

Kidney vacuity (*shen xu* 肾虚)

Signs & symptoms: Bleeding with a sinking sensation, lower back pain

Tongue: In case of kidney yin vacuity, red, cracks, and scanty fur; in case of kidney yang vacuity, pale and enlarged with moist fur

Pulse: Deep, weak

Treatment principles: Supplement the kidney

Formula: Shou Tai Wan (Fetal Longevity Pill)

Tu Si Zi (Cuscutae Semen)
Sang Ji Sheng (Taxilli Herba)
Xu Duan (Dipsaci Radix)
E Jiao (Asini Corii Colla)

Modifications:

- For more qi vacuity, add Dang Shen (Codonopsis Radix) and Huang Qi (Astragali Radix).

- For spleen vacuity, add Bai Zhu (Atractylodis Macrocephalae Rhizoma) and Shan Yao (Dioscoreae Rhizoma).

- For kidney yin vacuity, add Shan Zhu Yu (Corni Fructus) and Shu Di Huang (Rehmanniae Radix Praeparata).

- For kidney yang vacuity, add Bu Gu Zhi (Psoraleae Fructus) and Du Zhong (Eucommiae Cortex).

- For blood vacuity, add He Shou Wu (Polygoni Multiflori Radix), Gou Qi Zi (Lycii Fructus), and Huang Jing (Polygonati Rhizoma).

- For lower abdominal pain, add Bai Shao (Paeoniae Radix Alba) and Zhi Gan Cao (Glycyrrhizae Radix cum Liquido Fricta).

- For nausea, add Chen Pi (Citri Reticulatae Pericarpium) and Sha Ren (Amomi Fructus).

- For vomiting, add Sheng Jiang (Zingiberis Rhizoma Recens) and Ban Xia (Pinelliae Rhizoma).

- For bleeding due to vacuity heat, add Mo Han Lian (Ecliptae Herba).

- For bleeding due to vacuity cold, add Ai Ye (Artemisiae Argyi Folium).

- For bleeding due to replete heat, add Ce Bai Ye (Platycladi Cacumen), Huang Qin (Scutellariae Radix), and Di Yu (Sanguisorbae Radix).

Blood heat (*xue re* 血热)

Signs & symptoms: Bleeding with fresh red blood, excessive fetal movement

Tongue: Red, dry fur

Pulse: Rapid, deep, replete

Treatment principles: Clear heat, staunch bleeding, and nourish the fetus\

Formula: Bao Yin Jian (Yin-safeguarding Brew)

Sheng Di Huang (Rehmanniae Radix)
Shu Di Huang (Rehmanniae Radix Praeparata)
Huang Qin (Scutellariae Radix)
Huang Bai (Phellodendri Cortex)
Shan Yao (Dioscoreae Rhizoma)
Gan Cao (Glycyrrhizae Radix)
Bai Shao (Paeoniae Radix Alba)
Xu Duan (Dipsaci Radix)

Modifications:

- For yin vacuity, add Mai Men Dong (Ophiopogonis Radix).

- For blood vacuity, add He Shou Wu (Polygoni Multiflori Radix) and Huang Jing (Polygonati Rhizoma).

- For lower back pain, add Sang Ji Sheng (Taxilli Herba).

- For bleeding, add Mo Han Lian (Ecliptae Herba), Di Yu (Sanguisorbae Radix), and Ce Bai Ye (Platycladi Cacumen).

- For insomnia, add Suan Zao Ren (Ziziphi Spinosi Semen) and Wu Wei Zi (Schisandrae Fructus).

Traumatic injury (*shou shang* 受伤)

Tongue: Pale

Pulse: Weak

Treatment principles: Supplement the qi and nourish the blood, supplement the kidney

Formula: Modified Sheng Yu Tang (Sagacious Cure Decoction)

Sheng Di Huang (Rehmanniae Radix)/Shu Di Huang (Rehmanniae Radix
  Praeparata)
Dang Gui (Angelicae Sinensis Radix)
Bai Shao (Paeoniae Radix Alba)
Ren Shen (Ginseng Radix)
Huang Qi (Astragali Radix)
Tu Si Zi (Cuscutae Semen)
Sang Ji Sheng (Taxilli Herba)
Xu Duan (Dipsaci Radix)

Clinical Treatment

Although TCM gynecology textbooks describe the discrete disease mechanisms of qi vacuity, blood vacuity, kidney vacuity, blood heat, my clinical experience has shown that it is most efficacious to treat threatened miscarriage by treating the kidney as the root and modifying that to include other elements as necessary. This makes sense if you consider that the kidney, as the source of yin and yang for the body as well as the container of essence, is most intimately connected with conception and gestation. Successful initiation and development of pregnancy depends on an abundant supply of each of these elements and this depends on the health of the kidney. When the kidney is vacuous, there is difficulty holding the pregnancy and miscarriage can result. While qi and blood vacuity and blood heat definitely play a role in miscarriage, the role of the kidney is so fundamental that I believe it must be addressed before anything. It is like the foundation of the house. There may also be weak walls or a weak roof, but, ultimately, if the foundation is unable to support the structure, all other repairs are useless. Therefore, I begin clinical treatment for prevention of miscarriage by addressing this foundation.

Hence, my first step is to identify whether kidney yin or kidney yang vacuity is most prominent. In clinic, typically there will be either primarily kidney yang vacuity with spleen qi vacuity or kidney yin vacuity with blood vacuity.

Kidney yang vacuity (shen yang xu 肾阳虚)

For a patient who tends toward cold signs, we say there is primarily kidney yang vacuity. The basic formula for threatened miscarriage with a predominance of kidney yang vacuity signs is An Tai Fang (Fetus-quieting Formula). This formula also addresses blood, yin, and qi.

An Tai Fang (Fetus-quieting Formula)

Tu Si Zi (Cuscutae Semen)
Xu Duan (Dipsaci Radix)
Sang Ji Sheng (Taxilli Herba)
Shan Zhu Yu (Corni Fructus)
Bai Shao (Paeoniae Radix Alba)
Gou Qi Zi (Lycii Fructus)
Dang Shen (Codonopsis Radix)
Bai Zhu (Atractylodis Macrocephalae Rhizoma)

Formula analysis

Tu Si Zi and Xu Duan both supplement kidney yang and quiet the fetus. Tu Si Zi also fills the essence, while Xu Duan also stops uterine bleeding. These yang-supplementing agents are chosen over other warmer, more moving herbs such as Ba Ji Tian (Radix Morindae Officinalis) and Yin Yang Huo (Herba Epimedii). The last thing we want to do in case of threatened miscarriage is to move the blood or qi too much since this will only further threaten miscarriage. Sang Ji Sheng quiets the fetus and nourishes kidney yin which is important because yin and yang are mutually rooted or dependent. Shan Zhu Yu secures the essence and also stops bleeding. Bai Shao and Gou Qi Zi nourish the yin and blood without promoting the movement of blood. Dang Shen and Bai Zhu supplement qi, while Bai Zhu also quiets the fetus. Gan Cao supplements the qi and harmonizes all the other elements of the formula. In addition, with Bai Shao, it calms spasms such as uterine contractions (as in Shao Yao Gan Cao Tang [Peony & Licorice Decoction]).

Modification: In case of marked qi vacuity, Hu Tai Fang (Fetus-protecting Formula) is recommended. Hu Tai Fang (Fetus-protecting Formula) is An Tai Fang plus Huang Qi (Astragali Radix) to secure the exterior (and thus hold the the qi within the body) and Suan Zao Ren to quiet the spirit.

Hu Tai Fang (Fetus-protecting Formula)

Tu Si Zi (Cuscutae Semen)
Xu Duan (Dipsaci Radix)
Sang Ji Sheng (Taxilli Herba)
Shan Zhu Yu (Corni Fructus)
Bai Shao (Paeoniae Radix Alba)
Gou Qi Zi (Lycii Fructus)
Dang Shen (Codonopsis Radix)
Bai Zhu (Atractylodis Macrocephalae Rhizoma)
Huang Qi (Astragali Radix)
Suan Zao Ren (Ziziphi Spinosi Semen)

In the event that a patient shows great emotion or nervousness, Jing Tai Fang (Quiet the Fetus Formula) is recommended. Jing Tai Fang is An Tai Fang plus Wu Wei Zi (Schisandrae Fructus) and Suan Zao Ren (Ziziphi Spinosi Semen) to quiet the spirit. Suan Zao Ren also nourishes the heart, while Wu Wei Zi quiets the heart, supplements the kidney, and secures the essence.

Jing Tai Fang (Quiet the Fetus Formula)

Tu Si Zi (Cuscutae Semen)
Xu Duan (Dipsaci Radix)
Sang Ji Sheng (Taxilli Herba)
Shan Zhu Yu (Corni Fructus)
Bai Shao (Paeoniae Radix Alba)
Gou Qi Zi (Lycii Fructus)

Dang Shen (Codonopsis Radix)
Bai Zhu (Atractylodis Macrocephalae Rhizoma)
Suan Zao Ren (Ziziphi Spinosi Semen)
Wu Wei Zi (Schisandrae Fructus)

In the event that a patient with kidney yang vacuity is experiencing bleeding, Nuan Tai Zhi Xu Fang (Fetus-warming Vacuity-treating Formula) is the best approach. This is a modification of An Tai Fang that includes Huang Qi (Astragali Radix), E Jiao (Asini Corii Colla), Ai Ye (Artemisiae Argyi Folium), and Suan Zao Ren (Ziziphi Spinosi Semen).

Nuan Tai Zhi Xu Fang (Fetus-warming Vacuity-treating Formula)

Tu Si Zi (Cuscutae Semen)
Xu Duan (Dipsaci Radix)
Sang Ji Sheng (Taxilli Herba)
Shan Zhu Yu (Corni Fructus)
Bai Shao (Paeoniae Radix Alba)
Gou Qi Zi (Lycii Fructus)
Dang Shen (Codonopsis Radix)
Bai Zhu (Atractylodis Macrocephalae Rhizoma)
Huang Qi (Astragali Radix)
E Jiao (Asini Corii Colla)
Ai Ye (Artemisiae Argyi Folium)
Suan Zao Ren (Ziziphi Spinosi Semen)

Formula analysis

Within this formula, Ai Ye warms the uterus, quiets the fetus, and stops bleeding. E Jiao both stops bleeding and nourishes the blood. Huang Qi upbears the qi and supplements the spleen to help it contain the blood. Suan Zao Ren and Huang Qi both secure and astringe which is helpful when there has already been blood loss and fluids need to be conserved. Suan Zao Ren has the added benefit of quieting the spirit and nourishing the heart. This can relax the uterus and prevent further contractions. Ai Ye, Huang Qi, and Suan Zao Ren are all warm in nature. E Jiao is neutral.

Kidney yin vacuity (shen yin xu 肾阴虚)

A patient with primarily kidney yin vacuity often shows vacuity heat signs, such as night sweating and insomnia. The basic formula I use for threatened miscarriage with kidney yin vacuity signs is Yang Tai Fang (Formula to Nourish the Fetus).

Yang Tai Fang (Formula to Nourish the Fetus)

Tu Si Zi (Cuscutae Semen)
Shu Di Huang (Rehmanniae Radix Praeparata)
Shan Zhu Yu (Corni Fructus)
Shan Yao (Dioscoreae Rhizoma)
Bai Shao (Paeoniae Radix Alba)
Mai Men Dong (Ophiopogonis Radix)
Suan Zao Ren (Ziziphi Spinosi Semen)
Gan Cao (Glycyrrhizae Radix)

Formula analysis

Tu Si Zi supplements both kidney yang and essence and quiets the fetus. Shu Di Huang and Bai Shao nourish the blood without quickening it too much. Shan Zhu Yu secures the essence and stops uterine bleeding. Shan Yao supplements the qi and fortifies the spleen. It also supplements the kidney and secures the essence. Mai Men Dong and Bai Shao nourish yin. Mai Men Dong and Suan Zao Ren quiet the heart. Mai Men Dong clears heat as well. Gan Cao supplements the qi and harmonizes the other elements of the formula, and, together with Bai Shao, relaxes spasms, such as uterine contractions, as in Shao Yao Gan Cao Tang (Peony & Licorice Decoction).

Modification: If the patient shows more qi vacuity signs and symptoms, Zhi Tai Fang (Formula to Treat the Fetus) is recommended. This formula is Yang Tai Fang (Formula to Nourish the Fetus) plus Dang Shen (Codonopsis Radix) to supplement the qi and Wu Wei Zi (Schisandrae Fructus) to quiet the heart, supplement the kidney, and secure the essence. Wu Wei Zi is sweet and sour, and it nourishes yin by helping to engender fluids.

Zhi Tai Fang (Formula to Treat the Fetus)

Tu Si Zi (Cuscutae Semen)
Shu Di Huang (Rehmanniae Radix Praeparata)
Shan Zhu Yu (Corni Fructus)
Shan Yao (Dioscoreae Rhizoma)
Bai Shao (Paeoniae Radix Alba)
Mai Men Dong (Ophiopogonis Radix)
Suan Zao Ren (Ziziphi Spinosi Semen)
Dang Shen (Codonopsis Radix)
Wu Wei Zi (Schisandrae Fructus)

In the event that a patient with kidney yin vacuity is experiencing bleeding, I believe Liang Tai Zhi Xu Fang (Fetus-cooling Vacuity-treating Decoction) is the best approach. This is a modification of An Tai Fang with E Jiao (Asini Corii Colla), Mo Han Lian (Ecliptae Herba), and Wu Wei Zi (Schisandrae Fructus) added.

Liang Tai Zhi Xu Fang (Fetus-cooling Vacuity-treating Decoction)

Tu Si Zi (Cuscutae Semen)
Xu Duan (Dipsaci Radix)
Sang Ji Sheng (Taxilli Herba)
Shan Zhu Yu (Corni Fructus)
Bai Shao (Paeoniae Radix Alba)
Gou Qi Zi (Lycii Fructus)
Dang Shen (Codonopsis Radix)
Bai Zhu (Atractylodis Macrocephalae Rhizoma)
E Jiao (Asini Corii Colla)
Mo Han Lian (Ecliptae Herba)
Wu Wei Zi (Schisandrae Fructus)

Formula analysis

Mo Han Lian cools the blood and stops bleeding. It also nourishes kidney yin. E Jiao also stops bleeding and simultaneously nourishes the blood. Wu Wei Zi secures and astringes to prevent further loss of fluids. In addition, its sour nature combines with the sweet flavor of Dang Shen to engender yin. Wu Wei Zi also quiets the spirit to help relax the uterus.

Acupuncture formulas

Acupuncture can be an effective emergency treatment for threatened miscarriage. In one case, I treated a woman who was five months pregnant and experiencing severe abdominal cramping. She arrived at the hospital holding her stomach in pain. Examination revealed that she was dilated at four centimeters. I gave her Bai Shao (Paeoniae Radix Alba) to relax the uterus and needled the ear points Kidney and Shen Men as well as GV20 (Bai Hui) and Yin Tang (M-HN-3). The patient's cervix closed and she was then instructed to go home and rest.

The following acupuncture point prescription is useful in preventing miscarriage.

GV20 (Bai Hui), Yin Tang (M-HN-3), Ear Kidney, Spleen, Shen Men

Formula analysis

Primarily, we need to A) prevent the qi from falling downward, B) quiet the spirit, and C) encourage the spleen and kidney to hold the pregnancy. This is because the spleen contains the blood, while the kidney secures the essence. Quieting the spirit is vital because, when the spirit is disturbed, it affects the proper movement and distribution of the qi. Regulating and upbearing the qi is important in preventing abortion which is the untimely downward movement of the fetus. In this formula, GV20 upbears the qi to prevent it from falling downward. Yin Tang and ear Shen Men quiet the spirit. The ear points of the kidney and spleen encourage the containing and securing functions of these two viscera to maintain the pregnancy. Ear points are preferred in this case because the body points we would ordinarily use on the spleen and kidney channels are on the feet or lower leg and we wish to guide the qi upward as much as possible.

N.B. Do not use the points LI4 (He Gu) or SP6 (San Yin Jiao). These points can cause uterine contractions and, therefore, miscarriage.

Case Study

The patient was a 32-year-old woman with a history of three miscarriages. She was 29 days pregnant. She had been experiencing a small amount of vaginal bleeding for seven days that was red in color and without clots. The bleeding was accompanied by lower abdominal and lower back pain and a sinking sensation in the lower abdomen. She also was vomiting in the morning and was nauseous, dizzy, and fatigued throughout the day. Her appetite was poor. She was thirsty but did not feel the urge to drink. The patient's bowel movements were normal, but her urination was frequent. She felt anxious and worried constantly. Her pulse was slippery, bowstring, thin, and weak in both cubit positions. Her tongue was enlarged, slightly pale with a red tip, and had scanty fur.

Pattern identification: Spleen qi-kidney yin and yang vacuity with liver depression qi stagnation

Symptom analysis

Spleen qi vacuity was shown by the ongoing vaginal bleeding, the sinking sensation in the patient's abdomen, and the digestive and energy problems. This was further suggested by her thin and weak pulse. I believed the kidney was also involved because there was lower back pain and weakness in the cubit pulse positions. Her tongue was slightly enlarged and pale, suggesting an element of yang vacuity, but she also showed evidence of yin vacuity with the thirst, anxiety, and scanty tongue fur. Frequent urination is typically a manifestation of kidney qi vacuity (due to a loss of the kidney's securing function), and this was further supported by the fact that she had had three previous miscarriages (although the spleen is implicated in this also). Remembering that the kidney qi contains both yin and yang aspects, we can simply say that this patient presents with kidney yin and yang vacuity as well as spleen qi vacuity. Her bowstring pulse and anxious and worried mood suggested liver depression qi stagnation is also present.

Treatment principles: Supplement and nourish the kidney, fortify the spleen and boost the qi, course the liver and rectify the qi

Formula: Modified Nuan Tai Zhi Xu Fang (Fetus-warming Vacuity-treating Formula)

> Tu Si Zi (Cuscutae Semen)
> Xu Duan (Dipsaci Radix)
> Sang Ji Sheng (Taxilli Herba)
> Bai Shao (Paeoniae Radix Alba)
> Dang Shen (Codonopsis Radix)
> Bai Zhu (Atractylodis Macrocephalae Rhizoma)
> Gan Cao (Glycyrrhizae Radix)
> Huang Qi (Astragali Radix)
> Suan Zao Ren (Ziziphi Spinosi Semen)
> Ai Ye (Artemisiae Argyi Folium)

Formula analysis

In this case, several yin- and blood-nourishing medicinals have been removed from the original formula, such as Shan Zhu Yu (Corni Fructus), Gou Qi Zi (Lycii Fructus), and E Jiao (Asini Corii Colla). This is because these medicinals may be too slimy and enriching for this patient and also because her yin vacuity was not very significant. In my opinion, Bai Shao and Tu Si Zi provided enough yin nourishment and are not difficult to digest. Additionally, she was not bleeding heavily. Therefore, she did not require the strong blood-nourishing and blood-staunching action of E Jiao.

Tu Si Zi supplements both kidney yin and yang. Xu Duan supplements kidney yang. Sang Ji Sheng nourishes yin and blood and quiets the fetus. Bai Shao relaxes the uterus. Dang Shen and Huang Qi supplement the qi. Huang Qi also promotes the upbearing of the spleen qi. Bai Zhu also assists in fortifying the spleen and eliminating any dampness arising from vacuity. Suan Zao Ren quiets the spirit and, along with Huang Qi, has a securing and astringing effect. Ai Ye stops bleeding, warms the uterus, and quiets the fetus.

Acupuncture points:

GV20 (Bai Hui), Yin Tang (M-HN-3), Ear Kidney, Spleen, Shen Men

Formula analysis

GV20 upbears the qi and, thereby, helps the spleen qi contain the pregnancy.

Yin Tang and Ear Shen Men quiet the spirit to relax the uterus and prevent contractions. Ear Kidney and Spleen points supplement the two primary viscera responsible for maintaining the pregnancy according to Chinese medicine.

Outcome

Following treatment, the bleeding stopped. The patient was able to carry her pregnancy to term and gave birth to a healthy baby girl.

Miscarriage

Type	Premiscarriage	Incomplete miscarriage	Complete miscarriage
Bleeding	Light	Heavy	Light ---> Spotting ---> None
Cramps	Mild	Bad	Light ---> None
Uterus / Cervix	Loose	Open	Open ---> Loose ---> Closed (=normal)
Western treatment	Progesterone	D&C	Vitamins & Supplements
TCM treatment principles	Supplement K, Blood, Qi (to secure fetus), quiet spirit	Move Qi and Blood	Supplement K, Blood, Qi. Course LV
Medicinals	**K Yang vacuity:** Hu Tai Fang **K Yin and Yang vacuity:** Jing Tai Fang **K Yin vacuity:** Zhi Tai Fang	Gua Gong Fang **After HCG lowers:** Jing Gong Fang	Tiao Jing Fang
Acupuncture	Yintang, Du20, Ear: K, SP, Shenmen	SP10, Ren3, Ren4, LV3, SP6, LI4, Yintang	ST36, LI4, K3, Zigong, Yintang, Du20

11

Ectopic Pregnancy

Western Medical View

Ectopic pregnancy refers to the implantation of a fertilized egg outside the uterine cavity.

Most ectopic pregnancies (95%) occur within the fallopian tubes and are called tubal pregnancies. Rarely, an ectopic pregnancy occurs in the abdomen, ovary, or cervix. Ectopic pregnancies occur in approximately one out of every 60 pregnancies. Early detection of an ectopic pregnancy, especially for patients with difficulty conceiving, can preserve the reproductive organs, preserve fertility, and prevent the serious consequences of ectopic rupture.

Ruptured ectopic pregnancies are acute conditions that cause internal hemorrhage, are life-threatening, and require immediate surgical attention. They may result in infertility or loss of reproductive organs. Women with at least one normally functioning fallopian tube still have an approximately 40% chance of pregnancy.

Most ectopic pregnancies with very low levels of pregnancy hormones spontaneously resolve without medical or surgical intervention.

Causes:

- Fallopian tubes that have been damaged or blocked by infection, surgery or other trauma
- History of inflammation or infection, especially pelvic inflammatory disease (PID), usually results in scar tissue in and around the fallopian tubes
- Pelvic infections commonly result from intrauterine devices (IUDs), or sexually transmitted diseases (STDs, especially chlamydia) and often develop into PID
- Adhesions and scar tissue block the fallopian tubes

- Abnormal fallopian tube shape
- Endometriosis, a condition in which tissue that normally lines the uterus develops elsewhere in the abdominal cavity

Diagnosis:

- Ultrasound imaging to determine location of implanted fetus, uterine or elsewhere in the abdomen
- Pelvic exam to check for mass, tenderness and pain in the fallopian tube, ovary, or abdominal cavity
- Hysterosalpingogram (HSG) using dyes, fluoroscopy, and x-rays to determine if there are any blockages in the uterus or fallopian tubes
- Blood tests to determine if HCG and progesterone levels are rising slower than expected in a normal pregnancy
- Culdocentesis to detect blood in the vaginal fornix, thus confirming an acutely ruptured ectopic pregnancy
- Dull percussion detecting pooling of blood when patient lies on her side
- Rule out acute PID, threatened or incomplete abortion, ruptured cysts, pancreatitis, acute appendicitis and pyelonephritis

Symptoms:

- Normal signs of pregnancy: amenorrhea, breast tenderness, nausea, vomiting or frequent urination
- Abnormal vaginal bleeding, either heavier or lighter than normal menstruation
- Lower abdominal pain
- One-sided pelvic pain or cramps
- Lower back pain
- Sharp or stabbing pain in the pelvis, abdomen, shoulder or neck, which may vary in intensity
- Low blood pressure

Symptoms of acutely ruptured ectopic pregnancy:

- Weakness, dizziness, light-headedness or fainting
- Severe abdominal pain
- Shock (*i.e.*, pale face, dizziness, low blood pressure, sweating, rapid pulse)
- Sharp stabbing pain in the pelvis, abdomen or shoulder and neck, indicating internal hemorrhage

Risk factors:

- Maternal age over 35 years
- Previous ectopic pregnancy
- History of infertility problems
- History of fallopian tube, pelvic or abdominal surgery, induced abortions
- History of PID, inflammation of the fallopian tubes, ovaries or uterus (often caused by IUD use)
- Endometriosis
- Use of fertility medications that stimulate ovulation
- Use of progesterone-only contraceptives or the morning after pill
- Multiple sexual partners, resulting in STDs (especially gonorrhea or chlamydia)
- Pregnancy with concurrent use of contraceptive pills, IUD, or after tubal ligation
- Exposure to Diethylstilbestrol (DES)
- Smoking

Treatment:

- Removal of ectopic tissue
- Early detection

Medical intervention:

- Blood tests to monitor HCG levels once there is a positive pregnancy
- If levels remain low and decline, ectopic pregnancy may resolve itself
- Methyltrexate injections to stop cell growth and allow body to reabsorb existing pregnancy (70-80% success rate) and may save fallopian tube

Surgical intervention:

- Laparoscopic surgery to remove ectopic tissue, repair or remove fallopian tube
- Fallopian tube may heal without affecting future fertility

Ruptured ectopic pregnancy
Emergency surgery to:

- Promptly stop bleeding
- Remove ruptured fallopian tube
- Monitor HCG levels to ensure that all ectopic tissue has been removed

Prevention:

- Limit partners to help prevent transmission of Sexually Transmitted Diseases and reduce risk of PID
- Monitor HCG levels once there is a positive pregnancy
- Early medical or surgical treatment intervention to protect patient's fertility and health

Traditional Chinese Medical View

An ectopic pregnancy is a pregnancy located outside the uterine cavity, but the majority (95%) are located within the fallopian tubes.

Treatment based on pattern identification:

Ectopic pregnancy—blood stasis (*gong wai yun-xue yu* 宫外孕–血瘀)

Signs & symptoms:

Nonruptured: Absence of menses, low HCG on blood test but high HCG on urine sample, abdominal mass, irregular bleeding or spotting

Ruptured: Severe pain, shock (*i.e.,* pale face, cold extremities, sweating, low blood pressure), non-coagulating blood, positive percussion test

Tongue: Purple

Pulse: Rough or choppy

Treatment principles: Quicken the blood, transform stasis, and rectify the qi

Formula: Gong Wai Yin (Ectopic Pregnancy Beverage)

Chi Shao (Paeoniae Radix Rubra)
Dan Shen (Salviae Miltiorrhizae Radix)
Tao Ren (Persicae Semen)
San Leng (Sparganii Rhizoma)
E Zhu (Curcumae Rhizoma)

Prevention of future ectopic pregnancies:

Treatment principles: Supplement the spleen and disinhibit dampness, rectify the qi and quicken the blood

Formula: Man Pen Fang (Formula for Chronic Pelvic Infection)

Hei Lao Hu (Kadsurae Coccineae Caulis et Folium)
Ji Gu Xiang (Crotonis Crassifolii Radix)
Ji Xue Teng (Spatholobi Caulis)
Huang Qi (Astragali Radix)
Fu Ling (Poria)
Dan Shen (Salviae Miltiorrhizae Radix)
Yi Yi Ren (Coicis Semen)
Bai Jiang Cao (Patriniae Herba)

Clinical Treatment

Normally an egg and a sperm meet in the fallopian tube. There, the egg is fertilized and then travels back to the uterus to implant. However, sometimes a fertilized egg gets stuck at a narrow point in the fallopian tube. This may be due to a previous pelvic infection that has caused the tube to narrow or become damaged or may simply be due to an anatomical feature of that individual woman. In such cases, the embryo begins to develop in the tube. A very small percentage of fertilized eggs will even implant entirely outside both the uterus and tubes in the pelvic cavity. However, the fetus obviously cannot grow to full term in either of these locations. Usually within two months of conception, a tubal ectopic pregnancy will cause the fallopian tube to rupture depending on which part of the tube the embryo is stuck in. With an embryo implanted in the pelvic cavity, the signs and symptoms (as well as the timeline for discovery or rupture) will depend on the location of implantation and the surrounding structures and organs.

Because ectopic pregnancy may be a serious condition requiring emergency action, it is important to be able to recognize its signs and symptoms. These will vary depending on whether the ectopic pregnancy has ruptured or not. Therefore, it is worth recapping the clinical presentation of ectopic pregnancy:

Before rupture, the patient may report a missed period and/or vaginal bleeding. Laboratory tests will show raised HCG levels, and, after five weeks, distention may be detected in the fallopian tubes by palpation. An ultrasound should thus be performed. If an amniotic sac is not seen in the uterine cavity but serum HCG is elevated, the pregnancy may be in the fallopian tubes. A physician would do a gentle bimanual pelvic exam and may find a mass. Great care should be taken in any palpation because too much pressure may cause a rupture of the amniotic sac. A patient with a suspected ectopic pregnancy (prior to rupture) should always be immediately referred to her physician for examination.

After a rupture, the situation can rapidly become very serious, even life-threatening. Many blood vessels are present in the sac in order to nourish the embryo. Therefore, rupture usually causes extensive internal bleeding and very serious pain. Blood pressure will drop with the blood loss, and the patient will typically go into shock. Symptoms of shock include a pale face and rapid pulse. A blood test would show decreased hemoglobin and red blood cell count. A patient with a suspected ruptured ectopic pregnancy should be rushed to the emergency room immediately.

An examining physician may ask the patient to lie on the table on her side and then gradually change sides while the physician performs percussion to determine if there is free blood inside the body cavity. The physician may also insert a needle into the posterior fornix (the area posterior and inferior to the cervix) to determine whether there has been bleeding into the pelvic cavity. If there has, gravity and anatomy will cause blood to collect behind the fornix and a needle inserted there will extract blood.

During my years as a physician in China, I operated on a number of ruptured ectopic pregnancies. The situation was always very serious and, in many cases, we were unable to save the patient due to severe internal blood loss. In one happier case I recall, a woman came to me with an abdomen that was extremely bloated and swollen. She needed surgery immediately. When I made my incision, I saw that the uterine membrane was blue. In other words, the ectopic pregnancy had completely blocked the circulation. I had to excise an entire region of the fallopian tubes on one side where the ectopic pregnancy was located. Once I had done all I could surgically, I held my breath and the bleeding stopped. The following week, the patient's husband and son brought me a chicken as thanks! Unfortunately, not all cases of ectopic pregnancy end so well.

If the ectopic pregnancy is discovered before it has ruptured, Gua Tai Fang (Fetus-removing Formula) is the best choice. After surgery or administration of methyltrexate by injection, Gua Gong Yin (Uterine-scraping Beverage) works very well to resolve HCG levels and promote reabsorption of the mass. After recovery from an ectopic pregnancy or for the patient with a history of chronic pelvic infections, Man Pen Fang (Formula for Chronic Pelvic Infection) is recommended to protect against recurrence. It is important to follow up with Man Pen Fang because pelvic infections are usually bilateral. Therefore, if a patient has had one ectopic pregnancy, she is at risk for another in the future. Hence, it is very important to prevent another ectopic pregnancy from occurring in the fallopian tube on the opposite side.

In general, the Chinese medical method for treating this condition is to quicken the blood and disperse masses similar to the treatment of tumors.

Timing: Prior to Rupture

Treatment principles: Move the qi and blood downward, break stasis

Formula: Gua Tai Fang (Fetus-removing Formula)

San Leng (Sparganii Rhizoma)
E Zhu (Curcumae Rhizoma)
Wang Bu Liu Xing (Vaccariae Semen)
Dan Shen (Salviae Miltiorrhizae Radix)
Chi Shao (Paeoniae Radix Rubra)
Xiang Fu (Cyperi Rhizoma)
Qing Pi (Citri Reticulatae Pericarpium Viride)
Hong Hua (Carthami Flos)
Yi Mu Cao (Leonuri Herba)
Niu Xi (Achyranthis Bidentatae Radix)

Formula analysis

The name Gua Tai Fang means "Fetus-removing Formula." It is important to know that, as the name suggests, this formula will promote miscarriage as well as the termination and expulsion of an ectopic pregnancy. Because incomplete miscarriage can result in life-threatening hemorrhage, termination of any kind of pregnancy using this formula should never be attempted unless as part of a carefully managed integrative approach in conjunction with the patient's Western physician.

Within this formula, San Leng, E Zhu, and Wang Bu Liu Xing all enter the liver channel and strongly break blood stasis. San Leng and E Zhu also relieve pain and disperse accumulations. Dan Shen, Chi Shao, Hong Hua, and Yi Mu Cao all quicken the blood. Dan Shen, Chi Shao, and Yi Mu Cao also clear any heat which may arise as the result of blood stasis. Yi Mu Cao disperses masses and stimulates contraction of the uterus to promote expulsion. Xiang Fu and Qing Pi course the liver and rectify the qi. Niu Xi promotes the downward movement of the qi and blood, thus assisting with the expulsion of products of the ectopic pregnancy.

Timing: Following Surgery or Administration of Methyltrexate

Treatment principles: Move the qi and blood, disperse accumulations

Formula: Gua Gong Fang (Uterine-scraping Formula)

Ji Xue Teng (Spatholobi Caulis)
San Leng (Sparganii Rhizoma)
E Zhu (Curcumae Rhizoma)
Mu Dan Pi (Moutan Cortex)
Dan Shen (Salviae Miltiorrhizae Radix)
Chi Shao (Paeoniae Radix Rubra)
Tao Ren (Persicae Semen)
Fu Ling (Poria)
Zhi Ke (Qiao) (Aurantii Fructus)
Bai Zhu (Atractylodis Macrocephalae Rhizoma)
Yi Mu Cao (Herba Leonuri Heterophylli)
Niu Xi (Radix Achyranthis Bidentatae)

Formula analysis

In my opinion, Gua Gong Fang is the best formula for absorbing the mass left over following an ectopic pregnancy. In my clinical experience, this formula is also highly effective at bringing HCG levels back to baseline. These levels are typically carefully monitored after an ectopic pregnancy to ensure that the pregnancy has fully resolved and the tissue been moved out or reabsorbed by the body.

Within this formula, Ji Xue Teng moves the blood in the channels. San Leng and E Zhu powerfully break blood stasis, disperse accumulations, and relieve pain. Mu Dan Pi, Dan Shen, and Chi Shao quicken the blood and clear any heat that may arise from blood stasis. Tao Ren and Chi Shao also disperse congealed blood and, like San Leng and E Zhu, are useful for dispersing masses. Fu Ling and Bai Zhu fortify the spleen and supplement the qi without contributing to the existing stagnation. Zhi Ke moves stagnant qi in the abdomen to help the reabsorption of the ectopic mass. This helps to decrease adhesions and scarring due to surgery.

It is worthwhile to note that the channels entered in this formula are predominantly the liver, heart, and spleen. These are the viscera that respectively regulate, govern, and control the blood, which is fitting since the accumulation of blood stasis in the lower burner is the central disease mechanism addressed in this case.

Timing: After Resolution (for protection from future ectopic pregnancies)

Treatment principles: Move qi and blood, dispel phlegm-damp, and clear heat

Formula: Man Pen Fang (Formula for Chronic Pelvic Infection)

Hei Lao Hu (Kadsurae Coccineae Caulis et Folium)
Ji Gu Xiang (Crotonis Crassifolii Radix)
Fu Ling (Poria)
Dan Shen (Salviae Miltiorrhizae Radix)
Yi Yi Ren (Coicis Semen)
Bai Jiang Cao (Patriniae Herba)
Huang Qi (Astragali Radix)
Ji Xue Teng (Spatholobi Caulis)

Formula analysis

The name Man Pen Fang means "Formula for Chronic Pelvic [Infection]." Ectopic pregnancy has a significant rate of recurrence, possibly from anatomical anomalies, such as naturally narrow fallopian tubes or from residual scar tissue. Chronic pelvic infections can also narrow the fallopian tubes due to scarring, thus increasing the likelihood of future ectopic pregnancies. Prevention, therefore, focuses on maintaining free flow of the qi and blood through the channels and preventing the accumulation of stagnation of any kind, including dampness and phlegm.

Within this formula, Hei Lao Hu and Ji Gu Xiang move the qi and relieve pain. Fu Ling and Yi Yi Ren fortify the spleen and disinhibit dampness, helping to keep the channels clear of phlegm. Dan Shen nourishes and quickens the blood. Bai Jiang Cao clears heat and resolves toxins which is helpful in cases of chronic infection or inflammation. Huang Qi supplements the qi and promotes circulation. In China, Wu Zao Long is used in place of Huang Qi, as it has a similar function but also promotes circulation in the channels.

Before trying to conceive again, it is necessary to do a hysterosalpingogram (HSG) to help open or dilate the fallopian tubes and assist in preventing another ectopic pregnancy.

Acupuncture protocol:

LR14 (Qi Men), LR3 (Tai Chong), SP10 (Xue Hai), SP9 (Yin Ling Quan), SP6 (San Yin Jiao), CV4 (Guan Yuan), KI13 (Qi Xue)

Formula analysis

This combination of points first aims to move the qi since, no matter what kind of other obstruction is present (blood, phlegm-damp), the qi must be freely flowing in order to break the blockage. LR14 and LR3 together course the liver channel, being the mu points and stream points of the liver respectively. SP10 and SP6 both quicken the blood, while SP9 disinhibits dampness. CV4 is a local point to free qi and blood flow in the area. KI13 is also a local point that should be drained to remove obstruction.

Modifications:

- For blood stasis, add LR8 (Qu Quan) to improve the movement of blood to the lower burner.

- For dampness and phlegm, add ST40 (Feng Long) and TB5 (Wai Guan).

Case Study

The patient was a 36-year-old woman who complained of lower abdominal pain that had been present for a year but had intensified in the last seven days. Prior to the onset of the pain, the patient had had an ectopic pregnancy followed by abdominal surgery. She stated that her menses came three days late and now she had experienced spotting for four days. Prior to this, her menstruation had been normal. She also reported heart palpitations and dizziness and appeared pale. She had one child, a 6-year-old boy. Her tongue was pale and purplish with teethmarks on its edges a red tip with white, slimy fur. Her pulse was fast, small, bowstring, slippery, and weak.

Pattern identification: Blood vacuity, spleen qi vacuity, qi stagnation, blood stasis, and damp-heat

Symptom analysis

This was a case of mixed repletion and vacuity. The timeline and intensity of the pain, along with the patient's history of ectopic pregnancy and abdominal surgery, suggest blood and qi stagnation. This is supported by the purplish tongue and bowstring pulse as well as her delayed menstruation. She also showed signs of underlying blood and spleen qi vacuity, evidenced by the pale, teethmarked tongue (the purplish color may also point to blood vacuity as well as stagnation), and the vacuity aspects of the pulse (*i.e.*, small and weak). Heart palpitations, a pale face, and dizziness also suggest blood or qi vacuity (likely both). Finally, the slimy tongue fur, red tongue tip, and rapid, slippery pulse suggest that damp-heat had also accumulated due to the stagnation in the lower abdomen.

Treatment principles: Nourish the blood, fortify the spleen and supplement the qi, move the qi and quicken the blood, clear and eliminate dampness and heat

Treatment:

I first recommended that the patient be treated by surgery. This was a case of chronic pelvic infection. Following surgery, I prescribed:

Formula: Modified Man Pen Fang (Formula for Chronic Pelvic Infection)

> Hei Lao Hu (Kadsurae Coccineae Caulis et Folium)
> Ji Gu Xiang (Crotonis Crassifolii Radix)
> Fu Ling (Poria)
> Dan Shen (Salviae Miltiorrhizae Radix)
> Yi Yi Ren (Coicis Semen)
> Bai Jiang Cao (Patriniae Herba)
> Huang Qi (Astragali Radix)
> Dang Gui (Angelicae Sinensis Radix)
> Gou Qi Zi (Lycii Fructus)

Formula analysis

What had occurred in this case was blockage of the lower burner due to accumulation of blood and qi following surgery. Man Pen Fang would help the patient to recover from the surgery and open the fallopian tubes to prevent the recurrence of blockage as described above. I added Dang Gui (Angelicae Sinensis Radix) and Gou Qi Zi (Lycii Fructus) to this formula to nourish the blood. Dang Gui also quickens the blood, while Gou Qi Zi supplements liver and kidney yin and blood, thus helping to promote the overall health of the reproductive system. Gou Qi Zi is a good choice for nourishing the blood in this case because it is much easier to digest than many of the richer blood-nourishing agents, such as Shu Di Huang (Rehmanniae Radix Praeparata). This patient's spleen was not strong enough to assimilate such medicinals.

Outcome

After three months of treatment, a hysterosalpingogram (an ultrasound image of the uterus and fallopian tubes) was performed to confirm that the fallopian tubes were open. After five months of treatment, the patient became pregnant with twins. She carried these twins to term without complications and gave birth to a boy and a girl.

Ectopic pregnancy

Type	Before rupture	After rupture
Cramps	Mild	Severe
Missed period	(+)	(+)
Bleeding	Vaginal spotting	Very heavy bleeding
Pregnancy test	(+)	(+)
Shock	(−)	(+)
Lower blood pressure	(−)	(+)
Lower hemoglobin	(−)	(+)
Western treatment	Surgery or Methyltrexate	
TCM treatment	First: Lower HCG, absorb tissue, prevent adhesions: Gua Gong Fang Then: Strengthen body and prevent adhesions: Qing Gong Fang	
Acupuncture	SP10, LV3, ST36, LI4, Ren3, Zigong, Yintang	

12

Postpartum Hemorrhage

Western Medical View

Postpartum hemorrhage (PPH) refers to abnormal uterine bleeding after delivery. It is traditionally defined as a blood loss greater than 500 milliliters in a vaginal delivery and greater than 1,000 milliliters in a cesarean delivery. This definition has recently been altered as studies have shown that an uncomplicated delivery often involves a blood loss greater than 500 milliliters with little or no harm to the mother. These findings resulted in a broader definition for PPH. Now, any bleeding that results in or could potentially result in signs and symptoms of shock is considered PPH. The importance of a given volume of blood loss varies with the woman's hemoglobin level. A woman with a normal hemoglobin level will tolerate blood loss that would be fatal for an anemic woman. Typically, a blood loss of greater than 1,000 milliliters with a vaginal delivery or a decrease in postpartum hematocrit level greater than 10% of the prenatal value can be considered PPH.

Postpartum hemorrhage can be divided into two subcatagories:

1. Early PPH refers to PPH that occurs within 24 hours after delivery
2. Late PPH refers to PPH that occurs 24 hours to six weeks after delivery

Causes:

The most frequent cause of PPH is uterine atony, a condition in which the muscles of the uterus do not contract properly. This allows continued blood loss from the placental site. Uterine atony can occur in any of the following situations:

- The uterus is obstructed due to a retained placenta or other tissue
- The uterus is overdistended due to delivery of multiple infants, a large infant, or an excess of amniotic fluid

- The uterus is fatigued due to prolonged labor

The second most frequent cause is trauma to the uterus, cervix, and/or vagina. The risks for trauma include the following:

- Tearing due to delivery of a large infant
- Episiotomy
- Injury from the instruments used during childbirth
- Vaginal birth after a woman has had a C-section in a previous delivery
- Trauma during delivery can also result in hematomas in the perineum or pelvis. The patient will have unstable vital signs and little or no external bleeding.

Other causes of PPH include:

- Disorders in blood coagulation and thrombocytopenia
- Previous PPH
- Preeclampsia
- Uterine inversion
- Uterine rupture

Signs & symptoms:

- Excessive and severe uterine bleeding
- Complete blood count and other blood tests indicating severe blood loss:
- Hemoglobin & hematocrit level decrease

Shock, which may cause any of the following symptoms:

- Confusion or decreasing alertness
- Clammy skin
- Dizziness or light-headedness
- Low blood pressure
- Paleness
- Rapid pulse, increased heart rate
- Shortness of breath
- Weakness

Symptoms of internal bleeding may also include:

- Abdominal pain
- Abdominal swelling
- Chest pain

Treatment:

Treatment depends on the cause of PPH and the severity of the blood loss. In extreme conditions, blood transfusions and resuscitative measures may be needed. Ideally, treatment should begin at the beginning of the birthing process by obtaining a thorough medical history and a complete blood workup. After the delivery, the placenta detaches from the uterus and the doctor administers oxytocin to assist the uterus in contraction and to reduce blood loss. If the placenta does not detach on its own, the doctor will manually remove it.

If the uterus is atonic, the doctor will massage the uterus to help the muscles contract and the patient will be given oxytocin continuously. A prostaglandin may also be given to help the uterine muscles contract. The cervix and vagina will be thoroughly inspected for any trauma. Direct pressure over lacerations in the perineum, cervix, vagina, or uterus may help control bleeding; lacerations are repaired. If uterine inversion occurs, the uterus is gently pushed back into position. A salt solution is then administered into the uterus to re-inflate it. A ruptured uterus requires prompt surgery to repair it.

Traditional Chinese Medical View

After delivery of a newborn, the uterus is still stretched to many times its usual size. After a period of time, the uterus will contract back to its original size. A typical uterus is approximately the size of a hen's egg. Postpartum, the ligaments around the uterus will also contract back into place. This can result in pain. Sometimes there is also postpartum bleeding. All bleeding should resolve within two weeks. Bleeding that occurs after this point in time is considered pathological.

Treatment based on pattern identification:

Qi & blood vacuity (*qi xue xu* 气血虚)

Signs & symptoms: Postpartum uterine cramping which may be either dull or mild in nature and is better with pressure, profuse hemorrhage during delivery, pale face, fatigue, unformed bowel movements, dizziness, blurred vision, slight fever, night sweating, may be accompanied by long-term, nonstop pale colored bleeding that lasts up to a month

Tongue: Pale, teethmarks, thin body

Pulse: Slow, thin

Treatment principles: Warm and supplement the qi and blood, relieve pain

Formula: Chang Ning Tang (Calm the Intestine Decoction)

Dang Gui (Angelicae Sinensis Radix)
Shu Di Huang (Rehmanniae Radix Praeparata)
E Jiao (Asini Corii Colla)
Ren Shen (Ginseng Radix)
Shan Yao (Dioscoreae Rhizoma)
Xu Duan (Dipsaci Radix)
Mai Men Dong (Ophiopogonis Radix)
Rou Gui (Cinnamomi Cortex)
Gan Cao (Glycyrrhizae Radix)

Blood stasis (*xue yu* 血瘀)

Signs & symptoms: Postpartum uterine cramping which is sharp, stabbing, and worse with pressure, retention of placenta or tissue, constipation, may be accompanied by heavy bleeding with clots, may spot for up to one month. These symptoms may also be caused by D&C or a natural abortion.

Tongue: Dark purple

Pulse: Deep, bowstring, replete

Treatment principles: Quicken and supplement blood, warm the channels, supplement the spleen

Formula: Sheng Hua Tang (Engendering Transformation Decoction)

Dang Gui (Angelicae Sinensis Radix)
Chuan Xiong (Chuanxiong Rhizoma)
Tao Ren (Persicae Semen)
Pao Jiang (Zingiberis Rhizoma Praeparatum)
Zhi Gan Cao (Glycyrrhizae Radix cum Liquido Fricta)

Clinical Treatment

After birth, women often experience cramps for a whole month as the uterus shrinks back to its normal size. This can be exacerbated by breast-feeding. During this time, there will also usually be light bleeding. Because the body has been taxed by pregnancy and birth, much qi and blood has been consumed. Qi and blood vacuity is, therefore, the norm postpartum, and the bleeding is usually of a vacuity nature (light or pale in color with mild pain that responds favorably to pressure and possibly large blood loss due to the spleen being unable to contain the blood). If some of the placenta has been retained, there may also be blood stasis as the retained blood and tissue blocks the cervix from closing fully. In this case, there will be strong pain that is worse with pressure, dark bleeding with clots, and a tendency to spotting. In practice, I always combine support for vacuity with blood-quickening medicinals, as follows.

If there is light bleeding, I use:

Qing Gong Fang (Clear the Uterus Formula)

> Dang Gui (Angelicae Sinensis Radix)
> Chuan Xiong (Chuanxiong Rhizoma)
> Tao Ren (Persicae Semen)
> Yi Mu Cao (Leonuri Herba)
> San Qi (Notoginseng Radix)
> Dang Shen (Codonopsis Radix)
> Niu Xi (Achyranthis Bidentatae Radix)
> Xiang Fu (Cyperi Rhizoma)
> Zhi Gan Cao (Glycyrrhizae Radix cum Liquido Fricta)

Formula analysis

Light bleeding is usually due to mild qi and blood vacuity (which is standard after giving birth). The primary ingredient in this formula is Dang Gui which nourishes and also quickens the blood. Quickening the blood is important because it ensures that all products of pregnancy are expelled and there is no blood stasis (such as partial retention of the placenta) since this will prolong the bleeding. Chuan Xiong, Tao Ren, Yi Mu Cao, and San Qi all assist with quickening the blood and help with relieving pain. Gan Jiang warms the middle burner and helps supplement the spleen. Dang Shen supplements the spleen qi. This helps the spleen contain the blood and stop the bleeding. Zhi Gan Cao assists Gan Jiang and Dang Shen in supplementing the middle burner. It also harmonizes all the other the ingredients in the formula.

Modification: If there is heavy bleeding, use:

Zhi Beng Fang (Check Flooding Formula)

> Dang Shen (Codonopsis Radix)
> Bai Zhu (Atractylodis Macrocephalae Rhizoma)
> Xu Duan (Dipsaci Radix)
> Shan Zhu Yu (Corni Fructus)
> Yi Mu Cao (Leonuri Herba)

San Qi (Notoginseng Radix)

Huang Qi (Astragali Radix)

Formula analysis

As mentioned above, heavy postpartum bleeding is often due to significant damage of spleen qi and, thus, the spleen's function of containing the blood. In this formula, Dang Shen and Bai Zhu are the primary medicinals. They fortify the spleen and supplement the qi. Huang Qi supports them in this action. In such cases, it is also important to quicken the blood for the reasons noted above. However, in this case, Xu Duan is chosen because it also nourishes the blood and yin. Yi Mu Cao and San Qi stop bleeding without causing stasis. These medicinals help relieve pain. Shan Zhu Yu nourishes the blood and yin and secures and astringes, thus helping to hold in the blood and qi as much as possible.

Acupuncture formula:

Ear (Kidney, Spleen, Shen Men), GV20 (Bai Hui), ST36 (Zu San Li)

Formula analysis

I find these three ear points useful throughout pregnancy for balancing the endocrine system and calming the nervous system (which promotes overall balance as well). Ear Kidney promotes the healthy readjustment of hormone levels following the pregnancy. Ear Spleen assists in the engenderment and transformation of the qi and blood, helping to return the patient's constitution to strength after giving birth. GV20 upbears the qi to stop bleeding. ST36 supplements the qi and blood and supports the spleen's function of engendering and containing the blood.

Case Study

A 41-year-old woman came for treatment of vaginal bleeding three weeks after delivering a baby girl. The bleeding was intermittent and contained clots and a small amount of tissue. She also reported intermittent lower abdominal pain, dizziness, and fatigue. She said she had frequent heart palpitations as well as feelings of anxiety and stress. Her hands and feet were often cold and numb. Her urination was frequent and bowel movements alternated between unformed stool and constipation. Her tongue was pale with teethmarks on its edges and a slightly red tip with white fur. Her pulse was slippery, small, and weak in the cubit position. Her Western medical diagnosis via ultrasound showed some placental retention in the uterus.

Her physician had recommended D & C but the patient wanted to try acupuncture and herbs first.

Pattern identification: Blood stasis and qi stagnation, spleen qi and kidney vacuity

Treatment principles: Quicken the blood and rectify the qi, fortify the spleen and supplement the qi, supplement the kidney

Formula: Modified Qing Gong Fang (Clear the Uterus Formula)

Dang Gui (Angelicae Sinensis Radix)
Chuan Xiong (Chuanxiong Rhizoma)
Gan Jiang (Zingiberis Rhizoma)
Tao Ren (Persicae Semen)
Yi Mu Cao (Leonuri Herba)
San Qi (Notoginseng Radix)
Dang Shen (Codonopsis Radix)
Zhi Gan Cao (Glycyrrhizae Radix cum Liquido Fricta)
San Leng (Sparganii Rhizoma)
Ji Xue Teng (Spatholobi Caulis)
Zhi Ke (Qiao) (Aurantii Fructus)
Niu Xi (Achyranthis Bidentatae Radix)

Outcome

Initially, the patient was prescribed seven days' worth of the above formula. After treatment, the patient's vaginal bleeding and lower abdominal cramps increased, and subsequently a large clot passed (*i.e.*, the remains of the placenta). The bleeding and cramps were then greatly reduced. The next formula I prescribed was Qing Gong Fang (Clean the Uterus Formula), also for seven days. After taking this formula, the vaginal bleeding and cramps ceased completely. The patient was then given Tiao Jing Fang (Menstruation-regulating Formula) for three weeks. During this time, the patient's energy returned to normal, her dizziness ceased, and all her other symptoms resolved.

13

Insufficient Lactation

Western Medical View

Insufficient lactation is the inability of the mother to produce enough milk to provide adequate nutrition for the growth of her newborn. Most cases of insufficient lactation resolve naturally. However, some women are persistently unable to produce sufficient milk to nourish their infant.

Normal lactation

The production of breast milk (lactogenesis) begins immediately after delivery. High levels of the pituitary hormone prolactin (produced in the hypothalamus) stimulate the synthesis of lactose, the main component of breast milk. Other hormones are also involved: placental lactogen, cortisol, insulin, and oxytocin. During the first five days after delivery, deep lemon-colored colostrum is produced that contains more minerals and protein than mature milk as well as less sugar and fat.

Colostrum gradually converts to mature milk over the next month. Breast milk is also rich in minerals, protein, sugar, and fat. It contains all necessary vitamins (except vitamin K) and important immune system components such as IgA and T- and B-lymphocytes.

The release of the hormone oxytocin from the hypothalamus stimulates "the letdown" reflex as breast epithelial cells contract to squeeze milk from the ducts. When an infant suckles, prolactin levels rise. Each nursing stimulates the intensity and duration of subsequent lactation. Even the sound of a crying infant stimulates the let down of milk. If there is no initial letting-down of milk, the suckling stimulus is often enough to normalize milk production over the course of time. Correct positioning of mother and infant for proper feeding can increase the suckling stimulus which encourages milk let down and continued synthesis. Average milk production is approximately 600 milliliters of milk per day.

Diagnosis:

Insufficient lactation is diagnosed by failure of the infant to thrive. If milk production per feeding is below normal (at least 60 milliliters per feeding), the infant may not show expected weight gain. Frequent newborn weight checks, even before and after each feeding during a 24-hour period, can also help diagnose insufficient lactation.

General treatment:

The Western medical treatment of this condition addresses the underlying cause of insufficient lactation. During treatment, use of an unaffected breast or supplementation with formula is suggested. Patients are usually advised to increase their intake of food and liquids. Specific treatment protocols are discussed below.

Causes:

Persistent insufficient lactation can be caused by:

- Physical blockages
- Hormonal imbalance
- Psychological causes

Physical causes:

Galactocele

A galactocele is a milk-filled cyst caused by a blocked mammary duct.

Treatment: Frequent cleaning of the areola prevents the accumulation of dried milk, which minimizes obstruction of the ducts. Expression of milk before each feeding, either manually or with a breast pump, may relieve engorgement and congestion.

Depressed/inverted nipples

When the nipples have an inverted or depressed shape, the correct suckling position may be difficult or impossible.

Treatment: Manual manipulation of the nipples may be sufficient to draw out the inverted nipple, thus allowing the infant access to the milk ducts.

Fissures

Fissures are painful cracks in the areola that make nursing difficult and decrease milk secretion. Fissures are prone to infection and may become purulent.

Treatment: Nipple shields can be used to protect the fissured area. Pump breast milk until the lesion heals.

Mastitis

Mastitis is a purulent infection that appears in the third or fourth week of nursing. This condition affects approximately 33% of breastfeeding women. Aversion to cold, fever, severe pain, and increased heart rate accompany a hard, red breast.

Treatment: Treating mastitis usually requires a 10-14 day course of antibiotics. Self-care to speed recovery includes application of warm compresses, increased fluid intake, and, if possible, continuing to nurse with the affected breast.

Milk fever

Milk fever is a self-limiting condition that occurs in the first 24 hours after delivery. The breast is distended, firm, and nodular. The mother may have a fever of 100°F or higher.

Treatment: Use a breast pump until the symptoms subside.

Ineffective suckling

Some infants are unable to sufficiently empty the breast of its milk. Others show little interest in food. Physical aberrations such as a cleft palate also make suckling difficult. Breasts become engorged, hot, painful, hard, and knotty. Congestion and pressure on the ducts prevents proper flow of milk.

Treatment: Continue to regularly express milk. If both breasts are affected, supplement the infant's nutrition with pumped milk.

Postpartum hemorrhage

Postpartum hemorrhage can result in blood loss that affects prolactin production, and consequently, maternal milk production.

Treatment: Seek immediate medical care.

Hormonal causes:

Birth control pills

Women taking combination estrogen/progestin contraceptive pills have a decreased volume of milk. Progestin-only contraceptives are typically recommended.

Sheehan syndrome

This is a rare condition (occurring in approximately one in every 10,000 deliveries) in which the pituitary fails. Consequently, production of prolactin stops, leading to lactation failure. This condition is often caused by severe hemorrhaging (in utero or postpartum), which deprives the pituitary of oxygen, leading to pituitary necrosis. Other symptoms of Sheehan syndrome may develop over future years, including amenorrhea, breast atrophy, hypothyroidism, pubic and axillary hair loss, adrenal cortex insufficiency, hypotension, hypoglycemia, and increased heart rate.

Pituitary macroadenoma

This is a benign brain tumor that can compress the pituitary, inhibit prolactin production, and cause strokes.

Psychological causes:

Fright and stress

Emotional upset can cause a decrease in oxytocin production, resulting in subsequent inhibition of the milk let-down reflex.

Traditional Chinese Medical View

Some women have difficulty producing milk after the delivery of the baby. Typically, the process of milk production should begin by the second day after delivery. However, premature delivery or cesarean section delivery may delay lactogenesis for a few days. The average woman should be able to produce about 600 milliliters of milk per day for feeding the infant. If milk production is scanty and is not due to a physical or anatomical blockage, Chinese medicine may be able to assist in the production of more milk through medicinal therapy and acupuncture.

Treatment based on pattern identification:

Qi & blood dual vacuity *(qi xue liang xu 气血两虚)*

Signs & symptoms: Scanty or no milk. In addition, what milk there is has a thin consistency and may leak from the breasts. The breasts are soft, not bloated, and not tender to the touch. Other symptoms include a pale facial complexion, poor appetite, fatigue, blurred vision, vertigo, tinnitus, heart palpitations, night sweats, five center heat, malar flushing, and dry skin.

Tongue: Pale with scanty, white fur

Pulse: Weak, thin

Treatment principles: Supplement the qi and blood, free the flow of the network vessels of the breasts and promote lactation

Formula: Tong Ru Dan (Lactation Elixir)

Ren Shen (Ginseng Radix)
Huang Qi (Astragali Radix)
Dang Gui (Angelicae Sinensis Radix)
Mai Dong (Ophiopogonis Radix)
Mu Tong (Akebiae Trifoliatae Caulis)
Jie Geng (Platycodonis Radix)
Zhu Ti (pig's feet, Suis Pes)

Modifications:

- For severe qi depression, add Qing Pi (Citri Reticulatae Pericarpium Viride), Zhi Ke (Aurantii Fructus), and Yu Jin (Curcumae Radix).

- For qi depression with heat, add Mu Dan Pi (Moutan Cortex), Zhi Zi (Gardeniae Fructus), Xia Ku Cao (Prunellae Spica), Lou Lu (Rhapontici Radix), and/or Pu Gong Ying (Taraxaci Herba).

- For painful, swollen breasts, consider medicinals such as Tong Cao (Tetrapanacis Medulla), Mu Tong (Akebiae Trifoliatae Caulis), Jie Geng (Platycodonis Radix), Wang Bu Liu Xing (Vaccariae Semen), Gua Lou (Trichosanthis Fructus), Chuan Shan Jia (Manis Squama), Si Gua Luo (Luffae Fructus Retinervus), and Lu Lu Tong (Liquidambaris Fructus).

Caution: If breast lumps are palpable and are accompanied by high fever and aversion to cold, these are signs that mastitis may be present. In that case, immediate treatment is necessary.

Liver depression transforming heat *(gan yu hua re* 肝郁化热*)*

Signs & symptoms: Scanty or no milk. The breasts, chest, or nipples are bloated and tender, and there is emotional depression and/or irritability. Additional symptoms include belching, distention or pain in the rib-sides, nausea and headache, and a hot sensation in the breasts.

Tongue: Purplish, red on the sides, with yellow fur

Pulse: Bowstring, rapid

Treatment principles: Course liver and rectify the qi, free the flow of the network vessels of the breasts and promote lactation

Formula: Xiao Yao San (Rambling Powder)

Chai Hu (Bupleuri Radix)
Dang Gui (Angelicae Sinensis Radix)
Bai Shao (Paeoniae Radix Alba)
Bai Zhu (Atractylodis Macrocephalae Rhizoma)
Fu Ling (Poria)
Gan Cao (Glycyrrhizae Radix)
Sheng Jiang (Zingiberis Rhizoma Recens)
Bo He (Menthae Herba)

Clinical Treatment

When a mother cannot produce enough milk to feed her baby, the baby cries. Naturally, this is difficult for the mother as well. Insufficient lactation may simply be due to lack of milk production, or it may be the result of galactorrhea. This is when the milk leaks out of the breasts all the time and the flow cannot be controlled.

From a TCM perspective, milk is closely related to the blood. Blood is important during a woman's entire life. It is created and shed on a cyclical basis as part of the menstrual cycle, while, during pregnancy, it nourishes the growing fetus. Following delivery, blood continues to be important in nourishing the baby because it is the basis for the engenderment of milk. If there is insufficient blood, there will be insufficient milk. Like blood, milk is controlled by the qi. Therefore, milk can leak out in cases of qi vacuity. Similarly, the flow of milk can be impeded by qi stagnation. Thus, there are two possibilities for insufficient lactation: qi and blood vacuity or qi stagnation (possibly leading to heat).

Differentiation between these two patterns may be made by examining the breasts and milk. In vacuity cases, the breasts will feel soft and the milk will be thin in consistency. The patient will experience no pain in the breasts. If there is stagnation, the breasts will feel tender, bloated, and hot to the touch. The milk will be thick in consistency, and the patient may experience pain in the breasts.

Qi & blood dual vacuity (qi xue liang xu 气血两虚)

The formula I use in my clinic for insufficient lactation due to qi and blood vacuity is:

Formula: Zeng Ru Fang (Correct the Milk Formula)

Huang Qi (Astragali Radix)
Dang Gui (Angelicae Sinensis Radix)
Lu Rong (Cervi Cornu Pantotrichum) [Ba Ji Tian (Morindae Officinalis Radix) can be used if Lu Rong is too expensive]
Gou Qi Zi (Lycii Fructus)
Shu Di Huang (Rehmanniae Radix Praeparata)
Wang Bu Liu Xing (Vaccariae Semen)
Tong Cao (Tetrapanacis Medulla)
Bai Zhi (Angelicae Dahuricae Radix)

Formula analysis

This formula contains Huang Qi to supplement the qi. Dang Gui, Shu Di Huang, and Gou Qi Zi nourish the blood. Lu Rong (or Ba Ji Tian) supplements the kidneys and warms yang. Tong Cao, Bai Zhi, and Wang Bu Liu Xing free the flow of the breasts.

Eating fish is also very good for milk production. Fish soup, in particular, may be a good dietary addition to nourish the milk. The fish can be fried on both sides and then cooked down in a soup until the broth becomes milky white. A few slices of ginger may be added.

Modifications:

• If worry is a problem, causing liver qi depression and binding, effective additions include Zhi Ke (Aurantii Fructus), Bai Shao (Paeoniae Radix Alba), and Jie Geng (Platycodonis Radix). Zhi Ke rectifies the qi. Because it enters the stomach channel, it is especially useful for coursing qi in the breasts. Bai Shao emolliates the liver, and Jie Geng acts as a courier to the upper burner, the area of the breasts. Zhi Ke and Jie Geng work particularly well together because one moves upward and one moves downward. This regulates the flow of qi in both directions.

- When significant pallor indicates blood vacuity, add Huang Jing (Polygonati Rhizoma) and He Shou Wu (Polygoni Multiflori Radix). These medicinals both boost the essence. Huang Jing also supplements the spleen and nourishes yin, while He Shou Wu nourishes blood and secures and astringes. These two medicinals form a powerful pair. In cases in which kidney yang vacuity is pronounced, Rou Cong Rong (Cistanches Herba) should be added. Unlike many warming ingredients, Rou Cong Rong has a moist nature and warms yang without damaging fluids.

Qi stagnation (*qi zhi* 气滞)

The formula I prefer for insufficient lactation caused by qi stagnation is:

Formula: Xiao Yao Fang (Rambling Formula) with appropriate modifications, for instance:

Chai Hu (Bupleuri Radix)
Dang Gui (Angelicae Sinensis Radix)
Bai Shao (Paeoniae Radix Alba)
Bai Zhu (Atractylodis Macrocephalae Rhizoma)
Fu Ling (Poria)
Gan Cao (Glycyrrhizae Radix)

Recall that Xiao Yao Fang is Xiao Yao San (Rambling Powder) with Sheng Jiang (Zingiberis Rhizoma Recens) and Bo He (Menthae Herba) removed. This formula courses liver and rectifies the qi, fortifies the spleen and nourishes the blood. (For a detailed explanation of the individual herbs and their interactions in this formula, see the discussion of Xiao Yao Fang in the clinical treatment section of dysmenorrhea.)

Modifications:

- More qi-rectifying medicinals should be added in cases of more significant qi stagnation. The best medicinals to consider in this case are Qing Pi (Citri Reticulatae Pericarpium Viride), Zhi Ke (Aurantii Fructus), and Yu Jin (Curcumae Radix). Both Qing Pi and Zhi Ke rectify the qi. However, the former enters the liver channel, while the latter enters the stomach channel. These two channels are the primary channels that traverse the breasts. Yu Jin moves (liver) blood. This is often important since lack of free-flowing qi tends to produce blood stasis.

- If heat is present, appropriate additions include Mu Dan Pi (Moutan Cortex), Zhi Zi (Gardeniae Fructus), Xia Ku Cao (Prunellae Spica), Pu Gong Ying (Taraxaci Herba), Jin Yin Hua (Lonicerae Flos), Ju Hua (Chrysanthemi Flos), and/or Huang Qin (Scutellariae Radix). Clearly, not all of these need to be added, although it may be useful to include either Xia Ku Cao or Pu Gong Ying since these two specifically affect the breasts. Mu Dan Pi is indicated for vacuity heat. Zhi Zi is a good addition if there is evidence of heat elsewhere in the body since it clears heat from all three burners. Xia Ku Cao clears fire for cases of infection with redness and a burning sensation.

- Jin Yin Hua is indicated for heat toxins and enters the stomach channel. Pu Gong Ying is also used for heat toxins and it enters the liver channel. These two agents are a powerful combination to cover the breast area in heat toxin patterns, such as an infection in which the breasts are hot, red, swollen, and painfully hard. Huang Qin clears heat and damp-heat in the upper burner and may be a good choice when the breasts are congested, aching and heavy, and exuding a discharge. Ju Hua clears heat in the liver channel and downbears yang. Therefore, it is a good choice in cases of simple qi depression with heat and signs of ascendant liver yang hyperactivity, such as headache, irritability, or hypertension.

- If the breasts are extremely painful or swollen, add Si Gua Luo (Luffae Fructus Retinervus), Lou Lu (Rhapontici Radix), Tong Cao (Tetrapanacis Medulla), Jie Geng (Platycodonis Radix), Bai Zhi (Angelicae Dahuricae Radix), Lu Lu Tong (Liquidambaris Fructus), Zhi Ke (Aurantii Fructus), Jie Geng (Platycodonis Radix), and/or Wang Bu Liu Xing (Vaccariae Semen). These medicinals disperse obstruction in the breast area in different ways. Si Gua Luo is useful for obstruction due to hot phlegm, whereas Lou Lu is more useful in cases of pure heat. It is important to note that it is often most effective to combine two or three medicinals to achieve an amplified effect. For example, Lou Lu is heat-clearing and causes the milk to descend, while Wang Bu Liu Xing quickens the blood in the liver and stomach channels and encourages the smooth flow of milk. Together, these two free the flow of the milk and are a good combination for obstruction due to stagnation and heat in the breasts.

- For tender breasts, quicken the blood by adding Chuan Xiong (Chuanxiong Rhizoma), Chi Shao (Paeoniae Radix Rubra), Dan Shen (Salviae Miltiorrhizae Radix), and/or Wang Bu Liu Xing (Vaccariae Semen). All of these medicinals enter the liver channel. Wang Bu Liu Xing is a neutral medicinal that also enters the stomach channel and has a special empirical effect on the breasts and lactation. This makes it suitable in combinations with any of the other medicinals. Chi Shao is cool and can be used when heat is present. By contrast, Chuan Xiong is warm and acrid and has an additional action of moving the qi.

- If the patient shows evidence of blood and yin vacuity, Sheng Di Huang (Rehmanniae Radix Exsiccata seu Recens), Dang Gui (Angelicae Sinensis Radix), Chi Shao (Paeoniae Radix Rubra), and/or Chuan Xiong (Chuanxiong Rhizoma) may be added. Note that this is similar to the formula Si Wu Tang (Four Materials Decoction) with Chi Shao and Sheng Di Huang substituted for Bai Shao (Paeoniae Radix Alba) and Shu Di Huang (Rehmanniae Radix Praeparata). Both Chi Shao and Sheng Di Huang are cooling, which may be important if there is a pattern of vacuity heat in the blood.

Acupuncture formulas:

Qi & blood dual vacuity

CV17 (Dan Zhong), ST36 (Zu San Li), SP6 (San Yin Jiao), CV6 (Qi Hai), SP10 (Xue Hai)

Formula analysis

Since the conception vessel is the meeting of yin, it is useful to choose points on this channel when treating the yin areas of the body, such as the front of the torso. CV6 is named Sea of Qi, and it both rectifies and supplements the qi. The qi-rectifying effect of CV6 especially affects the middle and lower burners, while CV17 tends to rectify the qi of the upper burner. Together, these two points rectify the qi in all three burners to free the flow of the breasts. CV6 and ST36 supplement the qi to support milk production. SP 6 is the crossing point of the three yin channels of the leg. The kidney, liver, and spleen are the three viscera that are primarily involved in the production of milk. Finally, SP10 nourishes the blood to support the production of milk.

Liver qi depression & binding

CV17 (Dan Zhong), SP6 (San Yin Jiao), LR3 (Tai Chong), PC6 (Nei Guan), GB34 (Yang Ling Quan), LR14 (Qi Men)

Formula analysis

CV17 rectifies qi in the upper burner. Together with PC6, it powerfully frees the flow of the chest area. PC6 is also a spirit-quieting point. This is especially important because emotional stress is common with insufficient lactation. SP6 is the crossing point for the three yin channels of the leg and can be used to move both the qi and blood. LR3 and GB34 rectify the qi in the liver and gallbladder channels. If heat is present, LR2 may be substituted for LR3 to clear heat. LR14 is a good local point to move the qi in the breast area and promote lactation.

Case Study

A 38-year-old woman gave birth via Cesarean section at six months and four days of gestation. Her baby was born weighing less than two pounds and was placed in an incubator in the neonatal intensive care unit. Eight days after delivery, she was still only able to produce less than an ounce of milk every three hours (approximately 3-4 ounces per day). The mother was under a great deal of emotional stress from worrying about her baby's health. Examination revealed her breasts were soft and without distention. She reported no breast pain. Her tongue was pale and purplish with a slightly red tip and white fur. Her pulse was small and bowstring and weak at the cubit positions.

Pattern identification: Kidney qi vacuity, blood vacuity, binding depression of the liver qi

This was a case of mixed vacuity and repletion which is common. In fact, after childbirth, it is almost impossible to imagine a case without some element of vacuity given the physical and emotional costs involved in carrying a pregnancy and giving birth. In this case, we see signs of vacuity in the breasts themselves. The tissues are soft and feel empty without pain or fullness. This suggests a lack of qi and/or blood. Her tongue is pale and purple, and there are no signs of spleen qi vacuity. This suggests that this is primarily a blood vacuity. Her cubit pulses are weak, indicating kidney vacuity. Specifically, the preterm labor and delivery (as well as a lack of clear yin or yang vacuity signs) suggests kidney qi vacuity, manifesting in a failure of the kidney qi to secure the fetus. A repletion aspect is present as well. Emotional stress in combination with the bowstring pulse suggests liver qi depression and binding.

Treatment principles: Supplement the kidneys and nourish the blood, course the liver, rectify the qi, and promote lactation

Formula:

Xiao Yao Fang (Rambling Formula) plus Huang Qi (Astragali Radix), Shu Di Huang (Rehmanniae Radix Praeparata), Gou Qi Zi (Lycii Fructus) and Chen Pi (Citri Reticulatae Pericarpium)

Acupuncture formula:

SP6 (San Yin Jiao), ST36 (Zu San Li), CV17 (Dan Zhong), GV20 (Bai Hui), Yin Tang (M-HN-3), LR8 (Qu Quan), SP10 (Xue Hai)

Treatment:

Because this is a case of mixed repletion and vacuity, we must choose a base formula that addresses one or the other and then modify. In this case, Xiao Yao Fang was chosen as the base formula despite the fact that the breasts themselves presented with vacuity signs. This formula was used because of the very emotional nature of the situation. It was important for this patient to be able to have some relief from her feelings of stress and worry since continued emotional distress would tend to exacerbate her liver depression. Huang Qi was added to supplement the qi and blood. Shu Di Huang was chosen to supplement the kidneys and nourish the blood. Gou Qi Zi nourishes the blood. Chen Pi was added to fortify the spleen and stomach. It also reduces the possibility of stagnation from the use of slimy, enriching medicinals.

SP6 and ST36 together supplement the qi and blood and further support the spleen's function of engendering the blood. CV17 frees the flow in the breast area. GV20 and Yin Tang are used to calm the emotions. LR8 and SP10 nourish the blood.

Outcome

One week later, the patient reported a 50% increase in her milk production. Within three weeks, she was producing approximately 14 ounces of milk per day, and her baby was thriving at nearly three pounds.

It is worth mentioning that many women have difficulty with lactation after having a premature delivery. This can be due to a number of factors, but one issue with very small babies can be weak suckling. Weak suckling may not provide the breasts with sufficient stimulation to increase milk production. The support that Chinese medicine may provide in these situations is, therefore, especially important. Chinese medicine can be combined with other supportive approaches, such as mechanical stimulation (pumping, breast massage), proper hydration, and nutrition. An International Board Certified Lactation Consultant (IBCLC) can be a valuable resource, and they can also help to ensure the baby is latching on properly. Most IBCLCs are very supportive of combining Western and TCM therapies.

14

Vaginal Itching

Western Medical View

Vaginal itching also known as vaginal pruritis or vulvovaginitis, is an infection of the vulva and/or vagina leading to itching, burning, and possible vaginal discharge.

General Signs & Symptoms:

- Redness, swelling and irritation of the vagina and surrounding vulva
- Leukorrhea or excess vaginal discharge with or without a foul odor and color
- Pain during urination (dysuria) and intercourse (dyspareunia)

Pathology:

- Candidiasis or yeast infections
- Most common in women with diabetes
- Virus infections
- Human papillomavirus (HPV) and herpes virus
- Bacterial vaginosis
- Gardnerella vaginalis
- Protozoans
- Trichomonas vaginalis
- Sexually transmitted diseases
- Chlamydia, gonorrhea
- Poor hygiene
- Allergic reactions & chemical irritants
- Detergents, soaps, spermicides, feminine products
- Postmenopausal atrophic vaginitis

- Drop in estrogen levels causing thinning of vaginal wall and less lubrication
- Foreign bodies
- IUD, diaphragm, condom, forgotten tampon
- Tumors and abnormal tissue

Diagnostic tests:

- Culture and microscopic exam of vaginal discharge
- Pap smear and pelvic exam
- Skin biopsies of the vulvar area
- Urine and blood studies (including hormone levels)

Treatments:

- Antibiotics for bacterial vaginal infections, including sexually transmitted diseases
- Antifungal drugs for yeast infections
- Benzodiazepines or antihistamines for nighttime relief
- Ointments containing hormones
- Steroid creams or lotions to reduce inflammation

Traditional Chinese Medical View

Vaginitis is a condition presenting with severe itching in the vagina, possibly accompanied by anal itching. There often is increased vaginal discharge that will present differently depending on the cause of the vaginal infection.

Damp heat (*shi re* 湿热)

Signs & symptoms: Yellow purulent vaginal discharge

Tongue: Red with yellow greasy fur

Pulse: Slippery, rapid

Treatment principles: Clear heat, disinhibit dampness

Formula: Bei Xie Sheng Shi Tang (Fish Poison Yam Dampness-Overcoming Decoction)

Bi Xie (Dioscoreae Hypoglaucae Rhizoma)
Yi Yi Ren (Coicis Semen)
Chi Fu Ling (Poria Rubra)

Ze Xie (Alismatis Rhizoma)
Tong Cao (Tetrapanacis Medulla)
Hua Shi (Talcum)
Mu Dan Pi (Moutan Cortex)
Huang Bai (Phellodendri Cortex)

Add:

Bai Xian Pi (Dictamni Cortex)
Chen Pi (Citri Reticulatae Pericarpium)
Qing Tian Kui (Nerviliae Fordii Folium)
Jin Yin Hua (Lonicerae Flos)
Ju Hua (Chrysanthemi Flos)

Exterior wash formula for damp heat:

Di Fu Zi (Kochiae Fructus)
She Chuang Zi (Cnidii Fructus)
Huang Bai (Phellodendri Cortex)
Ku Shen (Sophorae Flavescentis Radix)
Bai Bu (Stemonae Radix)
Jing Jie (Schizonepetae Herba)
Bo He (Menthae Herba)

(10 qian each; 20 cups water cooked down to 10 cups, soak or douche as slowly as possible)

Exterior wash formula for cold damp:

Gan Jiang (Zingiberis Rhizoma)
Xi Xin (Asari Radix)
He Shi (Carpesii Fructus)
Gui Zhi (Cinnamomi Ramulus)
Bai Bu (Stemonae Radix)

(10 qian each; prepare and use same as above)

Kidney yin & liver blood deficiency (*shen yin xu he gan xue xu* 肾阴虚和肝血虚)

Signs & symptoms: Dry, rough, chafed vaginal area, worse at night, burning, red and inflamed

Tongue: Red with scanty fur, cracks on tongue body

Pulse: Thin, rapid

Treatment principles: Nourish liver and kidney yin stop itch

Formula: Zhi Bai Di Huang Wan (Anemarrhena, Phellodendron, and Rehmannia Pill)

Shan Yao (Dioscoreae Rhizoma)
Shan Zhu Yu (Corni Fructus)
Ze Xie (Alismatis Rhizoma)
Mu Dan Pi (Moutan Cortex)
Fu Ling (Poria)
Zhi Mu (Anemarrhenae Rhizoma)
Huang Bai (Phellodendri Cortex)

More damp-heat, add:

Yin Chen (Artemisiae Scopariae Herba)
Zhi Zi (Gardeniae Fructus)
Tu Fu Ling (Smilacis Glabrae Rhizoma)
Di Fu Zi (Kochiae Fructus)
Bai Xian Pi (Dictamni Cortex)
Ku Shen (Sophorae Flavescentis Radix)

Nourish blood, add:

Bai Shao (Paeoniae Radix Alba)
Gou Qi Zi (Lycii Fructus)
Ji Xue Teng (Spatholobi Caulis)
He Shou Wu (Polygoni Multiflori Radix)
Dang Gui (Angelicae Sinensis Radix)
Hei Da Dou Pi (Glycines Testa Atra)

Clinical Treatment

The clinical treatments of vaginal itch that are discussed here are topical. This is not to imply that it is always enough to treat this condition topically, but rather to suggest that vaginal itch is a manifestation that is usually connected to another deeper condition such as pelvic infection or leukorrhea. The root will be treated by treating the central condition (this may be damp-heat, or chronic deficiency, for example). However, these topical washes should be used as adjunct therapies to address the branch (the itching itself).

As in the case of abnormal vaginal discharge, when vaginal itching is acute we primarily think of damp-heat. In biomedicine, for example, this may be diagnosed as a yeast infection or other bacterial imbalance of the vagina such as bacterial vaginosis (BV). In chronic cases there is usually an element of yin and/or blood vacuity, giving rise to internal dryness leading to wind and therefore itching.

The following exterior wash should be prescribed for itching due to a yeast infection. Use 10 qian (30 g) of each herb except for Jing Jie and Bo He, of which use 5 qian (15 g) each. Soak or douche the vagina with the cool tea, or soak clean cotton in the tea and insert into the vagina. Soak at least 30 minutes per day. Treat for at least one week; if there is a stubborn and recurrent infection the treatment may need to be continued for several months, possibly up to one year. This formula is very cold and bitter, and should only be used externally.

> Huang Bai (Phellodendri Cortex)
> Ku Shen (Sophorae Flavescentis Radix)
> Bai Bu (Stemonae Radix)
> Jing Jie (Schizonepetae Herba)
> Bo He (Menthae Herba)
> Bai Hua She She Cao (Oldenlandiae Diffusae Herba)
> Ban Zhi Lian (Scutellariae Barbatae Herba)
> She Chuang Zi (Cnidii Fructus)
> Di Fu Zi (Kochiae Fructus)

The combination in this formula includes herbs which vent the surface and release wind, clear heat and damp-heat, and resolve fire toxin. Several of the herbs are specifically able to soothe the skin and relieve itching, such as Ku Shen, Di Fu Zi, Jing Jie, and She Chuang Zi. Huang Bai, Ku Shen and Di Fu Zi drain damp-heat. Huang Bai, Bai Hua She She Cao and Ban Zhi Lian relieve heat and fire toxin. Bai Bu is helpful for skin rash from wind. Bo He and Jing Jie together vent rashes and alleviate itching. She Chuang Zi is effective for genital area itching and infections, especially when dampness is an issue.

If the patient is an elderly woman, the following wash is beneficial. The herbs in this prescription are gentle surface-venting herbs that soothe the skin, combined with herbs that quicken and cool the blood. As before, use 10 qian (30 g) of each herb except Jing Jie and Bo He, of which use 5 qian (15 g) each.

> Jin Yin Hua (Lonicerae Flos)
> Ju Hua (Chrysanthemi Flos)

Mu Dan Pi (Moutan Cortex)
Chi Shao (Paeoniae Radix Rubra)
Bo He (Menthae Herba)
Jing Jie (Schizonepetae Herba)

Jin Yin Hua, Ju Hua, Bo He and Jing Jie together disperse wind, vent rashes and relieve itching. Jin Yin Hua additionally clears heat and fire toxin. Mu Dan Pi and Chi Shao together move and cool the blood. For elderly females, yin and blood vacuity is often the central factor; for this reason, no damp-disinhibiting herbs are used in this wash.

This wash is also good for bacterial infection, skin infection, and rash. It can be taken internally for rash but the dosage of herbs should be decreased.

Acupuncture Points

Acupuncture points should be chosen according to the root focus; for example, if there is pelvic infection or leukorrhea, the point protocol should follow that given for these conditions. Sp10 (Xue Hai) can be included no matter what the etiology of the itching is. This point moves and cools the blood and helps to ease the itching.

Case Study

A 28-year-old woman presented with intermittent vaginal itching for the last two years. She is anxious, under a great deal of stress and irritable due to the itching. Her sleep is also poor and disturbed by the itching. She has a moderate amount of white and yellow vaginal discharge. She feels tired easily. Her appetite is poor and she experiences bloating and gas following meals. Her bowel movements are typically loose and her urination is yellow. Her tongue is slightly pale with teethmarks and red sides, and a greasy yellow coat. Her pulse is slippery, slightly weak and somewhat bowstring on the left.

Signs and symptoms: Damp-heat in the lower burner with spleen qi vacuity and liver qi depression

The combination of itching and yellow discharge suggests the presence of both dampness and heat in the genital region (the lower burner). The issue has become chronic because the patient has an underlying spleen qi deficiency that has impaired her ability to transform dampness. This is clear from her digestive difficulties and energy level. Additionally, liver involvement is suggested by her irritable mood and feelings of stress. Damp is a yin pathogen and tends to settle in the lower burner; the obstruction of the lower burner by both dampness and qi stagnation (since the liver channel courses through the genital region) has perpetuated the accumulation of heat in this area.

Treatment principles: Drain dampness, clear heat, fortify the spleen, smooth liver qi

Formula (Internal): Er Chen Tang modified (Two Matured Ingredients Decoction)

Ban Xia (Pinelliae Rhizoma)
Chen Pi (Citri Reticulatae Pericarpium)
Fu Ling (Poria)
Gan Cao (Glycyrrhizae Radix)
Bi Xie (Dioscoreae Hypoglaucae Rhizoma)
Yi Yi Ren (Coicis Semen)
Huang Bai (Phellodendri Cortex)
Jing Jie (Schizonepetae Herba)
Tu Fu Ling (Smilacis Glabrae Rhizoma)
Bai Shao (Paeoniae Radix Alba)

Ku Shen Tang modified (Flavescent Sophora Decoction):

Ku Shen (Sophorae Flavescentis Radix)
Bai Bu (Stemonae Radix)
Jing Jie (Schizonepetae Herba)
She Chuang Zi (Cnidii Fructus)
Huang Bai (Phellodendri Cortex)
Ban Zhi Lian (Scutellariae Barbatae Herba)
Bai Hua She She Cao (Oldenlandiae Diffusae Herba)
Di Fu Zi (Kochiae Fructus)

Acupuncture Points: CV3 (Zhong Ji), SP9 (Yin Ling Quan), ST36 (Zu San Li), LR5 (Li Gou)

Treatment analysis

Er Chen Tang (Two Matured Ingredients Decoction)

Here the basic internal formula is Er Chen Tang, which addresses the dampness (Ban Xia, Chen Pi, Fu Ling, Gan Cao). Bi Xie, Jing Jie and Tu Fu Ling help to relieve the itching. Yi Yi Ren helps to disinhibit dampness by promoting urination and fortifying the spleen. Huang Bai clears heat in the lower burner. Bai Shao soothes the liver.

The external herbs help to soothe the itching when applied with a douche or as a sitz bath. Ku Shen clears heat, dampness and wind from the skin. Jing Jie releases exterior wind to relieve itching. Bai Bu and She Chuang Zi are used to kill worms and are good for dermal itching. Huang Bai and Ban Zhi Lian clear heat, while Bai Hua She She Cao and Ban Zhi Lian both clear heat toxin. Di Fu Zi also clears heat and relieves itching.

Needling CV3 clears lower burner repletion such as dampness and heat. SP9 disinhibits dampness and supports the spleen, in conjunction with ST36. LR5 circulates to the genital region and clears heat.

Outcome

After treatment for 21 days, the itching was gone. The patient reported that her energy has returned and her vaginal discharge was now back to normal. Her bowel movements were regular and formed, and her digestion had greatly improved. Her appetite was good and she enjoyed eating once again. She felt comfortable and happy.

15

Abnormal Vaginal Discharge

Western Medical View

Leukorrhea (more commonly called vaginitis in the U.S.) refers to an abnormal or excessive vaginal discharge. It is suspected if the normal volume of discharge increases, has an odor, or shows changes in consistency and color. Usually, it is accompanied by itching, rash, soreness, and burning. Occasionally, painful urination (dysuria) and light vaginal bleeding may occur. Abnormal vaginal discharge is often a sign of bacterial infection, sexually transmitted disease (STD), or yeast overgrowth.

Normal vaginal discharge

All women have a normal physiologic vaginal discharge. Such a normal discharge cleanses the vagina and maintains the acidic pH that promotes the growth of infection-fighting flora. In this case, the discharge is thin, odorless, and appears clear, milky white, or yellowish on clothing. It contains mucus from the cervix, endometrium, epithelial cells, and microflora.

Normal vaginal discharge varies with cyclic hormonal changes. As estrogen levels rise, discharge increases. At ovulation, vaginal discharge continues to increase and is clear, thin, and stretchy. Discharge also increases during times of stress, sexual arousal, pregnancy, and with use of oral contraceptives. As estrogen levels drop after menopause, vaginal discharge decreases and may change in character.

Causes:

The most common causes (90%) of leukorrhea/vaginitis are:

- Bacterial vaginosis (BV) (*Gardnerella vaginalis*)
- Vaginal yeast infection (*Vulvovaginal candidiasis*)

- Trichomoniasis (*Trichomonas vaginalis*)
- *Atrophic vaginitis* (Postmenopausal)

Less common, but more serious causes include:

- Chlamydia
- Gonorrhea
- Neoplasms

Causes of noninfectious vaginitis include:

- Foreign bodies
- IUD, diaphragm, condom or forgotten tampon
- Allergic reactions and chemical irritants
- Spermicides
- Detergents, fabric softeners or soaps
- Feminine sprays, ointments, and creams
- Excessive douching
- Vitamin B-complex deficiency
- Uncontrolled diabetes

Common causes of leukorrhea:

Bacterial vaginosis

Bacterial vaginosis (BV) is the most common cause of vaginitis. Overgrowths of microorganisms such as *Gardnerella vaginalis*, anaerobic bacteria, and genital mycoplasmas upset the normal balance of the vaginal environment. Half of women with BV are asymptomatic. When symptoms do present, vaginal discharge is profuse, thin, and watery. It also may be a milky, grayish white discharge with a foul fishy odor. Sexual intercourse and menses often aggravate symptoms. Usually there is no vulvar or vaginal inflammation.

Vaginal yeast infection (*Candida vaginitis*)

The second most common cause of vaginitis is an overgrowth of fungal yeast (predominantly *Candida albicans*) in the vagina. Presenting symptoms include thick, white, clumpy (cottage cheese-like) discharge that is odorless and accompanied by vulvar or vaginal redness, itching, and burning. Urination and sexual intercourse are often painful. Twenty-five percent of women with this condition are asymptomatic. Yeast infections are most often caused by use of antibiotics, oral estrogen or contraceptives, by increased stress, and a diet high in sugars. Spermicides used with diaphragms, pregnancy, uncontrolled diabetes, or a weakened immune system can also cause yeast infections.

Trichomoniasis

Trichomonas vaginalis is a sexually transmitted one-celled parasite that causes a yellowish gray or green, frothy discharge together with intense itching. There is also a foul, musty odor, increased urinary frequency (which is sometimes painful), and vulvar or vaginal inflammation.

Approximately 50% of cases are asymptomatic. Because the parasite can survive for up to 24 hours in a moist environment, contact with wet towels or bathing suits can also be vectors of transmission.

Atrophic vaginitis

Atrophic vaginitis is the most common cause of vaginal irritation in post-menopausal women. In this case, reduced estrogen levels due to menopause cause atrophy of the vaginal epithelium and results in a secondary infection that presents as irritation of the vulva, a clear or yellow vaginal discharge, urinary frequency, and stress incontinence.

A dark brown or blood-tinged foul odor can be a sign of malignancy and requires immediate medical attention.

Sexually transmitted diseases

Chlamydia trachomatis infection is the most common sexually transmitted bacterial infection in the U.S. Seventy percent of infected females have no symptoms. Symptomatic cases present with increased yellowish discharge (possibly blood-tinged), dysuria, and lower abdominal pain. Chlamydia often results in PID, chronic pelvic pain, ectopic pregnancy, and infertility.

Gonorrhea (*Neisseria gonorrhea*) is the second most common sexually transmitted infection. Most women are asymptomatic. The remainder present with a purulent, yellow or bloody vaginal discharge, bleeding with intercourse, pain or burning with urination, pelvic pain or cramping, fever, vomiting, and intermenstrual bleeding. Gonorrhea is a common cause of PID.

Neoplasms

Common neoplasms that present with vaginitis include endometrial cancer, cervical cancer, and vaginal/vulvar cancers. Generally, the discharge is dark brown or blood-tinged with a foul odor.

Endometrial cancer is signaled by an offensive brown, watery, blood-tinged discharge or by abnormal vaginal bleeding. Postmenopausal women with these symptoms should be checked immediately.

Late-stage cervical cancer presents with persistent vaginal discharge, bleeding after intercourse, between menstruation, and after menopause, urinary frequency, pelvic pain, and lower extremity edema.

Vaginal or vulvar cancers often are accompanied by a dark, watery, blood-tinged, offensively smelling discharge together with cauliflower-like lesions in the vulva or vagina.

Complications of vaginitis:

BV & trichomoniasis are associated with low birth weight or premature birth, if contracted during pregnancy and are linked to a higher risk of acquiring other STD infections and HIV. There may also be transmission of STDs (trichomoniasis, chlamydia, gonorrhea) to partners.

Risks factors:

- Multiple sex partners
- Oral contraceptives and IUDs
- Douching
- Pregnancy
- Menopause
- Compromised immune system

Diagnosis:

Vaginitis is diagnosed by:

- Type, color, consistency, and odor of the discharge
- Examination of cervical or vaginal fluid under a microscope
- Pelvic exams; for example, red sores on the cervix or inside the vagina suggests trichomoniasis
- Yeast infections can be mistaken for other types of vaginitis and should be carefully diagnosed

Treatment:

In all cases of vaginitis, avoid sex until the full course of treatment is completed.

BV & trichomoniasis

- Partners are usually treated in cases of *Trichomonas vaginalis*.
- Oral antibiotics, *e.g.*, metronidazole (Flagyl)
- Intravaginal and topical antibiotic creams, *e.g.*, metronidazole (MetroGel), clindamycin (Cleocin)

Yeast infections

- Over-the-counter or prescription antifungal creams or vaginal suppositories, such as miconazole (Monistat), clotrimazole (Gyne-Lotrimin)
- Oral medication, including fluconazole (Diflucan), ketoconazole (Nizoral), miconazole (Monistat), butoconazole (Femstat), and tioconazole (Vagistat)
- Eat foods containing live lactobacillus cultures (yogurt)
- Apply cold compresses to labia to ease discomfort until medication takes effect

Atrophic vaginitis

- Oral estrogen
- Estradiol vaginal creams
- Estrogen rings

Neoplasms

- Surgery
- Chemotherapy

Prevention:

- Use a latex condom
- Avoid irritants such as scented tampons, harsh or antibacterial soaps
- Wipe from front to back after bowel movements
- Do not douche
- Wear underclothes with a cotton lining

Traditional Chinese Medical View

Abnormal vaginal discharge is defined as excessive vaginal discharge with or without odor, tingling sensation, and yellow or green color. Sometimes it may present with blood, pus, and/or pain.

Treatment based on pattern identification:

Damp-heat toxin (*shi re du* 湿热毒)

Signs & symptoms: Foul odor, yellow, green, purulent pus (possibly with blood), sticky, turbid discharge with lower abdominal pain and cramps

Tongue: Red with yellow, slimy fur

Pulse: Rapid, bowstring

Treatment principles: Clear heat and resolve toxins, eliminate dampness

Formula: Zhi Dai Tang (Check Discharge Decoction)

Zhu Ling (Polyporus)
Fu Ling (Poria)
Che Qian Zi (Plantaginis Semen)
Ze Xie (Alismatis Rhizoma)

Modifications:

• To clear heat, add Yin Chen Hao (Artemisiae Scopariae Herba), Zhi Zi (Gardeniae Fructus), and Huang Bai (Phellodendri Cortex).

• To quicken the blood, break stasis, and relieve pain, add Chi Shao (Paeoniae Radix Rubra), Mu Dan Pi (Moutan Cortex), and Niu Xi (Achyranthis Bidentatae Radix).

Spleen qi vacuity (*pi qi xu* 脾气虚)

Signs & symptoms: White or slightly yellow discharge with no odor, copious or scanty amount, thick consistency

Tongue: Pale with white, sticky fur

Pulse: Slow, weak

Treatment principles: Fortify the spleen and supplement the qi, dry dampness and upbear yang

Formula: Wan Dai Tang (Discharge-ceasing Decoction)

Ren Shen (Ginseng Radix)
Shan Yao (Dioscoreae Rhizoma)
Bai Zhu (Atractylodis Macrocephalae Rhizoma)
Bai Shao (Paeoniae Radix Alba)

Chai Hu (Bupleuri Radix)
Cang Zhu (Atractylodis Rhizoma)
Chen Pi (Citri Reticulatae Pericarpium)
Che Qian Zi (Plantaginis Semen)
Hei Jing Jie (Schizonepetae Herba)
Gan Cao (Glycyrrhizae Radix)

Modifications:

- For chronic pain due to blood stasis, add qi- and blood-moving medicinals, such as Yu Jin (Curcumae Radix), Xiang Fu (Cyperi Rhizoma), Chuan Xiong (Chuanxiong Rhizoma), Chi Shao (Paeoniae Radix Rubra), and/or Mu Dan Pi (Moutan Cortex).

- For lower back pain, add Du Zhong (Eucommiae Cortex), Xu Duan (Dipsaci Radix), Ba Ji Tian (Morindae Officinalis Radix), and Tu Si Zi (Cuscutae Semen).

- To secure the essence and supplement the kidney, add Fu Pen Zi (Rubi Fructus), Lian Zi (Nelumbinis Semen), Qian Shi (Euryales Semen), Shan Zhu Yu (Corni Fructus), Hai Piao Xiao (Sepiae Endoconcha), Wu Wei Zi (Schisandrae Fructus), and/or Jin Ying Zi (Rosae Laevigatae Fructus).

- For even more securing and astringing, add Long Gu (Mastodi Ossis Fossilia), Mu Li (Ostreae Concha), and/or Hai Piao Xiao (Sepiae Endoconcha).

Kidney yang vacuity (*shen yang xu* 肾阳虚)

Signs & symptoms: Clear white discharge, odorless with watery quality, continuous profuse discharge, sore lower back

Tongue: Pale with thin fur

Pulse: Deep

Treatment principles: Supplement the kidney, secure the essence, check vaginal discharge

Formula: Nei Bu Wan (Internal Supplementation Pill)

Lu Rong (Cervi Cornu Pantotrichum)
Tu Si Zi (Cuscutae Semen)
Sha Yuan Zi (Astragali Complanati Semen)

Rou Cong Rong (Cistanches Herba)
Rou Gui (Cinnamomi Cortex)
Huang Qi (Astragali Radix)
Ci Ji Li (Tribuli Fructus)
Sang Piao Xiao (Mantidis Ootheca)
Zhi Fu Zi (Aconiti Carmichaeli Radix Praeparata)
Zi Wan (Asteris Radix)

Modifications: If there is diarrhea, add the ingredients of Si Shen Wan (Four Spir-its Pill), *i.e.*, Bu Gu Zhi (Psoraleae Fructus), Wu Zhu Yu (Evodiae Fructus), Rou Dou Kou (Myristicae Semen), and Wu Wei Zi (Schisandrae Fructus), plus Sheng Jiang (Zingiberis Rhizoma Recens) and Da Zao (Jujubae Fructus).

Acute pelvic infection

Signs & symptoms: High WBC count, pus, discharge, severe cramps and pain, fever

Formula: Modified Long Dan Xie Gan Tang (Gentian Liver-draining Decoction)

Long Dan Cao (Gentianae Radix)
Huang Qin (Scutellariae Radix)
Zhi Zi (Gardeniae Fructus)
Ze Xie (Alismatis Rhizoma)
Mu Tong (Akebiae Trifoliatae Caulis)
Che Qian Zi (Plantaginis Semen)
Sheng Di Huang (Rehmanniae Radix)
Chai Hu (Bupleuri Radix)
Dang Gui Wei (Angelicae Sinensis Radicis Extremitas)
Gan Cao (Glycyrrhizae Radix)
Xiang Fu (Cyperi Rhizoma)
Qing Pi (Citri Reticulatae Pericarpium Viride)
Zhi Ke (Qiao) (Aurantii Fructus)
Hei Lao Hu (Kadsurae Coccineae Caulis et Folium)
Ji Gu Xiang (Crotonis Crassifolii Radix)

As an external wash, use:

Da Huang (Rhei Radix et Rhizoma)
Huang Lian (Coptidis Rhizoma)
Huang Bai (Phellodendri Cortex)
Huang Qin (Scutellariae Radix)

Clinical Treatment

In our previous discussions of theory and diagnosis, we have treated vaginal itching and vaginal discharge separately. However, it is important to note that they often coexist clinically and, therefore, may be treated with a combined approach. Most commonly, both of these conditions result from either acute or chronic pelvic infection. In acute cases, we are often dealing with damp-heat and toxins. When the situation is chronic, there is usually vacuity of some kind. This may include vacuity of yin, blood, or spleen qi as well as kidney qi, yin, or yang vacuities. Clinically, treatment can be divided into acute and chronic approaches, with appropriate modifications to reflect the individual pattern of each patient.

Treatment of acute pelvic infection:

In Western medicine, this is also referred to as pelvic inflammatory disease (PID). From a Chinese medical perspective, this is thought of as a replete condition related to damp-heat and toxins. In such cases, the patient may have a high fever, vaginal discharge, lower abdominal pain, and possibly laboratory tests showing a high white blood cell (WBC) count. The basic formula of choice is:

Long Dan Xie Gan Tang (Gentian Liver-draining Decoction)

> Long Dan Cao (Gentianae Radix)
> Huang Qin (Scutellariae Radix)
> Zhi Zi (Gardeniae Fructus)
> Ze Xie (Alismatis Rhizoma)
> Mu Tong (Akebiae Trifoliatae Caulis)
> Che Qian Zi (Plantaginis Semen)
> Chai Hu (Bupleuri Radix)
> Sheng Di Huang (Rehmanniae Radix)
> Gan Cao (Glycyrrhizae Radix)

This is an excellent base or guiding formula for addressing damp-heat and toxins but modifications specific to the patient will be necessary.

Modifications:

- For symptoms of bloating and gas due to qi stagnation, qi-moving medicinals such as Qing Pi (Citri Reticulatae Pericarpium Viride), Zhi Ke (Qiao) (Aurantii Fructus), Xiang Fu (Cyperi Rhizoma), or Yu Jin (Curcumae Radix) may be added. These medicinals specifically enter the liver channel which circles the genitalia.

- If the patient experiences pain, Hei Lao Hu (Kadsurae Coccineae Caulis et Folium), Ji Gu Xiang (Crotonis Crassifolii Radix), Yan Hu Suo (Corydalis Rhizoma), and/or San Qi (Notoginseng Radix) are good choices. If the pain is specifically related to blood stasis, the following herbs may be helpful in addition to the Yan Hu Suo and San Qi: Mu Dan Pi (Moutan Cortex), Chi Shao (Paeoniae Radix Rubra), Niu Xi (Achyranthis Bidentatae Radix), Dan Shen (Salviae Miltiorrhizae Radix), and/or Da Huang (Rhei Radix et Rhizoma). When using Da Huang as a blood-quickening substance, it should be cooked along with the other medicinals rather than adding it near the end of the decoction.

- If there is significant dampness, urination may be promoted with damp-disinhibiting medicinals such as Tong Cao (Tetrapanacis Medulla), Bi Xie (Dioscoreae Hypoglaucae seu Semptemlobae Rhizoma), Yi Yi Ren (Coicis Semen), Che Qian Zi (Plantaginis Semen), and/or Ze Xie (Alismatis Rhizoma).

- If there are more signs of heat toxins, strong heat-clearing agents may be added, including Jin Yin Hua (Lonicerae Flos), Chuan Shan Jia (Manis Squama), Zi Hua Di Ding (Violae Herba), Ju Hua (Chrysanthemi Flos), Bai Hua She She Cao (Oldenlandiae Diffusae Herba), Huang Bai (Phellodendri Cortex), Huang Qin (Scutellariae Radix), Huang Lian (Coptidis Rhizoma), Tian Kui Zi (Semiaquilegiae Radix), Pu Gong Ying (Taraxaci Herba), or Bai Jiang Cao (Patriniae Herba).

Treatment of chronic pelvic infection:

Most women recover from PID, but there can be serious complications if the infection is not identified and treated early. It can increase the risk of ectopic pregnancy, infertility, and chronic pelvic pain. Once a woman has developed PID, there is an increased risk of developing it again even after resolution.

The most common sequela affecting women who have recovered from PID is chronic pelvic pain. This is due to scars resulting from the infection, also known as adhesions. Adhesions can cause the organs and tissues to stick together and pull on each other, thus causing pain. Some adhesions can be treated surgically to help ease the pain. If scarring is severe enough, it can cause infertility. This is especially true if the adhesions block or constrict the fallopian tubes. The likelihood that a woman will develop infertility increases with each incidence of PID.

Scarred fallopian tubes also increase the chance of ectopic pregnancy since the egg has increased difficulty moving through the tube. If the egg is fertilized while lodged in the tube, the embryo will continue to grow and will potentially rupture the tube. When this occurs, it can be life-threatening.

Some women develop PID repeatedly. This happens either because a previous infection has not completely resolved or as a result of reinfection. On occasion, an abscess may develop from a PID infection. An abscess in the reproductive organs is very difficult to clear with antibiotics and may rupture, causing a life-threatening situation. In some cases a physician may recommend surgery to remove the abscess.

Nevertheless, the usual course of treatment for PID is antibiotics. Occasionally surgery is indicated if the PID is recurrent, the pelvic pain is severe, or an incurable abscess develops.

From a Chinese medical perspective, in cases of chronic pelvic infection it is important to consider spleen and/or kidney vacuity. In my experience, a good basic formula for this situation is:

Liu Jun Zi Tang (Six Gentlemen Decoction) with appropriate modifications to reflect the individual patient's condition.

> Ren Shen (Ginseng Radix) or Dang Shen (Codonopsis Radix)
> Bai Zhu (Atractylodis Macrocephalae Rhizoma)
> Fu Ling (Poria)
> Gan Cao (Glycyrrhizae Radix)
> Chen Pi (Citri Reticulatae Pericarpium)
> Ban Xia (Pinelliae Rhizoma)

Modifications:

- For qi stagnation, one can add Xiang Fu (Cyperi Rhizoma), Zhi Ke (Qiao) (Aurantii Fructus), Hei Lao Hu (Kadsurae Coccineae Caulis et Folium), or Ji Gu Xiang (Crotonis Crassifolii Radix).

- If there are signs of blood stasis, good choices include Dan Shen (Salviae Miltiorrhizae Radix), Chi Shao (Paeoniae Radix Rubra), Mu Dan Pi (Moutan Cortex), Gui Zhi (Cinnamomi Ramulus), and/or Xiao Hui Xiang (Foeniculi Fructus). The last two medicinals are warm and are particularly good if there are cold signs.

- In case of heat signs, Bai Jiang Cao (Patriniae Herba), Jin Yin Hua (Lonicerae

Flos), and/or Chuan Shan Jia (Manis Squama) may be used. It is important that heat-clearing medicinals are chosen carefully because, in this situation, some cooling medicinals can damage an already delicate spleen, such as Huang Qin (Scutellariae Radix), Huang Bai (Phellodendri Cortex), and Huang Lian (Coptidis Rhizoma).

Western medicine usually prescribes antibiotics for acute pelvic infection. When this is the case, we do not want to give cold medicinals because the antibiotics are already very cold and damaging to the spleen. In such cases, Chinese medicine is still very useful. We can help by giving medicinals to protect the spleen. This will also help prevent yeast infection which is a common side effect of antibiotic therapy. Liu Jun Zi Tang is a good choice for this. If no antibiotics are used, we can use cold medicinals as described above.

Acupuncture formula:
Acute PID

SP10 (Xue Hai), SP9 (Yin Ling Quan), CV3 (Zhong Ji)

Formula analysis

Typically, in acute cases, there is damp-heat. SP9 is especially useful for clearing and eliminating dampness and heat from the lower burner. SP10 quickens and cools the blood to help with the itching and clear inflammation. CV3 is an effective local point to clear damp-heat.

Chronic PID

SP10 (Xue Hai), ST36 (Zu San Li)

Modifications:

- If there is cold-damp, SP9 (Yin Ling Chuan) may also be used with moxibustion.

- If there is kidney vacuity also, KI3 (Tai Xi) is a good addition.

Formula analysis

In chronic cases of PID, there may be elements of damp-heat or cold-damp. SP10 is again used to quicken and cool the blood to ease itching and clear inflammation from the system. ST36 is used to boost the middle burner and for its ability to control dampness in the body. Also, it is important to supplement the qi and blood in chronic conditions because there is a tendency for the body to become weakened over time. Moxibustion on SP9 will help to warm and support the spleen's transformation function to eliminate the dampness. KI3 is the source point of the kidney channel and helps supplement all aspects of the kidney.

Case Study

The patient was a 32-year-old woman whose chief complaint was excessive vaginal discharge for more than two years. She had to change pads three times a day on average. The discharge was usually clear or white but sometimes slightly yellow. The patient reported that she was fatigued and had little energy. Sometimes she had asthma or allergies. She had some phlegm in her throat in the mornings. Her lower back was sore and she felt bloated. She was thirsty but only liked to drink hot ginger tea. Her bowel movements varied between being constipated and unformed, and her urination was frequent. She reported a high degree of stress in her life. Her tongue was pale and enlarged with thick, wet fur that was slightly yellow. Her pulse was slippery, slightly bowstring, and weak in the cubit positions.

Pattern identification: Kidney yang vacuity, lung-spleen qi vacuity, liver depression qi stagnation, and damp stagnation in all three burners

Symptom analysis

In addition to the copious, clear or pale-colored discharge, this patient's frequent urination, sore lower back, and the quality of her tongue and cubit pulses point to kidney yang vacuity. Additionally, she desired hot ginger tea to drink, suggesting an interior vacuity cold condition. Her tendency to asthma and allergies is indicative of lung qi vacuity. In tandem with the lung qi vacuity, there is an element of spleen qi vacuity. This we see from the low energy and the phlegm in her throat. It is said, "The spleen is the root of phlegm engenderment; the lung is the place where phlegm is stored." In other words, phlegm arises from spleen vacuity and is then contained in the throat which is connected to the lung in TCM. The spleen qi also seemed to be vacuous due to liver depression qi stagnation. The patient reported stressful feelings, and her changeable bowel movements are a hallmark of liver assailing the spleen. Her bowstring pulse confirms liver involvement. Dampness as a result of impairment of the spleen's transformation function is evident in the phlegm as well as the vaginal discharge and slippery pulse. The fact that her discharge and tongue fur both have a slightly yellow color can be taken as a further indication of dampness. The yellow color can indicate either dampness or heat, but there is no evidence of heat here, and the shade of yellow is also very pale, thus pertaining to the spleen.

Treatment principles: Supplement the kidney and warm yang, supplement the lung and spleen, course the liver and rectify the qi, eliminate dampness

Formula: Modified Wan Dai Tang (Discharge-ceasing Decoction)

Ren Shen (Ginseng Radix)
Shan Yao (Dioscoreae Rhizoma)
Cang Zhu (Atractylodis Rhizoma)
Chen Pi (Citri Reticulatae Pericarpium)
Tu Si Zi (Cuscutae Semen)
Lu Rong (Cervi Cornu Pantotrichum)
Huang Qi (Astragali Radix)
Rou Gui (Cinnamomi Cortex)
Sang Piao Xiao (Mantidis Ootheca)

Acupuncture Points:

SP9 (Yin Ling Quan), ST36 (Zu San Li), KI3 (Tai Xi), CV3 (Zhong Ji)

Treatment analysis

The quality and quantity of the discharge as well as the patient's other signs and symptoms (lack of energy, frequent urination, sore lower back, abdominal bloating, and allergies) indicate that this patient's basic picture is one of vacuity. However, there are also replete elements, such as dampness and qi stagnation, that complicate treatment. Therefore, I began with Wan Dai Tang as my base formula. I then removed Bai Zhu (Atractylodis Macrocephalae Rhizoma), Che Qian Zi (Plantaginis Semen), Bai Shao (Paeoniae Alba Radix), Chai Hu (Bupleuri Radix), and Jing Jie Sui (Schizonepetae Spicae), leaving Ren Shen, Shan Yao, Cang Zhu, and Chen Pi as my core ingredients to fortify the spleen, supplement the qi, and eliminate dampness. Next, I added Huang Qi to further supplement the qi and specifically supplement the lungs. Then I added Tu Si Zi, Lu Rong, and Rou Gui to warm and supplement kidney yang. Finally, I added Sang Piao Xiao to both secure the essence to stop the "leakage" of vaginal discharge and supplement the kidney.

In terms of acupuncture, needling SP9 and CV3 was meant to eliminate dampness by promoting urination. ST36 supplements the qi and promotes the dampness-transforming function of the spleen. As the source point of the kidney, KI3 supplements both kidney yin and yang.

Outcome

After one month of treatments, the patient's discharge returned to normal, she had more energy and her asthma symptoms had subsided. She was so satisfied with her treatments that she decided to go to acupuncture school.

16

Pelvic Masses

Western Medical View

Pelvic masses refer to a mass or masses in the pelvis found by physical examination or found incidentally during diagnostic imaging studies (*i.e.*, ultrasound, MRI). Such masses may be cystic or solid and occur in any age group. They may originate from the cervix, uterus, adnexa, and from other organs, such as the bowel, musculoskeletal, vascular, lymphatic, or nervous systems. The two main types of benign pelvic masses specific to gynecology are ovarian cysts and uterine myomas.

Ovarian cysts

Ovarian cysts are fluid-filled sacs that develop on the ovaries as a normal part of the menstrual cycle. They are quite common in women during their childbearing years. Usually they are benign, small, asymptomatic and harmless. They go away on their own within a few months and are rarely cancerous. If they become large, they may cause abdominal discomfort. Occasionally, they may twist their own blood supply, the ovaries or the fallopian tubes, or may bleed or rupture. This causes sudden acute abdominal pain that requires emergency attention. Some ovarian cysts, especially in women over 35 (and particularly in Postmenopausal years), can signal ovarian cancer. Cysts are less common in women who do not ovulate regularly, for example those on birth control pills or who are menopausal. Ovarian cysts can also develop during pregnancy. Usually, they disappear without treatment.

Types of ovarian cysts

- Functional cysts are the most common type and develop during the normal process of ovulation. They usually shrink and dissolve naturally within a few months. They are harmless.

- Follicular cysts develop when a normal ovarian follicle fails to release an egg during the menstrual cycle (anovulation) and instead fills with fluid, initiating cyst formation.

- Corpus luteum cysts form when a normal follicle does release an egg but the follicular sac (now called the corpus luteum) fails to disintegrate normally. Instead, the opening of the ruptured sac closes off. Fluid or blood accumulates inside to form a cyst. The sac usually disappears within a few weeks. Occasionally, they may grow large (up to four inches in diameter) and cause pelvic or abdominal pain. If they twist or rupture, they may cause internal bleeding and a sudden sharp pain. Fertility drugs that are used to induce ovulation increase the risk of a corpus luteum cyst.

- Hemorrhagic cysts are functional cysts that sometimes burst. Leaking blood may cause a burning sensation in the pelvic region. They usually resolve without treatment.

- Other ovarian cysts are less common and are usually benign. These cysts may grow large. Rapid growth or twisting of internal organs may cause pain and occasional rupture.

- Cystadenomas are cysts that develop from cells on the outer surface of the ovary. They are filled with watery fluid or mucus. If they grow particularly large, they may cause pain.

- Endometriomas are cysts that form from endometrial tissue that grows on or in the ovaries. Endometriomas can cause pain during intercourse or during menstruation.

- Dermoid cysts arise from embryonic germ cells that form many of our body tissues. Often, they contain some of these tissues, such as hair, skin or teeth. They can grow large and cause twisting of the ovary.

- Frequent small cysts developing on the ovary may indicate the hormonal disorder of polycystic ovarian syndrome (PCOS).

Risk factors:

- History of previous ovarian cysts
- Concurrent use of fertility drugs that stimulate ovulation
- History of endometriosis – more likely to develop endometriomas
- Irregular menstrual cycles

- Early menstruation
- Infertility
- Hormonal imbalances
- Tamoxifen therapy for breast cancer
- Ovarian cancer

Signs & symptoms: The majority of ovarian cysts have no symptoms. Cysts that may grow large (cystadenomas, endometriomas, or dermoid) may produce the following symptoms:

- Feeling of pain, fullness or pressure in the lower abdomen or pelvis
- Dull ache in the lower back and thighs
- Menstrual irregularities
- Constant dull aching pelvic pain
- Painful menstruation or abnormal uterine bleeding
- Pelvic pain during intercourse (dyspareunia), movement or strenuous exercise
- Incomplete urination
- Infertility
- Weight gain
- Breast tenderness

These symptoms may also be associated with other conditions such as endometriosis, ectopic pregnancy or PID. A doctor must be seen for a differential diagnosis.

Urgent symptoms requiring immediate emergency attention:
- Sudden onset of severe abdominal or pelvic pain
- Persistent fever
- Nausea and vomiting
- Weakness, dizziness or fainting
- Excessive thirst or urination
- Rapid breathing
- Signs of shock

Diagnosis:
- Routine pelvic exam
- Ultrasound
- Laparoscopy
- Blood tests to rule out ectopic pregnancy, hormonal abnormalities, and ovarian cancer

- MRI
- CT scan
- Biopsy

Treatment:

- Regular monitoring of asymptomatic cysts
- Oral contraceptives to prevent ovulation and thus the formation of follicles
- Laparoscopic cystectomy to remove persistently large cysts or those that cause symptoms (in this case, fertility is preserved)
- Laparotomy if there is significant risk for a malignancy
- Removal of affected ovary or complete hysterectomy (removal of both ovaries and the uterus)
- Salpingo-oophorectomy for neoplasms and emergency twisting or rupture of a cyst

Uterine myomas (a.k.a. fibroids)

Uterine myomas are benign tumors that develop from the smooth muscle tissue of the uterus (myometrium). Also called leiomyomas or fibromyomas, they are thought to affect one in every four women of childbearing age in the United States. These may grow as a single tumor, in clusters, or with stems. (Those with stems are called pedunculated.) Size varies from less than one inch to eight inches or more. They are rarely cancerous.

Fibroids are classified according to where they grow:

- Submucosal fibroids grow just underneath the uterine lining
- Intramural fibroids grow within the muscle of the uterus
- Subserosal fibroids grow on the outside wall of the uterus

Most women who have fibroids are able to become pregnant.

Risk factors:

- Genetics
- Obesity
- Nulliparity

Cause: To date, the cause of fibroids is unknown. However, they may be affected by estrogen levels. This is what my experience suggests. Fibroid tissue has more receptors for these hormones than other uterine smooth muscle cells. During pregnancy, when estrogen levels are high, fibroids may grow rapidly. After menopause, estrogen levels decline. Fibroids usually stop growing or often shrink.

Signs & symptoms: Most fibroids, even very large ones, cause no symptoms.

Approximately 25-50% of fibroid patients present with the following symptoms:

- Abnormal uterine bleeding
- Heavy or painful menstruation
- Bleeding between menstruation
- Prolonged spotting
- Feeling of pain, pressure or fullness in the lower abdomen and pelvic area
- Frequent urination
- Pain during sex (dyspareunia)
- Lower back pain
- Enlarged uterus or abdomen
- Infertility, multiple miscarriages or early labor

Diagnosis:

- Routine pelvic exam
- Ultrasound
- Hysteroscopy
- Laparoscopy
- MRI
- X-rays
- CT scan

Treatment: Asymptomatic women need no treatment. Treatments for symptomatic women include:

Medication:

- Pain medication
- Hormone therapy

Surgery:

- Myomectomy
- Uterine artery embolization (UAE)
- Hysterectomy

Some relatively new treatments, with unknown long-term effects, include:

- Endometrial ablation
- Cryomyolysis
- Focused ultrasound

Traditional Chinese Medical View

In TCM, women's tumors are categorized under the term *zheng jia*, concretions and conglomerations. Concretions (*zheng*) refer to a true mass that is hard, fixed, and localized. Conglomerations (*jia*) refer to a movable, formless body that is not fixed or hard. Together, they describe two different pathological conditions which often manifest as uterine fibroids (*zheng* 癥) and ovarian cysts (*jia* 瘕).

Treatment based on pattern identification:

Qi stagnation (*qi zhi* 癥滯)

Signs & symptoms: Abdominal pain that moves or feels like pressure or bloating, irregular or delayed menstrual cycles, possibly with PMS or dysmenorrhea, depression or irritability

Tongue: Purple

Pulse: Bowstring

Treatment principles: Rectify the qi, quicken the blood, and disperse concretions

Formula: Xiang Leng Wan (Cyperus & Sparganium Pill)

Mu Xiang (Aucklandiae Radix)
Ding Xiang (Caryophylli Flos)
Qing Pi (Citri Reticulatae Pericarpium Viride)
Chuan Lian Zi (Toosendan Fructus)
Zhi Ke (Qiao) (Aurantii Fructus)
San Leng (Sparganii Rhizoma)
E Zhu (Curcumae Rhizoma)
Xiao Hui Xiang (Foeniculi Fructus)

Modifications:

- If there is more qi stagnation, add Chai Hu (Bupleuri Radix), Bai Shao (Paeoniae Radix Alba), Yu Jin (Curcumae Radix), Xiang Fu (Cyperi Rhizoma), and/or Fo Shou (Sacrodactylis Fructus).

- Several seeds are used clinically as well: Ju He (Citri Reticulatae Semen), Li Zhi He (Litchi Semen), and Pi Pa He (Eriobotryae Semen).

To supplement the kidney, add Xu Duan (Dipsaci Radix).

Blood stasis (*xue yu* 血瘀)

Signs & symptoms: Abdominal pain that is fixed, sharp, and worse at night, delayed menstruation, painful menstruation with dark blood and clots

Tongue: Purplish, purple spots

Pulse: Rough or choppy

Treatment principles: Quicken the blood, break stasis, and course the qi

Formula: Gui Zhi Fu Ling Wan (Cinnamon Twig & Poria Pill)

Gui Zhi (Cinnamomi Ramulus)
Fu Ling (Poria)
Tao Ren (Persicae Semen)
Chi Shao (Paeoniae Radix Rubra)
Mu Dan Pi (Moutan Cortex)

Modifications:

- If there is more blood stasis, add medicinals such as Yu Jin (Curcumae Radix), Dan Shen (Salviae Miltiorrhizae Radix), Dang Gui (Angelicae Sinensis Radix), Yi Mu Cao (Leonuri Herba), Mu Xiang (Aucklandiae Radix), Hong Hua (Carthami Flos), Chuan Xiong (Chuanxiong Rhizoma), San Leng (Sparganii Rhizoma), E Zhu (Curcumae Rhizoma), Shui Zhi (Hirudo), Zhe Chong (Eupolyphaga seu Steleophaga), Ji Xue Teng (Spatholobi Caulis), Yan Hu Suo (Corydalis Rhizoma), Wang Bu Liu Xing (Vaccariae Semen), Meng Chong (Tabanus), and/or Ji Nei Jin (Galli Gigeriae Endothelium Corneum).

- For phlegm fibroids, add medicinals such as Chen Pi (Citri Reticulatae Pericarpium), Ban Xia (Pinelliae Rhizoma), Cang Zhu (Atractylodis Rhizoma), Dan Xing (Arisaema cum Bile), Zhe Bei Mu (Fritillariae Thunbergii Bulbus), Lian Qiao (Forsythiae Fructus), Hai Zao (Sargassum), Kun Bu (Laminariae/Eckloniae Thallus), and/or Xia Ku Cao (Prunellae Spica).

- For ovarian cysts, add medicinals such as Mu Tong (Akebiae Trifoliatae Caulis), Yi Yi Ren (Coicis Semen), Che Qian Cao (Plantaginis Herba), Zhu Ling (Polyporus), Deng Xin Cao (Junci Medulla), Dong Kui Zi (Malvae Semen), Qu Mai (Dianthi Herba), and/or Ze Xie (Alismatis Rhizoma).

- For uterine bleeding, add medicinals such as San Qi (Notoginseng Radix), Pu Huang (Typhae Pollen), Yi Mu Cao (Leonuri Herba), Shan Zhu Yu (Corni Fructus), charred Shan Zha (Crataegi Fructus), Xue Yu Tan (Crinis Carbonisatus), Hai Piao Xiao (Sepiae Endoconcha), Ce Bai Ye (Platycladi Cacumen), and/or Wu Ling Zhi (Trogopteri Faeces).

Clinical Treatment

As described above, the term concretions and conglomerations includes gynecological masses of various types, such as uterine fibroids and ovarian cysts (also commonly related to endometrio- sis). In Western medicine, these conditions are often associated with hormonal imbalance, such as high relative levels of estrogen or unopposed estrogen.

From a Chinese medicine perspective, we must distinguish between concretions and conglomerations. Concretions refer to masses that are immobile and hard to the touch. Conglomerations refer to masses that are movable and softer to the touch. Therefore, according to the logic of Chinese medicine, concretions are primarily related to blood stasis, whereas conglomerations are primarily indicative of qi stagnation. Theoretically, these are two separate disease mechanisms. However, clinically, these two are always combined to some degree. Therefore, in the case of pelvic masses in females, the treatment principles are always to move both qi and blood.

Myomas (fibroids)

Is immediate surgery always necessary? Is Chinese medicine always an appropriate intervention? The answer to both questions is no, and the distinction depends on the location of the fibroid. As stated above, there are three types of fibroids: sub-serous (outside the uterus), myometrial (in the muscular layer of the uterine walls), and submucosal (in the cavity of the uterus).

Subserous fibroids can grow very large and obstruct nearby structures. The presenting symptoms typically include urinary frequency or constipation (depending on the location of the fibroid) and possibly even nephritis due to obstruction of the ureter. In cases of nephritis or severe bowel or bladder obstruction, surgery is necessary and urgent. Subserous fibroids will usually not affect menstruation. Assessment of this type of fibroid depends on the size and location.

Myometrial fibroids can cause heavy bleeding due to engorgement of local uterine blood vessels as well as the loss of the uterine cavity due to impingement as the fibroid grows into the uterus. Sometimes, myometrial fibroids are small and completely contained in the muscular layer and their symptoms are minimal. The necessity for surgery again depends upon the size and location of the fibroid. If it is large enough to cause significant bleeding or to impair fertility, surgery may be the best option.

Submucosal fibroids occur on the inside of the uterine wall, and these may be treated with Chinese medicine depending upon their location. If the fibroid is at the base of the uterus and blocking the cervix, there is a risk of significant bleeding.

If we determine the fibroid is suitable for treatment with Chinese medicine, I recommend using the following formula:

Formula: Xiao Zheng Fang (Concretion-dispersing Formula)

Ji Xue Teng (Spatholobi Caulis)
San Leng (Sparganii Rhizoma)
E Zhu (Curcumae Rhizoma)
Mu Dan Pi (Moutan Cortex)
Dan Shen (Salviae Miltiorrhizae Radix)
Chi Shao (Paeoniae Radix Rubra)
Tao Ren (Persicae Semen)
Fu Ling (Poria)
Bai Zhu (Atractylodis Macrocephalae Rhizoma)
Zhi Ke (Qiao) (Aurantii Fructus)

Formula analysis

The first six medicinals in this formula all quicken the blood. San Leng and E Zhu are especially strong at breaking blood stasis. Mu Dan Pi, Chi Shao, and Dan Shen also cool the blood. Fu Ling and Bai Zhu eliminate the dampness that is often a component of congealed masses. They also fortify the spleen's transformative function to prevent further damp stagnation. Zhi Ke moves the qi downward, thus helping rid the body of the mass.

Modification: If the mass is an ovarian cyst rather than a fibroid, there is often an element of damp stagnation as well. This is because cysts are fluid-filled. Therefore, we also want to dry dampness and/or promote urination in such cases. Hence, we should add appropriate medicinals for these purposes. Cang Zhu (Atractylodis Rhizoma) is an excellent medicinal for strongly drying damp-heat in the lower burner despite its warm nature. Cang Zhu has the added advantage that it fortifies the spleen's transformative function. In addition, several other medicinals clear heat by promoting urination: Hai Zao (Sargassum), Yi Yi Ren (Coicis Semen), Che Qian Zi (Plantaginis Semen), Tong Cao (Tetrapanacis Medulla), Zhu Ling (Polyporus), and Ze Xie (Alismatis Rhizoma). Hai Zao also softens hardness and disapates nodules. In this case, one should combine this ingredient with Kun Bu (Laminariae/Eckloniae Thallus). Yi Yi Ren also fortifies the spleen. Chuan Bei Mu (Fritillariae Cirrhosae Bulbus) clears heat and transforms phlegm while nourishing yin. For more replete conditions with stronger heat, Zhe Bei Mu (Fritillariae Thunbergii Bulbus) may be used instead. Qu Mai (Dianthi Herba) has the ability to also break blood stasis and has a downward moving action. Dan Nan Xing (Arisaema cum Bile) and Ban Xia (Pinelliae Rhizoma) are both acrid and bitter and strongly transform phlegm. Dan Nan Xing is good for hot phlegm, while Ban Xia is good for cold phlegm. So, together, they can be used as a strong temperature-neutral combination.

Surgery

Even if it is determined that surgery is the best option, Chinese medicine can be used as a powerful adjunctive therapy as follows.

Before the surgery:

Tiao Jing Qian Fang (Menstruation-regulating Early Formula)

Dang Gui (Angelicae Sinensis Radix)
Bai Shao (Paeoniae Radix Alba)
Chai Hu (Bupleuri Radix)
Fu Ling (Poria)
Bai Zhu (Atractylodis Macrocephalae Rhizoma)
Gan Cao (Glycyrrhizae Radix)
Shu Di Huang (Rehmanniae Radix Praeparata)
Chen Pi (Citri Reticulatae Pericarpium)
Dang Shen (Codonopsis Radix)
Suan Zao Ren (Ziziphi Spinosi Semen)

Formula analysis

This formula strikes an appropriate balance. Although we want to supplement the patient's qi and blood to facilitate recovery from the impending surgery, we do not want to supplement too much because we do not want to encourage any further growth of the fibroids. Similarly, although we want to quicken the blood to prevent blood stasis from the mass itself and the local trauma from surgery, we do not want to quicken too strongly because this can cause more bleeding during surgery.

Readers should note that this formula is a modification of Xiao Yao Fang (Relaxed Wanderer Formula). This base formula soothes the liver qi and fortifes the spleen. To this, Shu Di Huang has been added to supplement the blood. Chen Pi has been added to move the qi of the middle burner. Dang Shen supplements the qi, and Suan Zao Ren quiets the spirit. I like to add this last ingredient because patients are often anxious prior to surgery.

After surgery:

Bei Luan Fang (Prepare the Egg Formula)

Dang Gui (Angelicae Sinensis Radix)
Bai Shao (Paeoniae Radix Alba)
Chai Hu (Bupleuri Radix)
Fu Ling (Poria)
Bai Zhu (Atractylodis Macrocephalae Rhizoma)
Dan Shen (Salviae Miltiorrhizae Radix)
Zhi Ke (Qiao) (Aurantii Fructus)
Gan Cao (Glycyrrhizae Radix)
Shu Di Huang (Rehmanniae Radix Praeparata)
Suan Zao Ren (Ziziphi Spinosi Semen)

Formula analysis

After surgery, we want to prevent adhesions and scars as well as the recurrence of fibroids. Therefore, we want to quicken the blood but also want to supplement be-cause of loss of blood and qi during the surgical procedure. For this, we can use Bei Luan Fang. Again, this formula is a modification of Xiao Yao Fang (Relaxed Wan-derer Formula) to which Zhi Ke, Dan Shen, Shu Di Huang, and Suan Zao Ren have been added. Zhi Ke is a strong qi-moving agent. Dan Shen quickens the blood and also enters the liver channel. Additionally, Dan Shen gathers in the heart and, like Suan Zao Ren, has the ability to quiet the spirit. This is also important in the recovery phase. When the body experiences trauma, the spirit often becomes unsettled. Shu Di Huang richly nourishes the blood. It also supplements kidney essence which is the substance that fundamentally allows for the body's reconstruction after injury.

Modifications:

- For pain, we can add San Qi (Notoginseng Radix). Not only is this ingredient a good analgesic but, because it strongly breaks blood stasis, it is good for preventing scars and adhesions that can be a result of the recovery process. Yan Hu Suo (Corydalis Rhizoma) is a particularly potent qi- and blood-moving substance that may also be added to enhance pain relief and prevent scarring.

- If the patient is very weak due to qi vacuity, add Huang Qi (Astragali Radix) and Dang Shen (Codonopsis Radix) to boost the qi. If the patient is also very pale, add medicinals to nourish the blood, such as Gou Qi Zi (Lycii Fructus) and He Shou Wu (Polygoni Multiflori Radix). Both of these also benefit kidney essence, especially He Shou Wu. He Shou Wu also has a securing and astringing function that helps to restrain leakage of vital substances. This is very important during recovery. However, this slimy, enriching medicinal can be difficult to digest. So attention should be paid to the strength of the patient's spleen function if it is included.

Acupuncture formulas:

Liver depression qi stagnation:

LR14 (Qi Men), LR3 (Tai Chong), SP10 (Xue Hai), SP9 (Yin Ling Quan), SP6 (San Yin Jiao), CV4 (Guan Yuan), KI13 (Qi Xue)

Formula analysis

LR14 is the front *mu* point of the liver and an intersection point of the spleen and liver channels. It promotes the smooth flow of liver qi and can also be used to cool heat in the blood. This latter may be useful because qi and blood stagnation often result in heat. LR3 is the source point of the liver. It is used to course the liver and rectify the qi as well as to drain patterns of liver repletion. If there is evidence of strong heat, LR2 (Xing Jian) may be substituted for LR3. SP10 is used to quicken and eliminate blood stasis, especially in the uterus. This point also cools the blood and, thus, helps with any heat that may arise from stagnation. SP6 is most frequently thought of as a primary yin-supplementing point due to its being the intersection point of the three leg yin channels (spleen, liver, and kidney). However, it also has the function of quickening and cooling blood, eliminating blood stasis (especially in the uterus), and promoting the smooth flow of liver qi. CV4 is also an intersection point of the three leg yin channels, and, although it is also thought of as a supplementing point, it can (through its association with the leg yin channels) be used to regulate the flow of qi and blood to and in the uterus. Finally, KI13 is a local point that is helpful in freeing the flow of the qi and blood from the area.

Blood stasis: Same as liver depression qi stagnation with the addition of LR8 (Qu Quan)

Formula analysis

From the above description, we can see that most of the points in this formula move not only qi but blood. LR8 is added as a point to strengthen the movement of blood specifically through the liver channel since this channel goes through and around the uterus.

It is important to remember that qi and blood are interdependent for their smooth flow. So both elements should be addressed in either case. This is especially true for the case of concretions and conglomerations because, even when the root disease mechanism is qi stagnation, there is a tip or branch of uterine blood stasis.

Phlegm-damp stagnation: Same as liver depression qi stagnation with the addition of ST40 (Feng Long) and TB4 (Yang Chi)

Formula analysis

Points for liver depression qi stagnation essentially course and quicken the qi and blood in the uterine area. Therefore, these points are appropriate for the manifestation of concretions and conglomerations even when there is an underlying etiology of phlegm-dampness congesting the channels. However, in this case, we need to add points to directly deal with these pathological substances. For this, I recommend ST40 for phlegm accumulation and TB4 to promote fluid transformation (especially for fluid accumulation in the lower burner). It should also be mentioned that several points in the original formula, such as SP6, SP9, and CV4, supplement the spleen and fortify the spleen's function of transforming dampness.

Case Study

The patient was a 50-year-old woman who was diagnosed with uterine fibroids three years previously. She reported hot flashes and sweating as well as insomnia and constant thirst. Although this woman was prone to depression, she felt emotionally labile and her moods were up and down. She said she did not have much energy. She also experienced constipation and frequent urination. The woman had not menstruated for one year. Her tongue was red with multiple cracks and scanty fur. Her pulse was small, bowstring, and weak in the cubit positions (particularly on the left). Western diagnostic findings included a biopsy of the fibroids which showed abnormal cells. Therefore, surgery had been recommended by her physician.

Pattern identification: Kidney yin vacuity, liver depression qi stagnation, and blood stasis

Symptom analysis

As is common clinically with concretions and conglomerations, this was a case of mixed repletion and vacuity. We see evidence of an underlying kidney yin vacuity in her classic symptoms of hot flashes, sweating, insomnia, thirst, tongue, and pulse. Also, due to her age, we expect that the kidney yin was declining. Her mood swings, depression, and constipation as well as the bowstring pulse suggest liver depression qi stagnation. The diagnosis of fibroids tells us that there is blood stasis in her lower burner.

Treatment principles: Move the qi and quicken the blood

N.B. Because of the fibroids, we must not focus on nourishing her underlying vacuity. We must focus on moving the qi and quickening the blood. In my experience, the key to successful treatment with this particular type of mixed vacuity-repletion presentation is to address the repletion first.

Formula: Modified Xiao Zheng Fang (Concretion-dispersing Formula)

San Leng (Sparganii Rhizoma)
E Zhu (Curcumae Rhizoma)
Dan Shen (Salviae Miltiorrhizae Radix)
Tao Ren (Persicae Semen)
Zhi Ke (Aurantii Fructus)
Mu Li (Ostreae Concha)
Gui Ban (Testudinis Plastrum)/Bie Jia (Trionycis Carapax)
Sheng Di Huang (Rehmanniae Radix)
Xuan Shen (Scrophulariae Radix)
Mai Men Dong (Ophiopogonis Radix)

Treatment analysis

Together, San Leng and E Zhu strongly break blood stasis. In this, they are assisted by the blood-quickening agents Dan Shen and Tao Ren. Dan Shen, which also enters the heart, will help to quiet the patient's spirit. Zhi Ke moves the qi and also promotes the movement of stool downwards. This will help with the patient's bowel movements. Mu Li quiets the spirit and, like Bie Jia, dissipates nodules. Both Gui Ban and Bie Jia are potent yin-supplementing medicinals. Gui Ban is particularly effective in extreme heat due to yin vacuity (steaming bone). Sheng Di Huang, Xuan Shen, and Mai Men Dong also nourish yin and clear heat. This is important since the patient showed signs of vacuity heat.

Readers should note that Zhi Ke is the only true qi-moving substance included in this formula, and it does not enter the liver. Here, I was focusing on moving the qi through moving the blood. This is because I believed that the underlying condition was due to kidney yin vacuity causing heat. This then had caused the blood to stagnate in the yin areas which then lead to qi stagnation. This is different from someone who reports symptoms of emotional and psychological stress as precursors to the development of concretions and conglomerations. Of course, it is difficult to know whether there was an element of liver depression qi stagnation that was already present due to personality or lifestyle. In such a case, if the mood issues persist, we can add a medicinal such as Xiang Fu (Cyperi Rhizoma) to directly address the liver.

Outcome

In this case, the above formula resolved the menopausal and mood symptoms. Examination by a physician three months later revealed the fibroids were shrinking and no surgery was required.

Mass: Female

Type	Fibroids			Ovarian cyst
	Subserosal	Intramural	Submucosal	
Bleeding	(−) No	(+ / −) Maybe	(+) Heavy	(−) No
Cramps	(−)	(−)	(+ / −) Maybe	(+) Twisting
Pressure	(+) Constipation or frequent urination	(+ / −) Maybe	(−)	(−)
Period	(−) Normal	(+ / −) Maybe heavy	(+) Heavy	(+ / −) Maybe irregular
Infertility	(−)	(+ / −) Maybe	(+)	(+)
Pelvic exam	Fibroid: Hard, enlarged	Uterus: Hard, enlarged	Uterus: normal	Ovary: Soft, moving
Western treatment	Surgery or Lupron (to decrease mass)			
TCM treatment principle	Move qi and blood			Supplement qi and blood, drain damp
Herbs	Xiao Jing Fang			Xiao Nang Fang
Acupuncture	SP10, LV3, LI4, ST36, UB17, UB18, Zigong, Yintang			Same as fibroids treatment, plus SP9

17

Infertility

Infertility is also one area where the integration of TCM and Western biomedicine may be especially useful and effective. Therefore, I have spent some time focusing on the details of biomedical interventions so that we may describe in detail how and when TCM may be added to the treatment plan.

Western Medical View

One of the challenging aspects of pinpointing causes of infertility in women is that the conception process may go awry at a great number of points. Below is an overview of the four main classes of biophysical factors: ovarian, fallopian, uterine, and cervical.

Ovarian factors

At around 41 years of age, the function of the woman's ovaries starts to decline. (Although this is a natural cycle of a woman's development, for the purposes of achieving pregnancy, it is considered pathological here.) This decline results in lower quality eggs. Fertilization of these eggs is more difficult, and, generally, they do not develop as well after fertilization. When the ovaries decline in function, follicle-stimulating hormone (FSH) levels increase in order to induce ovulation. Follicle-stimulating hormone levels above 10 at most laboratories indicate that the ovarian function has declined, making pregnancy more difficult to achieve. Even when pregnancy does occur, it is usually more difficult for the woman to carry the embryo to term, and miscarriage often results. In addition, estrogen and progesterone levels decrease, causing a thinning of the endometrium. All of these factors affect the implantation of the embryo.

Another problematic condition is the occasional or total failure to ovulate. This may be due to hormonal changes causing irregular menstruation, amenorrhea, or heavy uterine bleeding. Pituitary hormone insufficiency, usually from an absent or infrequent release of (GnRH), leads to decreased levels of FSH and (LH) and anovulation. This can be seen in cases of injury, tumors, excessive exercise, and starvation. Hyperprolactinemia is a condition where a woman will have elevated levels of the hormone prolactin which stimulates milk production. In women who are not pregnant or nursing, high levels will inhibit ovulation or progesterone production and are often seen in women with pituitary tumors. Anovulation also occurs in women who have polycystic ovary syndrome (PCOS). In PCOS, the body produces too many androgen hormones, which affects ovulation.

Hypothyroidism can also cause anovulation and, thereby, lead to infertility. The hypothalamus and pituitary gland can sense an underactive thyroid gland and will try to maintain homeostasis by increasing levels of the hormones thyroid-releasing hormone (TRH) and thyroid-stimulating hormone (TSH). Thyroid-releasing hormone prompts the pituitary to release TSH to stimulate the thyroid gland. However, TRH also prompts the pituitary to release more prolactin. As stated above, elevated levels of prolactin can interfere with ovulation by suppressing the release of the hormones LH and FSH.

Fallopian tube factors

Fallopian tube damage or blockage can cause infertility by hindering or blocking the transport of the sperm to the egg and/or the fertilized egg to the uterus. Fallopian tube damage usually results from inflammation of the fallopian tube (salpingitis). The inflammation results in adhesions or scar tissue forming in and around the fallopian tubes. Chlamydia and pelvic inflammatory disease (PID) are common causes of salpingitis. Endometriosis may also lead to the occlusion of the fallopian tubes. Tubal inflammation may go unnoticed or cause pain and fever. Tubal damage is the major risk factor of a pregnancy in which the fertilized egg is unable to make its way through the fallopian tube to implant in the uterus, thus leading to an ectopic pregnancy. One episode of tubal infection may cause fertility difficulties. The risk of ectopic pregnancy increases with each occurrence of tubal infection.

Uterine factors

Uterine myomas (a.k.a. fibroids) or endometrial polyps distort the uterine cavity or block the interstitial parts of the tubes, thus preventing the embryo from moving to the uterus. Sometimes, a uterine fibroid or endometrial polyp may be the cause of first trimester miscarriages. Scar tissue or adhesions can also inhibit the growth of a healthy uterine lining and inhibit embryo implantation, leading to infertility. Other problems arise when the uterus is too small, is abnormally shaped, or has a septum or dividing wall within the uterus that prevents the embryo from growing and developing to full term.

Cervical factors

Cervical infertility involves the inability of the sperm to pass through the opening of the uterus. Causes include the following:

- Inadequate or inhospitable cervical mucus

- Cervical narrowing (stenosis)

- Infections of the cervix with common sexually transmitted diseases (chlamydia, gonorrhea, or trichomona)

- The presence of antibodies that attack the sperm

Traditional Chinese Medical View

Female infertility is the inability to conceive after one year of unprotected intercourse due to female factors.

Treatment based on pattern differentiation:

Kidney vacuity or blood vacuity (*shen xu* 肾虚, *xue xu* 血虚)

Signs & symptoms: Infertility, fatigue, lack of strength, low back and/or knee pain, fear of cold, dry skin, scanty, pale-colored menstruation, late menstruation, low libido, a pale facial complexion, and pale lips, nails, and tongue

Tongue: Pale, enlarged

Pulse: Deep, weak, thin

Treatment principles: Supplement the kidneys or nourish the blood

Formulas: For kidney yang vacuity, use:

Yu Lin Zhu (Unicorn-rearing Pill)

Ren Shen (Ginseng Radix)
Bai Zhu (Atractylodis Macrocephalae Rhizoma)
Fu Ling (Poria)
Zhi Gan Cao (Glycyrrhizae Radix cum Liquido Fricta)
Shu Di Huang (Rehmanniae Radix Praeparata)

Dang Gui (Angelicae Sinensis Radix)
Chuan Xiong (Chuanxiong Rhizoma)
Bai Shao (Paeoniae Radix Alba)
Tu Si Zi (Cuscutae Semen)
Du Zhong (Eucommiae Cortex)
Lu Jiao (Cervi Cornu)
Hua Jiao (Zanthoxyli Pericarpium)

Modifications:

- Other yang supplementing and warming medicinals can be added, such as Yin Yang Huo (Epimedii Herba), Ba Ji Tian (Morindae Officinalis Radix), Rou Cong Rong (Cistanches Herba), Fu Zi (Aconiti Radix Lateralis Praeparata), Rou Gui (Cinnamomi Cortex), Xian Mao (Curculiginis Rhizoma), and/or Fu Pen Zi (Rubi Fructus)

- For cases with a small uterus, add Fu Pen Zi (Rubi Fructus), Bu Gu Zhi (Psoraleae Fructus), Nu Zhen Zi (Ligustri Lucidi Fructus), Yi Zhi Ren (Alpiniae Oxyphyllae Fructus), Jin Ying Zi (Rosae Laevigatae Fructus), and/or Sha Yuan Zi (Astragali Complanati Semen).

For kidney yin vacuity use Yang Jing Zhong Ru Tang (Essence-nourishing Conception Decoction):

Dang Gui (Angelicae Sinensis Radix)
Shu Di Huang (Rehmanniae Radix Praeparata)
Bai Shao (Paeoniae Radix Alba)
Shan Zhu Yu (Corni Fructus)

Modifications:

- Other blood and yin supplementing medicinals can be added to this formula, such as Tu Si Zi (Cuscutae Semen), Gou Qi Zi (Lycii Fructus), He Shou Wu (Polygoni Multiflori Radix), Nu Zhen Zi (Ligustri Lucidi Fructus), Sang Shen (Mori Fructus), Mo Han Lian (Ecliptae Herba), Mai Men Dong (Ophiopogonis Radix), and/or Sha Shen (Adenophorae seu Glehniae Radix).

Another formula to consider is Wu Zi Zhong Zi Wan (Childless Seed-planting Pill):

Tu Si Zi (Cuscutae Semen)
Nu Zhen Zi (Ligustri Lucidi Fructus)

Gou Qi Zi (Lycii Fructus)
Sang Shen (Mori Fructus)
Ba Ji Tian (Morindae Officinalis Radix)
Shu Di Huang (Rehmanniae Radix Praeparata)
Dang Gui (Angelicae Sinensis Radix)
Bai Shao (Paeoniae Radix Alba)
Dan Shen (Salviae Miltiorrhizae Radix)
Dang Shen (Codonopsis Radix)
Fu Ling (Poria)
Gan Cao (Glycyrrhizae Radix)

Liver qi depression & binding (*gan qi yu jie* 肝气郁结)

Signs & symptoms: Infertility, irritability, moodiness, PMS, dysmenorrhea, irregular menstruation, hypochondriac pain, and breast tenderness

Tongue: Purplish

Pulse: Bowstring

Treatment principles: Course the qi and quicken the blood

Formula: Kai Yu Zhong Yu Tang (Stasis-opening Conception Decoction)

Dang Gui (Angelicae Sinensis Radix)
Bai Zhu (Atractylodis Macrocephalae Rhizoma)
Bai Shao (Paeoniae Radix Alba)
Mu Dan Pi (Moutan Cortex)
Xiang Fu (Cyperi Rhizoma)
Fu Ling (Poria)
Tian Hua Fen (Radix Trichosanthis)

Modifications:

- For more severe qi stagnation, add Zhi Qiao (Ke) (Aurantii Fructus), Xiang Fu (Cyperi Rhizoma), Yu Jin (Curcumae Radix), Wu Yao (Linderae Radix), Qing Pi (Citri Reticulatae Pericarpium Viride), and/or Chuan Lian Zi (Toosendan Fructus).

- For more severe blood stasis, add Dan Shen (Salviae Miltiorrhizae Radix), Tao Ren (Persicae Semen), Hong Hua (Carthami Flos), Yan Hu Suo (Corydalis Rhizoma), Yi Mu Cao (Leonuri Herba), Niu Xi (Achyranthis Bidentatae Radix), Chi Shao (Paeoniae Radix Rubra), San Qi (Notoginseng Radix), and/or Chuan Xiong (Chuanxiong Rhizoma).

- For blocked fallopian tubes, add Chuan Shan Jia (Manis Squama), Lu Lu Tong (Liquidambaris Fructus), Di Long (Pheretima), and Wang Bu Liu Xing (Vaccariae Semen).

Phlegm-dampness (*tan shi* 痰湿)

Signs & symptoms: Infertility, generalized heaviness, tendency to gain weight, history of ovarian cysts or PCOS, tendency to experience irregular menstruation or anovulatory cycles

Tongue: Pink or pale with thick, white fur

Pulse: Slippery

Treatment principles: Transform phlegm and eliminate dampness, move the qi and quicken the blood

Formula: Qi Gong Wan (Uterine Treatment Pill)

Ban Xia (Pinelliae Rhizoma)
Fu Ling (Poria)
Chen Pi (Citri Reticulatae Pericarpium)
Cang Zhu (Atractylodis Rhizoma)
Xiang Fu (Cyperi Rhizoma)
Shen Qu (Massa Medicata Fermentata)
Chuan Xiong (Chuanxiong Rhizoma)

Modifications:

- For more severe phlegm, add Dan Xing (Arisaema cum Bile), Zhe Bei Mu (Fritillariae Thunbergii Bulbus), and Tian Nan Xing (Arisaematis Rhizoma).

- For more severe dampness, add Mu Tong (Akebiae Trifoliatae Caulis), Huang Bai (Phellodendri Cortex), Zhu Ling (Polyporus), Tu Fu Ling (Smilacis Glabrae Rhizoma), Bi Xie (Dioscoreae Hypoglaucae Rhizoma), Che Qian Zi (Plantaginis Semen), and Yi Yi Ren (Coicis Semen).

- For more severe heat, add Huang Bai (Phellodendri Cortex), Hua Shi (Talcum), Bai Jiang Cao (Patriniae Herba), Ku Shen (Sophorae Flavescentis Radix), Long Dan (Gentianae Radix), and Zhi Zi (Gardeniae Fructus).

To relieve cervical infections, apply Zhen Zhu (Margarita) powder to the cervix.

Relationships Between Chinese & Western Medicine

Many findings, including absence or irregularity of ovulation, a small uterus, a thin endometrium, poor quality of eggs, a poor quantity of follicles, low estradiol, and low progesterone and high FSH typically correspond to vacuity of kidney yin, yang, or both. However, qi and blood vacuity may also be correlated to such signs. Conditions such as uterine myomas, ovarian cysts, adhesions, endometriosis, and blockage of the fallopian tubes often correspond to patterns such as liver depression, blood stasis, and phlegm-damp. (Infections of the cervix, vagina, pelvis, and fallopian tubes often correspond to damp heat or heat toxins with blood stasis.)

Traditional Chinese Medicine	Western Medicine
Kidney yin vacuity	Lack of ovulation
Blood vacuity	Small uterus
Kidney yang vacuity	Thin endometrium
Qi vacuity	Poor quality eggs
	Poor quality follicles
	Low estradiol
	Low progesterone
	High FSH
Qi stagnation	Blocked fallopian tubes
Blood stasis	Uterine myoma
Phlegm-damp obstruction	Ovarian cysts
	Endometriosis
	Adhesions
	Stress
Damp heat heat toxins blood stasis	Cervical infection
	Vaginal infection
	Pelvic infection
	Fallopian tube infection

Clinical Experience

In many Western countries, women study and work harder than ever before. With the move towards equality in the workplace, modern women are enjoying new opportunities and new challenges. They are busy, first in school earning a higher education, and then becoming successful in their chosen careers and businesses. This is a wonderful thing, but it also poses a potential sacrifice. Many women are waiting until later in life to marry and have children. While this has distinct advantages from the aspects of financial stability and even parental maturity, it has disadvantages from the physiological perspective.

Most women want to start having children at about 35 years old. Unfortunately, when women reach that age, their egg quality starts to suffer and the hormones estrogen and progesterone decline. These two hormones are important for the production of a thick uterine lining. If the egg quality is poor and the uterine lining is too thin, it is hard to conceive and maintain a healthy pregnancy. Therefore, it is vitally important to improve the ovarian function for these women in order to preserve and prolong their fertile years.

Step 1: Improving ovarian function with Chinese medicine alone

See the chart on page 257 for a visual representation of this. Improving ovarian function with medicinal therapy and acupuncture is a good first step when dealing with infertility. In some cases, a little nourishment and support will allow a woman to achieve natural pregnancy without any further intervention. Here is my protocol for this first step:

During menstruation (Days 1-5)

One of three possible formulas may be used for five days. Each formula helps to move the qi and quicken the blood, although they are used for slightly different patient presentations (as described below).

If the patient's menstrual bleeding is light, we need to nourish and move the blood. The appropriate formula is:

Tiao Jing Xing Fang (Regulate Menstrual Movement Formula)

Dang Gui (Angelicae Sinensis Radix)
Bai Shao (Paeoniae Radix Alba)
Shu Di Huang (Rehmanniae Radix Praeparata)
Chuan Xiong (Chuanxiong Rhizoma)
Niu Xi (Achyranthis Bidentatae Radix)
Dan Shen (Salviae Miltiorrhizae Radix)
Xiang Fu (Cyperi Rhizoma)
Gou Qi Zi (Lycii Fructus)
Xiao Hui Xiang (Foeniculi Fructus)
Yan Hu Suo (Corydalis Rhizoma)

Formula analysis

Note that this formula includes Si Wu Tang (Four Materials Decoction), the basic blood-nourishing formula of Chinese medicine. Si Wu Tang also has a gentle moving aspect, with Chuan Xiong and Dang Gui encouraging the movement of blood. Dan Shen and Yan Hu Suo help to move the blood more strongly. Niu Xi guides downward and Xiang Fu moves qi in the liver channel, together encouraging menstruation to flow. Gou Qi Zi supplements the liver and nourishes the blood. Xiao Hui Xiang warms and regulates the qi in the liver channel and, in this way, promotes menstruation.

Jing Tong Fang (Painful Menstruation Formula) is used for women who suffer from painful menstruation.

> Dang Gui (Angelicae Sinensis Radix)
> Bai Shao (Paeoniae Radix Alba)
> Chai Hu (Bupleuri Radix)
> Fu Ling (Poria)
> Bai Zhu (Atractylodis Macrocephalae Rhizoma)
> Gan Cao (Glycyrrhizae Radix)
> Xiao Hui Xiang (Foeniculi Fructus)
> Gui Zhi (Cinnamomi Ramulus)
> San Qi (Notoginseng Radix)
> Yan Hu Suo (Corydalis Rhizoma)

Formula analysis

Dang Gui encourages the blood to move. Bai Shao and Chai Hu together soothe the liver and help alleviate any qi stagnation that may be contributing to the pain. Fu Ling and Bai Zhu fortify the spleen since the spleen often suffers when there is liver depression. Bai Shao and Gan Cao together act to alleviate cramping and form the ingredients of Shao Yao Gan Cao Tang (Peony & Licorice Decoction). Xiao Hui Xiang and Gui Zhi are warm, acrid medicinals that encourage the movement of qi and blood respectively. San Qi and Yan Hu Suo are strong pain-relieving agents that break stasis.

For women with cold in the lower abdomen:

Wen Jing Xing Fang (Warm Menstrual Movement Formula) can be used.

> Dang Gui (Angelicae Sinensis Radix)
> Bai Shao (Paeoniae Radix Alba)

Shu Di Huang (Rehmanniae Radix Praeparata)
Chuan Xiong (Chuanxiong Rhizoma)
Niu Xi (Achyranthis Bidentatae Radix)
Dan Shen (Salviae Miltiorrhizae Radix)
Xiang Fu (Cyperi Rhizoma)
Gou Qi Zi (Lycii Fructus)
Xiao Hui Xiang (Foeniculi Fructus)
Gui Zhi (Cinnamomi Ramulus)

Formula analysis

This formula is almost the same as Tiao Jing Xing Fang discussed above. The main difference is that, in this case, there is cold. Therefore, Gui Zhi is substituted for Yan Hu Suo (Corydalis Rhizoma). Gui Zhi is acrid and warm and can warmly free the flow of the channels.

After menstruation

After menstruation, the primary goal is to supplement the kidneys and nourish yin, supplement the kidneys and invigorate yang, and supplement the qi and blood. One of the three following formulas should be taken for 13 days. The choice depends upon the exact presentation of the individual patient (as described below).

My basic formula for this time is:

Yang Luan Fang (Egg-nourishing Formula)

This formula is a modification of Ding Jing Fang (Stabilize Menstruation Formula), the basic regulating formula introduced earlier in the book.

Dang Gui (Angelicae Sinensis Radix)
Bai Shao (Paeoniae Radix Alba)
Chai Hu (Bupleuri Radix)
Fu Ling (Poria)
Shan Yao (Dioscoreae Rhizoma)
Dang Shen (Codonopsis Radix)
Ba Ji Tian (Morindae Officinalis Radix)
Tu Si Zi (Cuscutae Semen)
Shu Di Huang (Rehmanniae Radix Praeparata)
Zhi Gan Cao (Glycyrrhizae Radix cum Liquido Fricta)
Shan Zhu Yu (Corni Fructus)
Wu Wei Zi (Schisandrae Fructus)

Formula analysis

Shu Di Huang, Tu Si Zi, and Ba Ji Tian together supplement all aspects of the kidneys. Shu Di Huang supplements yin and essence, Tu Si Zi supplements yin, yang, and essence, and Ba Ji Tian supplements yang. Supplementing the kidneys is extremely important since (as discussed in the beginning of the book) we may think of the kidneys as the reproductive aspect of the endocrine system. Shan Zhu Yu and Wu Wei Zi help to astringe the essence, yin, and qi, preventing their dispersion.

Fu Ling, Zhi Gan Cao, and Dang Shen are three of the four components of Si Jun Zi Tang (Four Gentlemen Decoction), the basic formula to supplement spleen qi in Chinese medicine. The spleen is responsible for both engendering and controlling the blood, and blood is necessary to create an environment that is ripe for ovulation and conception. In addition to supporting the spleen's function of engendering the blood, Dang Gui and Shu Di Huang directly nourish the blood.

Chai Hu and Bai Shao harmonize the liver, meaning that, together, they both course and emolliate the liver. This allows the qi and blood to flow without obstruction, setting the stage for ovulation to occur on schedule.

If the menses are irregular, I use:

Tiao Jing Fang (Regulate Menstruation Formula)

This is almost the same formula as above. However, Xiang Fu (Cyperi Rhizoma) is included to more strongly course liver and rectify the qi, and the securing and astringing medicinals Shan Zhu Yu (Corni Fructus) and Wu Wei Zi (Schisandrae Fructus) are left out.

> Dang Gui (Angelicae Sinensis Radix)
> Bai Shao (Paeoniae Radix Alba)
> Chai Hu (Bupleuri Radix)
> Fu Ling (Poria)
> Shan Yao (Dioscoreae Rhizoma)
> Dang Shen (Codonopsis Radix)
> Ba Ji Tian (Morindae Officinalis Radix)
> Tu Si Zi (Cuscutae Semen)
> Shu Di Huang (Rehmanniae Radix Praeparata)
> Zhi Gan Cao (Glycyrrhizae Radix cum Liquido Fricta)
> Xiang Fu (Cyperi Rhizoma)

If there is marked kidney yin vacuity:

Zi Ru Fang (Conception Formula) may be used instead.

Shan Yao (Dioscoreae Rhizoma)
Shan Zhu Yu (Corni Fructus)
Shu Di Huang (Rehmanniae Radix Praeparata)
Fu Ling (Poria)
Mu Dan Pi (Moutan Cortex)
Ze Xie (Alismatis Rhizoma)
Bai Shao (Paeoniae Radix Alba)
Tu Si Zi (Cuscutae Semen)
Suan Zao Ren (Ziziphi Spinosi Semen)
Gan Cao (Glycyrrhizae Radix)

Formula analysis

This formula is a modification of Liu Wei Di Huang Wan (Six Flavors Rehmannia Pill), a basic formula for nourishing yin. Liu Wei Di Huang Wan includes six medicinals: Shan Yao, Shan Zhu Yu, Shu Di Huang, Fu Ling, Mu Dan Pi, and Ze Xie. The first three medicinals nourish yin. There is Shan Yao for the spleen, Shan Zhu Yu for the liver, and Shu Di Huang for the kidney. The second three medicinals are dispersing. They encourage urination to balance the richness of the yin-nourishing medicinals. These two sets of medicinals together make a wonderfully balanced design.

The additions to this formula include Bai Shao for nourishing the blood and Tu Si Zi for supplementing kidney yin, yang, and essence. Suan Zao Ren is included to further nourish the blood, specifically the heart blood, and to quiet the spirit. When there is extreme kidney yin vacuity, the heart often becomes agitated due to lack of cooling yin from the kidney. Finally, Gan Cao harmonizes all the other ingredients in the formula.

In cases of anovulation or delayed ovulation

If there is no ovulation or late ovulation, the patient should be switched to one of the following two formulas on day 12 of her cycle after taking six days of one of the above formulas. She should take the formula to promote ovulation for seven days. The formula I prefer and use most often is:

Wen Gong Fang (Warm the Uterus Formula)

Dang Gui (Angelicae Sinensis Radix)

Bai Shao (Paeoniae Radix Alba)

Chai Hu (Bupleuri Radix)

Fu Ling (Poria)

Shan Yao (Dioscoreae Rhizoma)

Dang Shen (Codonopsis Radix)

Ba Ji Tian (Morindae Officinalis Radix)

Tu Si Zi (Cuscutae Semen)

Shu Di Huang (Rehmanniae Radix Praeparata)

Zhi Gan Cao (Glycyrrhizae Radix cum Liquido Fricta)

Rou Gui (Cinnamomi Cortex)

Formula analysis

This formula is Ding Jing Fang (Stabilize Menstruation Formula) with the addition of Rou Gui. Dang Gui is the sovereign ingredient in this formula unlike in Ding Jing Fang where it occupies a lesser position. The reason is that, in order for ovulation to occur, the blood must be nourished and moving properly. Dang Gui both nourishes and gently quickens the blood, making it the primary medicinal in the formula. Shu Di Huang is used to further nourish the blood and kidney yin which is discussed next.

The fact that the ovulatory function has been disturbed, suggests that there is an endocrine imbalance. Therefore, we must focus on the kidney which, in a biomedical sense, can be considered the primary organ of endocrine regulation. Shu Di Huang, Ba Ji Tian, and Tu Si Zi are used to supplement both kidney yin and yang. Shu Di Huang and Tu Si Zi nourish yin, while Ba Ji Tian and Tu Si Zi supplement yang. Tu Si Zi is a seed. Therefore, it also supplements the essence. We want to address both kidney yin and kidney yang because each represents a different and vital aspect of the endocrine system. For example, estrogen may be thought of as part of the kidney yin, while progesterone is part of the kidney yang. Yin is more involved in the actual formation of the ova, while yang is necessary to promote the release of the egg.

Fu Ling, Zhi Gan Cao, and Dang Shen are three of the four components of Si Jun Zi Tang (Four Gentlemen Decoction), the basic formula to supplement spleen qi. This supports the spleen's function of engendering the blood, and blood is needed to nourish the developing egg.

Chai Hu and Bai Shao together regulate the smooth flow of the liver qi. It is important to disperse any qi stagnation in order for ovulation to occur. If the qi is stagnant, it may block nourishment to the egg (by restricting the movement of blood) and impact its development. Or it may make it difficult for the egg to release and travel to the fallopian tube.

Finally, Rou Gui warms and guides yang back to the life gate. In the context of ovulation, this can be thought of as stoking kidney yang for the process of ovulation.

If Wen Gong Fang (Warm the Uterus Formula) does not produce the desired result (ovulation), the following formula may be used:

Pai Luan Fang (Ovulation Formula)

> Dang Gui (Angelicae Sinensis Radix)
> Bai Shao (Paeoniae Radix Alba)
> Chai Hu (Bupleuri Radix)
> Fu Ling (Poria)
> Shan Yao (Dioscoreae Rhizoma)
> Dang Shen (Codonopsis Radix)
> Ba Ji Tian (Morindae Officinalis Radix)
> Tu Si Zi (Cuscutae Semen)
> Shu Di Huang (Rehmanniae Radix Praeparata)
> Zhi Gan Cao (Glycyrrhizae Radix cum Liquido Fricta)
> Yin Yang Huo (Epimedii Herba)

Formula analysis

This formula is Wen Gong Fang (Warm the Uterus Formula) with Rou Gui removed and Yin Yang Huo added instead. Like Rou Gui, Yin Yang Huo is a warm and acrid medicinal. However, Rou Gui guides to and reinforces the life gate fire, while Yin Yang Huo supplements the kidneys and invigorates yang. Yin Yang Huo is also dispersing and dispels dampness, and so may be useful if mild local dampness is restricting ovulation.

After ovulation

Once ovulation has occurred, I encourage the patient to have sexual intercourse with her partner. At this point, I hope and expect that conception may occur. In order to protect the fertilized egg, the patient should be given the following formula, called:

Pai Luan Hou Fang (After Ovulation Formula)

> Dang Gui (Angelicae Sinensis Radix)

Bai Shao (Paeoniae Radix Alba)
Shan Zhu Yu (Corni Fructus)
Shu Di Huang (Rehmanniae Radix Praeparata)
Shan Yao (Dioscoreae Rhizoma)
He Shou Wu (Polygoni Multiflori Radix)
Gou Qi Zi (Lycii Fructus)
Tu Si Zi (Cuscutae Semen)
Dang Shen (Codonopsis Radix)
Wu Wei Zi (Schisandrae Fructus)

The patient should begin taking this formula three days after ovulation (about day 18 of the cycle) and continue for five days.

Formula analysis

In this formula, Dang Gui, Shu Di Huang, and Bai Shao nourish the blood. These are three of the four components of Si Wu Tang (Four Materials Decoction), the basic blood-supplementing formula of Chinese medicine. Shan Zhu Yu, Shu Di Huang, and Shan Yao nourish yin. These three medicinals constitute half of Liu Wei Di Huang Wan (Six Flavors Rehmannia Pill), the basic yin-supplementing formula of Chinese medicine. He Shou Wu and Gou Qi Zi also assist in nourishing the blood and yin. He Shou Wu and Tu Si Zi supplement essence which is then secured with the assistance of Shan Zhu Yu and Wu Wei Zi. Dang Shen and Shan Yao together fortify the spleen and supplement the qi. This pair acts together with the securing and astringing Shan Zhu Yu and Wu Wei Zi to contain essence, qi, blood, and yin. This encourages the fertilized egg to be held and nourished.

After Pai Luan Hou Fang is taken, the patient should be given:

Tiao Jing Qian Fang (Regulate Menstruation Prior Formula) for five days.

Dang Gui (Angelicae Sinensis Radix)
Bai Shao (Paeoniae Radix Alba)
Chai Hu (Bupleuri Radix)
Fu Ling (Poria)
Bai Zhu (Atractylodis Macrocephalae Rhizoma)
Gan Cao (Glycyrrhizae Radix)
Shu Di Huang (Rehmanniae Radix Praeparata)
Chen Pi (Citri Reticulatae Pericarpium)
Dang Shen (Codonopsis Radix)
Suan Zao Ren (Ziziphi Spinosi Semen)

Formula analysis

I focus on nourishing the blood and kidney yin during this time in order to facilitate a viable, nutrient-rich environment in the uterus which will, in turn, encourage implantation. In fact, this formula is similar to Ding Jing Fang (Stabilize Menstruation Formula) without the focus on kidney yang. Here, the primary focus is to nourish the blood and yin while fortifying the spleen and supplementing the qi, coursing the liver and rectifying the qi. Suan Zao Ren nourishes the heart and liver blood and quiets the spirit. This is important because this is usually a very stressful time for patients since they are waiting to see whether they have conceived or not. It is during this time that the fertilized egg, if there is one, will reach the uterus and implant there.

After taking Tiao Jing Qian Fang, we next need to safeguard the potential newly implanted pregnancy. If tests have shown that the patient's progesterone is low (as is often the case as women age), the patient should use one of the pregnancy formulas. This will help to prevent miscarriage in the event that the patient has conceived. There are three possible choices of formulas. The decision on which to give will depend upon the patient's individual presentation as described below.

For kidney-spleen yang vacuity, I use:

Hu Tai Fang (Protect the Fetus Formula)

Sang Ji Sheng (Taxilli Herba)
Xu Duan (Dipsaci Radix)
Tu Si Zi (Cuscutae Semen)
Gou Qi Zi (Lycii Fructus)
Shan Zhu Yu (Corni Fructus)
Dang Shen (Codonopsis Radix)
Bai Shao (Paeoniae Radix Alba)
Bai Zhu (Atractylodis Macrocephalae Rhizoma)
Huang Qi (Astragali Radix)
Suan Zao Ren (Ziziphi Spinosi Semen)

Formula analysis

Sang Ji Sheng, the sovereign medicinal in this formula, supplements the liver and kidney and prevents miscarriage by quieting the fetus. Xu Duan and Tu Si Zi supplement kidney yang, while Gou Qi Zi and Shan Zhu Yu nourish kidney-liver yin. Here, Shan Zhu Yu also secures and astringes kidney essence. This is essential for securing and containing the pregnancy. Dang Shen, Bai Zhu, and Huang Qi fortify the spleen and supplement the qi. Huang Qi also has an upbearing function that assists with preventing miscarriage. Bai Shao nourishes liver blood and yin. Suan Zao Ren also nourishes the heart and liver blood and quiets the spirit. This is important for this time since many women become very anxious.

For vacuity of qi, blood and kidney yang, I think:

Jing Tai Fang (Quiet the Fetus Formula) is best.

> Sang Ji Sheng (Taxilli Herba)
> Xu Duan (Dipsaci Radix)
> Tu Si Zi (Cuscutae Semen)
> Gou Qi Zi (Lycii Fructus)
> Shan Zhu Yu (Corni Fructus)
> Dang Shen (Codonopsis Radix)
> Bai Shao (Paeoniae Radix Alba)
> Bai Zhu (Atractylodis Macrocephalae Rhizoma)
> Wu Wei Zi (Schisandrae Fructus)
> Suan Zao Ren (Ziziphi Spinosi Semen)

Formula analysis

Here we have a similar formula to Hu Tai Fang above but with Wu Wei Zi added instead of Huang Qi (Astragali Radix). Huang Qi is a drying medicinal and is not good for situations where the patient has prominent blood vacuity. Instead, Wu Wei Zi is used to nourish and secure the essence, engender fluids and quiet the spirit.

In the event of kidney yin vacuity:

Yang Tai Fang (Nourish the Fetus Formula) can be used instead.

> Tu Si Zi (Cuscutae Semen)
> Shu Di Huang (Rehmanniae Radix Praeparata)
> Shan Zhu Yu (Corni Fructus)
> Shan Yao (Dioscoreae Rhizoma)
> Bai Shao (Paeoniae Radix Alba)
> Mai Men Dong (Ophiopogonis Radix)
> Suan Zao Ren (Ziziphi Spinosi Semen)
> Gan Cao (Glycyrrhizae Radix)
> Dang Shen (Codonopsis Radix)
> Wu Wei Zi (Schisandrae Fructus)

Formula analysis

This formula contains Tu Si Zi which supplements both kidney yin and yang vacuity as well as the three primary yin-nourishing medicinals from Liu Wei Di Huang Wan (Six Flavors Rehmannia Pill): Shu Di Huang, Shan Zhu Yu, and Shan Yao. These three primarily nourish the yin of the kidney, liver, and spleen respectively. In addition, Bai Shao nourishes liver yin and blood, while Mai Men Dong engenders fluids and helps to clear any vacuity heat from the heart that is causing anxiety. Suan Zao Ren and Wu Wei Zi assist in quieting the spirit, and Dang Shen and Gan Cao supplement the spleen to help digest the slimy, enriching medicinals in the formula.

The patient should take one of the above formulas until they are certain they are not pregnant. It is important to note (and to remind the patient) that bleeding can occur even if the patient is pregnant. Hence, bleeding alone should never be taken as confirmation that there is no pregnancy. If laboratory results or other examinations confirm that a patient is not pregnant, then she should cycle back to the beginning of the protocol and begin taking the formula indicated during menstruation If she is pregnant, then she should continue to take the appropriate pregnancy formula.

The couple should be advised to try to have sex around the time of ovulation. Typically, a woman is most fertile three days before and on the day of ovulation. When a woman is not in that window of fertility, she and her partner should not have sex more than once every other day. This helps to store the semen and make the semen higher in both quality and quantity. It should be remembered that the cycle of maturation for sperm is on the order of two and a half months. It is possible to exhaust the supplies of highly potent semen.

Acupuncture formulas:

A. After menstruation: SP6 (San Yin Jiao), ST36 (Zu San Li), Zi Gong Xue (M-CA-18), GV20 (Bai Hui), LI4 (He Gu), Yin Tang (M-HN-3)

Formula analysis

SP6 and ST36 together supplement the spleen and nourish the blood. SP6 also nourishes the kidney. Zi Gong Xue stimulates circulation to the ovaries and uterus to help improve ovarian function and thicken the endometrial lining. LI4 courses the liver and thus helps to regulate menstruation. GV20 raises pituitary hormones (FSH and LH). Yin Tang quiets the spirit.

After ovulation (three days post-ovulation), replace Zi Gong Xue with KI13 (Qi Xue). This point supplements the kidney and encourages blood flow to the uterus.

B. Before menstruation: ST36 (Zu San Li), KI3 (Tai Xi), GV20 (Bai Hui), Yin Tang (M-HN-3), Ear points Kidney, Spleen, and Shen Men

Formula analysis

Since it is possible to be in the early part of pregnancy, I want to safeguard any potential fetus. ST36 supplements the spleen and engenders the blood. KI3 nourishes kidney essence to help nourish the embryo. GV20 upbears the qi to help hold the embryo in the uterus. Yin Tang relaxes the uterus to prevent contractions and also quiets the spirit. The ear points supplment the kidney and spleen and quiet the spirit, helping to prevent uterine contractions.

C. During menstruation: SP10 (Xue Hai), LI4 (He Gu), LR3 (Tai Chong), CV4 (Guan Yuan), SP6 (San Yin Jiao), Yin Tang (M-HN-3)

Formula analysis

If pregnancy has not occurred, menstruation will arrive. My goal during menstruation is to promote the smooth discharge of the blood. This can help with achieving pregnancy the next month. SP10 nourishes and quickens the blood, while LR3 and LI4 free the flow of the channels to encourage the qi and blood to flow smoothly. CV4 is a penetrating vessel intersection point that connects directly to the uterus. This point helps the uterine lining to shed smoothly and also helps to reduce or eliminate cramps. SP6 supplements the kidney and spleen and soothes liver. This point also helps to engender the blood and increase the flow of the menstruate, thus encouraging the uterus to contract and expel the blood completely. Yin Tang quiets the spirit.

Step 2: Assisted reproductive technology (ART) in conjunction with Chinese medicine

Pharmaceutical interventions

In some cases, a women may need to undergo assisted reproductive technology (ART) in order to boost her ability to ovulate. The first step in ART is drug therapy. Fertility drugs are given to stimulate follicular development and induce ovulation. Chinese herbal medicine is very helpful in conjunction with pharmaceutical ART. My clinical medicinal protocol is geared to assist the actions of the Western drugs for patients who attempt conception using the pharmaceuticals Clomid or other gonadotropins. At the same time, my formulas support and nourish the body so that conception can occur. This protocol must be timed with the pharmaceutical delivery as described below. See the chart on page 263 for a visual representation of Step 2.

A few days after the menstrual cycle begins, clomiphene (Clomid) or another gonadotropin is given to stimulate the development of multiple follicles. During this time, I prescribe:

Yang Luan Fang (Egg-nourishing Formula) This formula helps nourish the developing eggs, thickens the uterine lining, and increases the cervical mucus.

> Dang Gui (Angelicae Sinensis Radix)
> Bai Shao (Paeoniae Radix Alba)
> Chai Hu (Bupleuri Radix)
> Fu Ling (Poria)
> Shan Yao (Dioscoreae Rhizoma)
> Dang Shen (Codonopsis Radix)
> Ba Ji Tian (Morindae Officinalis Radix)
> Tu Si Zi (Cuscutae Semen)
> Shu Di Huang (Rehmanniae Radix Praeparata)
> Zhi Gan Cao (Glycyrrhizae Radix cum Liquido Fricta)
> Shan Zhu Yu (Corni Fructus)
> Wu Wei Zi (Schisandrae Fructus)

Formula analysis

This formula is Ding Jing Fang (Stabilize Menstruation Formula) with the addition of Shan Zhu Yu and Wu Wei Zi. Recall that Ding Jing Fang is our primary formula for regulating the female reproductive system by supplementing the kidney and supporting qi and blood. Shan Zhu Yu and Wu Wei Zi both engender and contain fluids.

If a patient's follicles develop slowly while using the drug Follistim, the formula Wen Gong Fang (Warm the Uterus Formula) is given instead. It is also based upon Ding Jing Fang but with the addition of Rou Gui (Cinnamomi Cortex) instead of Shan Zhu Yu and Wu Wei Zi. Rou Gui warms kidney yang which is comparable to the "motivating force" that causes the eggs to grow and develop. Rou Gui increases the movement of blood to the ovaries and uterus by freeing the flow of the channels and guiding the other medicinals to the local area.

Wen Gong Fang (Warm the Uterus Formula)

Dang Gui (Angelicae Sinensis Radix)
Bai Shao (Paeoniae Radix Alba)
Chai Hu (Bupleuri Radix)
Fu Ling (Poria)
Shan Yao (Dioscoreae Rhizoma)
Dang Shen (Codonopsis Radix)
Ba Ji Tian (Morindae Officinalis Radix)
Tu Si Zi (Cuscutae Semen)
Shu Di Huang (Rehmanniae Radix Praeparata)
Zhi Gan Cao (Glycyrrhizae Radix cum Liquido Fricta)
Rou Gui (Cinnamomi Cortex)

Once the follicles are fully developed and ovulation is ready to occur, an HCG injection is given to trigger ovulation. Approximately 36 hours after the HCG injection, ovulation should occur. I give either Pai Luan Fang (Ovulation Formula) or Wen Gong Fang during this time.

Pai Luan Fang (Ovulation Formula)

Dang Gui (Angelicae Sinensis Radix)
Bai Shao (Paeoniae Radix Alba)
Chai Hu (Bupleuri Radix)
Fu Ling (Poria)
Shan Yao (Dioscoreae Rhizoma)
Dang Shen (Codonopsis Radix)
Ba Ji Tian (Morindae Officinalis Radix)
Tu Si Zi (Cuscutae Semen)
Shu Di Huang (Rehmanniae Radix Praeparata)
Zhi Gan Cao (Glycyrrhizae Radix cum Liquido Fricta)
Yin Yang Huo (Epimedii Herba)

Formula analysis

The difference between these two formulas is simply Rou Gui (Cinnamomi Cortex) in Wen Gong Fang versus Yin Yang Huo in Pai Luan Fang. Rou Gui moves the blood more, while Yin Yang Huo directly supplements kidney yang and also lightly dispels dampness. Usually, Wen Gong Fang is better to try first.

Three days after ovulation has occurred, the patient should be given a formula to support pregnancy. If there is kidney yang vacuity, I use the formula Hu Tai Fang (Protect the Fetus Formula). If there is kidney yin vacuity, I prefer Zhi Tai Fang (Formula to Treat the Fetus). If there is both yin and yang vacuity, I then use Jing Tai Fang (Quiet the Fetus Formula). These three formulas are discussed in the previous section and have the same function here — to preserve pregnancy.

Hu Tai Fang (Protect the Fetus Formula)

Sang Ji Sheng (Taxilli Herba)
Xu Duan (Dipsaci Radix)
Tu Si Zi (Cuscutae Semen)
Gou Qi Zi (Lycii Fructus)
Shan Zhu Yu (Corni Fructus)
Dang Shen (Codonopsis Radix)
Bai Shao (Paeoniae Radix Alba)
Bai Zhu (Atractylodis Macrocephalae Rhizoma)
Huang Qi (Astragali Radix)
Suan Zao Ren (Ziziphi Spinosi Semen)

Yang Tai Fang (Formula to Nourish the Fetus)

Tu Si Zi (Cuscutae Semen)
Shu Di Huang (Rehmanniae Radix Praeparata)
Shan Zhu Yu (Corni Fructus)
Shan Yao (Dioscoreae Rhizoma)
Bai Shao (Paeoniae Radix Alba)
Mai Men Dong (Ophiopogonis Radix)
Suan Zao Ren (Ziziphi Spinosi Semen)
Gan Cao (Glycyrrhizae Radix)
Dang Shen (Codonopsis Radix)
Wu Wei Zi (Schisandrae Fructus)

Jing Tai Fang (Quiet the Fetus Formula)

Sang Ji Sheng (Taxilli Herba)
Xu Duan (Dipsaci Radix)
Tu Si Zi (Cuscutae Semen)
Gou Qi Zi (Lycii Fructus)
Shan Zhu Yu (Corni Fructus)
Dang Shen (Codonopsis Radix)
Bai Shao (Paeoniae Radix Alba)
Bai Zhu (Atractylodis Macrocephalae Rhizoma)

Wu Wei Zi (Schisandrae Fructus)
Suan Zao Ren (Ziziphi Spinosi Semen)

Acupuncture formula for drug ART: Refer to the acupuncture protocol for natural pregnancy in the previous section.

Intrauterine Insemination (IUI)

When the stimulating drugs alone do not work, the next step in ART is usually an IUI. During an IUI, the sperm are separated from the seminal fluid in the laboratory and deposited directly into the uterine cavity through the cervix. This procedure delivers a highly concentrated amount of the healthiest sperm directly into the uterus and can double the chance of conception. Intrauterine insemination is an ideal procedure for those with abnormal semen, cervical mucus problems, or sexual dysfunction. It is not indicated if there is anovulation or blocked fallopian tubes.

The sperm do not remain viable for as long as they do during regular intercourse and ejaculation. Therefore, it is important to inseminate as close to the time of ovulation as possible. One method to time an IUI uses an ovulation predictor kit that measures the LH surge. The surge peaks about 18 – 24 hours before the egg is released. A woman will test her urine in the morning or afternoon every day until the test is positive for the LH surge. When the test turns positive, the intrauterine insemination is scheduled for the following day.

A second method for timing an insemination is to artificially trigger ovulation. In this case, an ultrasound is used to determine when the follicles are mature enough to release an egg. An injection of HCG is given (as it is in the pharmaceutical protocol) to trigger the release of the egg. Ovulation usually occurs approximately 36-40 hours after the injection. The IUI is typically scheduled 1-1.5 days after the HCG trigger is given.

The sperm must be prepared before an IUI can occur. The ejaculate is composed of two main components: seminal fluid and sperm. Seminal fluid contains many types of hormones and chemicals. One group of chemicals (prostaglandins) can cause painful uterine contractions, nausea, vomiting, fever and diarrhea. The sperm are separated from the seminal fluid to avoid these problems. Preparation of the sperm can also increase the chances of conception because high concentrations of the strongest and healthiest sperm are used in the insemination.

In most cases, typical sperm processing involves the following steps: The semen is first collected and must sit for a while to allow it to liquefy. The semen is then mixed with a chemical solution called a sperm wash media. The semen and media mixture is rapidly spun in an instrument called a centrifuge. This causes the sperm to settle at the bottom in a small pellet. The fluid above the pellet contains the seminal fluid and can be separated out. The sperm pellet is then dissolved by adding more sperm wash media. The specimen is now ready for insemination. In some situations further preparation may occur that involves separating out dead or immobile sperm from the healthy sperm.

During the IUI procedure the physician draws the washed sperm specimen into a catheter attached to a syringe. The catheter tip is threaded through the vagina and cervix and into the uterus. The plunger on the syringe is pressed and this causes the sperm specimen to flow through the catheter into the uterus. Sometimes an ultrasound is used to guide the whole procedure. After the procedure is over, the patient may be asked to relax for about 30 minutes before leaving the doctor's office.

There are many factors that determine how successful an IUI procedure will be. These can be the same factors that apply to any fertility treatment such as the age, sperm count and motility, ovarian function, fallopian tube occlusion or scarring, pelvic adhesions, or other causes of infertility. Some women may be advised to take fertility drugs such as Clomid or FSH in conjunction with an IUI to improve their chances of success.

Acupuncture may be given to the patient to assist in the IUI process and increase the chances of success. The patient should receive acupuncture before and after the IUI procedure.

See page 259 for a chart presentation of treatment for patients doing IUI.

Acupuncture Formulas for IUI

Before IUI:

I use the following points prior to the IUI procedure to help increase the chances of success: ST36 (Zu San Li), SP6 (San Yin Jiao), KI13 (Qi Xue), LI4 (He Gu), Yin Tang (M-HN-3), GV20 (Bai Hui), Si Shen Cong (M-HN-1), Ear points Kidney, Spleen, and Shen Men.

Formula analysis

These points open the cervix to ease the injection of the semen and make it less painful. This protocol also helps the uterus to accept the semen. From a TCM point of view, ST36 and SP6 fortify the spleen to engender the qi and blood.

LI4 encourages the free flow of the qi, while KI13 moves the blood to the uterus. Yin Tang, GV20, and Si Shen Cong quiet the spirit. The ear points supplement the kidney and spleen and quiet the spirit.

After IUI:

The same or next day I use: ST36 (Zu San Li), KI3 (Tai Xi), KI13 (Qi Xue), GV20 (Bai Hui), Yin Tang (M-HN-3), Ear points Kidney, Spleen, and Shen Men.

Formula analysis

KI3 supplements kidney essence. In this formula, GV20 upbears the qi to retain the semen in the uterus and retain any fertilized eggs within the uterus. Taken as a whole, these points help the embryo transfer to the appropriate place in the uterus.

Three days afterward, I use: KI3 (Tai Xi), ST36 (Zu San Li), GV20 (Bai Hui), Yin Tang (M-HN-3), Ear points Kidney, Spleen, and Shen Men.

These points help the embryo implant in the uterus.

Once implantation has occurred, I use: GV20 (Bai Hui), Yin Tang (M-HN-3), Ear points Kidney, Spleen, and Shen Men.

These points help the uterus relax to prevent miscarriage.

If the patient is taking fertility drugs in preparation for IUI, the herbs given are the same as under pharmaceutical intervention above. If they are not taking fertility drugs, the formulas of choice are listed below.

For a patient with kidney yin vacuity, I find Zhi Ru Fang (Conception Formula) is the best choice. Kidney yin vacuity patients also tend to be more tense and anxious. Therefore, a few ingredients are used to relax the body and quiet the spirit.

Zhi Ru Fang (Conception Formula)

Shan Yao (Dioscoreae Rhizoma)
Shan Zhu Yu (Corni Fructus)
Shu Di Huang (Rehmanniae Radix Praeparata)
Fu Ling (Poria)

Mu Dan Pi (Moutan Cortex)
Ze Xie (Alismatis Rhizoma)
Bai Shao (Paeoniae Radix Alba)
Tu Si Zi (Cuscutae Semen)
Suan Zao Ren (Ziziphi Spinosi Semen)
Gan Cao (Glycyrrhizae Radix)

Formula analysis

This formula is a modification of Liu Wei Di Huang Wan (Six Flavors Rehmannia Pill). The first six medicinals comprise this classic formula which nourishes liver-kidney yin. Bai Shao is added to nourish the blood and yin. Tu Si Zi supplements the kidney, including the essence which is the source of yin. Suan Zao Ren quiets the spirit while also nourishing heart and liver blood. This time can be very stressful for a patient. So this is important. Gan Cao supplements the spleen so that the patient can digest the slimy, enriching medicinals in the formula. In addition, Gan Cao helps to quiet the spirit. Gan Cao and Bai Shao together relax the sinews to allow easier reception of the IUI.

If a patient shows predominantly yang vacuity, I use Wen Gong Fang (Warm the Uterus Formula) instead. As discussed above, this is Ding Jing Fang (Stabilize Menstruation Formula) with Rou Gui (Cinnamomi Cortex) added to enhance the movement of blood to the uterine area.

Wen Gong Fang (Warm the Uterus Formula)

Dang Gui (Angelicae Sinensis Radix)
Bai Shao (Paeoniae Radix Alba)
Chai Hu (Bupleuri Radix)
Fu Ling (Poria)
Shan Yao (Dioscoreae Rhizoma)
Dang Shen (Codonopsis Radix)
Ba Ji Tian (Morindae Officinalis Radix)
Tu Si Zi (Cuscutae Semen)
Shu Di Huang (Rehmanniae Radix Praeparata)
Zhi Gan Cao (Glycyrrhizae Radix cum Liquido Fricta)
Rou Gui (Cinnamomi Cortex)

For irregular menstruation, Tiao Jing Fang (Regulate Menstruation Formula) is appropriate. This is the same formula as above with Xiang Fu (Cyperi Rhizoma) substituted for Rou Gui in order to regulate and rectify the liver qi.

Tiao Jing Fang (Regulate Menstruation Formula)

Dang Gui (Angelicae Sinensis Radix)
Bai Shao (Paeoniae Radix Alba)
Chai Hu (Bupleuri Radix)
Fu Ling (Poria)
Shan Yao (Dioscoreae Rhizoma)
Dang Shen (Codonopsis Radix)
Ba Ji Tian (Morindae Officinalis Radix)
Tu Si Zi (Cuscutae Semen)
Shu Di Huang (Rehmanniae Radix Praeparata)
Zhi Gan Cao (Glycyrrhizae Radix cum Liquido Fricta)
Xiang Fu (Cyperi Rhizoma)

If stress is a central factor, Yang Luan Fang (Egg-nourishing Formula) should be used instead. This is also the same formula as above with Wu Wei Zi (Schisandrae Fructus) and Shan Zhu Yu (Corni Fructus) substituted for Xiang Fu. Wu Wei Zi quiets the spirit, and Shan Zhu Yu nourishes the liver.

Yang Luan Fang (Egg-nourishing Formula)

Dang Gui (Angelicae Sinensis Radix)
Bai Shao (Paeoniae Radix Alba)
Chai Hu (Bupleuri Radix)
Fu Ling (Poria)
Shan Yao (Dioscoreae Rhizoma)
Dang Shen (Codonopsis Radix)
Ba Ji Tian (Morindae Officinalis Radix)
Tu Si Zi (Cuscutae Semen)
Shu Di Huang (Rehmanniae Radix Praeparata)
Zhi Gan Cao (Glycyrrhizae Radix cum Liquido Fricta)
Shan Zhu Yu (Corni Fructus)
Wu Wei Zi (Schisandrae Fructus)

For a patient with digestive problems, I recommend trying Ji Luan Fang (Stimulate Ovulation Formula). This contains Chen Pi (Citri Reticulatae Pericarpium) to help regulate the stomach qi and digestion.

Ji Luan Fang (Stimulate Ovulation Formula)

Dang Gui (Angelicae Sinensis Radix)

Bai Shao (Paeoniae Radix Alba)

Chai Hu (Bupleuri Radix)

Fu Ling (Poria)

Shan Yao (Dioscoreae Rhizoma)

Dang Shen (Codonopsis Radix)

Ba Ji Tian (Morindae Officinalis Radix)

Tu Si Zi (Cuscutae Semen)

Shu Di Huang (Rehmanniae Radix Praeparata)

Zhi Gan Cao (Glycyrrhizae Radix cum Liquido Fricta)

Chen Pi (Citri Reticulatae Pericarpium)

Three days after IUI, I switch the formula to one of the three pregnancy formulas that are discussed above: Zhi Tai Fang (Formula to Treat the Fetus) for kidney yin vacuity, Hu Tai Fang (Protect the Fetus Formula) for kidney yang vacuity, or Jing Tai Fang (Quiet the Fetus Formula) for both yin and yang vacuity.

In vitro fertilization (IVF)

Human in vitro fertilization (IVF) is a process in which an egg and sperm are fertilized in vitro, meaning outside of the body in a petri dish (in vitro literally means "in glass"). The fertilized embryo is then implanted into the woman's uterus. In vitro fertilization was first successful in the United States in 1981. Since then, it has become a widely accepted method of treatment for infertile couples.

The initial step in IVF is regulation of the hormone levels. This is often achieved by having the female patient take oral contraceptive pills for one month. (Recently, there have been some physicians who do not give birth control pills to women over age 40 or if they have high FSH levels.) When trying to control ovulation, one common method is for the patient to take leuprolide acetate (Lupron) before or after stopping birth control pills. Another method is to give ganerelix (Antagon) three days prior to an HCG (human chorionic gonadotropin) injection to trigger ovulation.

Next, the goal is to stimulate ovulation. Even when the woman has normal ovulatory function, ovulation stimulation will be employed in almost all cases in order to induce development of the maximum number of follicles containing mature oocytes. There is no single approach to ovulation stimulation that works equally well for all patients. When determining the stimulation protocol best suited for each patient, physicians will be guided by the patient's medical history and their previous response to the drugs. Commonly used drugs, such as menotropins

(Menopur or Repronex), follitropin-beta (Follistim), and follitropin-alpha (Gonal-F), are given to stimulate the ovaries to produce more follicles and regulate the hormones. Pergonal, Repronex, and Menopur all contain LH (luteinizing hormone) and FSH (follicle-stimulating hormone), while Follistim and Gonal-F contain only FSH.

During the stimulation phase, the ovarian response is usually monitored with some combination of ultrasound examinations to track follicular development and blood tests to measure hormone levels (primarily estrogen and LH). As follicles mature, these tests may be performed daily over a 4-6 day interval.

During the final stage of follicular development and egg maturation, the patient will be given an HCG (human chorionic gonadotropin) injection. This is timed 34-36 hours prior to the egg retrieval (just before ovulation would naturally occur) and helps to change immature eggs into mature or metaphase II eggs, ready for conception.

Various techniques have been used for egg retrieval, also called oocyte aspiration. In the past, laparoscopy was often employed. This is a procedure that typically makes two or three small incisions on the abdomen. Currently, the most common method being used is the transvaginal ultrasound-guided (USG) approach. Guided by ultrasound scanning, a physician inserts a long, thin needle through the vagina and into the ovary, thereby emptying the follicles. The needle is connected to a suction pump and the fluid from each accessible follicle within the ovary is gently aspirated.

If the follicle is mature, a visible amount of granulosa cells will accompany the aspirated fluid in which the mature ovum is found. This fluid is examined by an embryologist under a microscope in order to identify and isolate the egg complex. The oocyte is identified and graded for its maturity, placed in an incubation medium within a petri dish, and finally transferred into the incubator. Eggs are usually cultured in the incubator for 3-6 hours depending on maturity before being exposed to sperm.

Not all the eggs retrieved will be mature or normal in appearance. The percentage of eggs achieving fertilization depends on many factors. Some eggs that appear to be mature and normal in appearance will not fertilize even when exposed to normal sperm. Not all fertilized eggs will go on to cell division (cleavage). As an example, a typical cycle may produce 12 eggs of which eight become fertilized and seven begin to divide in a satisfactory fashion. Depending on the female patient's age, 2-4 will be transferred to the uterus and 2-3 will be cryopreserved (frozen).

For semen, various forms of preparation can be used, from a simple washing and centrifugation similar to that used in the IUI process, to a more complicated "swim-up" procedure that separates out only motile sperm to be used for insemination. To perform insemination, between 50,000 and 500,000 motile sperm per milliliter are needed. When sperm quality and/or numbers are low, it may be necessary to hold the egg under the microscope and inject a single sperm into the interior of the egg (a procedure known as intracytoplasmic sperm injection or ICSI).

Once the oocyte has been fertilized with sperm, it is examined approximately 15-18 hours later for fertilization and switched from the incubation medium to a growth medium that contains twice the amount of protein. Next, the fertilized egg is returned to the incubator and kept there until the time of transfer, usually around 2-6 days after insemination. The fertilized egg is ordinarily in the four or eight-cell stage before transfer of the embryo can take place.

Approximately 2-6 days after insemination, the dividing embryos selected for re-placement in the uterus are loaded into a soft plastic catheter. Using a small volume of medium, the biologist loads the catheter and the physician passes it through the cervix into the uterine cavity. Most programs transfer two embryos in patients under age 35 undergoing their first cycle of treatment, and 3-4 in those ages 35-40 to maximize their chance of success while minimizing multiple pregnancies. Additional healthy embryos may be stored in liquid nitrogen to be used later if implantation and pregnancy do not occur.

After transfer has occurred, supplemental progesterone in the form of vaginal suppositories, injections, or micronized oral tablets may be prescribed. (In a natural pregnancy the corpus luteum, the remnants of the follicle, would be producing progesterone following conception.) Ultrasonography may be employed to measure ovarian size, particularly if hyperstimulation is suspected.

Pregnancy testing is usually performed 12-14 days after egg retrieval. If the results are positive, progesterone levels will be checked and the pregnancy test will be repeated in order to measure the rate of HCG rise that occurs in early pregnancy. Using vaginal ultrasonography, a fetal sac typically can be seen 25 days following egg retrieval, and by the 35th day, fetal heart motion can be observed.

I give the following Chinese medicinal formulas in conjunction with the drugs used in the IVF process as indicated. See page 260 for a visual chart presentation of treatment for IVF patients.

While the patient is on oral contraceptives, I use:

Bei Luan Fang (Prepare the Egg Formula)

> Chai Hu (Bupleuri Radix)
> Dang Gui (Angelicae Sinensis Radix)
> Bai Shao (Paeoniae Radix Alba)
> Bai Zhu (Atractylodis Macrocephalae Rhizoma)
> Fu Ling (Poria)
> Gan Cao (Glycyrrhizae Radix)
> Shu Di Huang (Rehmanniae Radix Praeparata)
> Dan Shen (Salviae Miltiorrhizae Radix)
> Suan Zao Ren (Ziziphi Spinosi Semen)
> Zhi Qiao (Ke) (Aurantii Fructus)

Formula analysis

This formula is based on Xiao Yao Fang (Rambling Formula) which courses the liver and rectifies the qi and helps to prevent liver depression qi stagnation. For many patients, the contraceptive pill and the stress associated with the IVF process can affect the normal flow of the liver qi. As we will see below, I use this formula again before the embryo transfer.

During ovarian stimulation:

If the follicles are growing too slowly, we need to nourish the kidney and blood while supplementing yang. For this, I use Wen Gong Fang (Warm the Uterus Formula). As discussed above, this is Ding Jing Fang (Stabilize Menstruation Formula) with Rou Gui (Cinnamomi Cortex) added to increase the movement of blood to the uterine area.

Wen Gong Fang (Warm the Uterus Formula)

> Dang Gui (Angelicae Sinensis Radix)
> Bai Shao (Paeoniae Radix Alba)
> Chai Hu (Bupleuri Radix)
> Fu Ling (Poria)
> Shan Yao (Dioscoreae Rhizoma)

Dang Shen (Codonopsis Radix)
Ba Ji Tian (Morindae Officinalis Radix)
Tu Si Zi (Cuscutae Semen)
Shu Di Huang (Rehmanniae Radix Praeparata)
Zhi Gan Cao (Glycyrrhizae Radix cum Liquido Fricta)
Rou Gui (Cinnamomi Cortex)

If the follicles are growing at a normal rate (1.5mm per day), I use Yang Luan Fang (Egg-nourishing Formula) to simply nourish their development. As discussed above, this formula is also based upon Ding Jing Fang (Stabilize Menstruation Formula) with two securing and astringing medicinals added, Wu Wei Zi (Schisandrae Fructus) and Shan Zhu Yu (Corni Fructus). These ensure that blood, essence, yin, and body fluids are contained.

Yang Luan Fang (Egg-nourishing Formula)

Dang Gui (Angelicae Sinensis Radix)
Bai Shao (Paeoniae Radix Alba)
Chai Hu (Bupleuri Radix)
Fu Ling (Poria)
Shan Yao (Dioscoreae Rhizoma)
Dang Shen (Codonopsis Radix)
Ba Ji Tian (Morindae Officinalis Radix)
Tu Si Zi (Cuscutae Semen)
Shu Di Huang (Rehmanniae Radix Praeparata)
Zhi Gan Cao (Glycyrrhizae Radix cum Liquido Fricta)
Shan Zhu Yu (Corni Fructus)
Wu Wei Zi (Schisandrae Fructus)

If the follicles are growing too fast, this indicates an excess of yang activity and we need to nourish kidney yin. In this case, I use:

Zhi Ru Fang (Conception Formula)

Shan Yao (Dioscoreae Rhizoma)
Shan Zhu Yu (Corni Fructus)
Shu Di Huang (Rehmanniae Radix Praeparata)
Fu Ling (Poria)
Mu Dan Pi (Moutan Cortex)
Ze Xie (Alismatis Rhizoma)
Bai Shao (Paeoniae Radix Alba)

Tu Si Zi (Cuscutae Semen)
Suan Zao Ren (Ziziphi Spinosi Semen)
Gan Cao (Glycyrrhizae Radix)

This formula nourishes yin to clear heat and slows down the rate of follicular growth.

Before the embryo transfer:

Bei Luan Fang (Prepare the Egg Formula) should be taken one time the night before and once on the morning of the transfer.

Bei Luan Fang (Prepare the Egg Formula)

Chai Hu (Bupleuri Radix)
Dang Gui (Angelicae Sinensis Radix)
Bai Shao (Paeoniae Radix Alba)
Bai Zhu (Atractylodis Macrocephalae Rhizoma)
Fu Ling (Poria)
Gan Cao (Glycyrrhizae Radix)
Shu Di Huang (Rehmanniae Radix Praeparata)
Dan Shen (Salviae Miltiorrhizae Radix)
Suan Zao Ren (Ziziphi Spinosi Semen)
Zhi Qiao (Ke) (Aurantii Fructus)

Formula analysis

This formula is Xiao Yao Fang (Rambling Formula), which courses the liver and rectifies the qi to decrease stress, plus Shu Di Huang to nourish heart blood, Dan Shen, and Suan Zao Ren to quiet the spirit, and Zhi Qiao (Ke) to assist in coursing the liver, rectifying the qi, and loosening the cervix.

After the embryo transfer and during pregnancy:

Once the embryo transfer has occurred, the patient should be treated as though she has conceived. Hence, a formula should be given to preserve the pregnancy. As stated above, there are three possible choices. For a patient showing signs of kidney yin vacuity, Zhi Tai Fang (Formula to Treat the Fetus) is appropriate. For kidney yang vacuity, Hu Tai Fang (Protect the Fetus Formula) is preferable. For a combination of yin and yang vacuity, Jing Tai Fang (Quiet the Fetus Formula) should be used.

Acupuncture formulas for IVF:

While taking the contraceptive pill: SP6 (San Yin Jiao), LI4 (He Gu), SP10 (Xue Hai), Zi Gong Xue (M-CA-18), Yin Tang (M-HN-3)

Formula analysis

The contraceptive pill is administered to give the ovaries a rest from ovulation. Therefore, we are not regulating the hormones at this time. Instead, we are circulating the blood flow to the ovaries to protect them from the suppression of the contraceptive pill. From a TCM point of view, LI4 and SP6 encourage the qi to flow smoothly, while SP10 nourishes and quickens the blood. Zi Gong Xue brings qi and blood to the ovaries and uterus. Yin Tang relaxes the uterus and quiets the spirit.

During ovarian stimulation:

ST36 (Zu San Li), SP6 (San Yin Jiao), KI3 (Tai Xi), Zi Gong Xue (M-CA-18), GV20 (Bai Hui), Yin Tang (M-HN-3)

Formula analysis

ST-36, SP-6, and KI3 together supplement the spleen qi and also supplement blood and the kidney to nourish the ovaries and uterus. This supports medication used to stimulate the growth of follicles and helps the uterine lining to thicken. Zi Gong Xue guides the qi and blood to the ovaries and uterus. GV20 stimulates the pituitary to raise FSH. This makes the ovaries more responsive to the stimulation medication and, therefore, produces more follicles. Yin Tang quiets the spirit and moderates medication side effects to reduce anxiety, irritability, and restlessness.

Before the IVF transfer:

ST36 (Zu San Li), SP6 (San Yin Jiao), LI4 (He Gu), KI13 (Qi Xue), GV20 (Bai Hui), Yin Tang (M-HN-3), Si Shen Cong (M-HN-1), Ear points Kidney, Spleen, and Shen Men

Formula analysis

Before IVF, it is very important to help relax the uterus and to loosen the cervix. This helps to more easily transfer the embryos into the uterus. Therefore, Si Shen Cong and KI13 loosen the cervix and relax the patient to prevent contraction of the uterus. If the uterus contracts, it can push all of the embryos out. The ear points and Yin Tang quiet the spirit and prevent contractions by relaxing the uterus. ST36 and GV20 together supplement and upbear the spleen qi to help hold the embryo within the uterus. ST36, KI3, and KI13 together supplement the kidney and nourish the blood which helps the uterine lining to thicken and be as receptive as possible to the implantation of the embryo.

After the IVF transfer:

ST36 (Zu San Li), KI3 (Tai Xi), GV20 (Bai Hui), Yin Tang (M-HN-3), Ear points Kidney, Spleen, and Shen Men

Formula analysis

ST36 and GV20 together supplement and upbear the spleen qi to help hold the embryo in the uterus. ST36 and KI3 supplement kidney essence and blood to provide nourishment for the embryo while building the endometrial lining. The ear points and Yin Tang quiet the spirit and discourage contractions of the uterus.

Once pregnancy is achieved: GV20 (Bai Hui), Yin Tang (M-HN-3), Ear points Kidney, Spleen, and Shen Men

Formula analysis

Once the patient is pregnant it is very important to prevent miscarriage. Therefore, GV20 supplements and upbears the spleen qi to hold the embryo within the uterus. The ear points and Yin Tang relax the uterus and quiet the spirit, discouraging contractions that might endanger the pregnancy. The ear points of the kidney and spleen supplement the kidney and spleen and encourage engenderment of blood to nourish the embryo.

Case 1: PCOS

A couple came in to see Dr. Liang after trying to get pregnant for about a year. The husband was 37 years old and had lost one testicle to cancer 20 years previously. As a result, his sperm count was low at eight million and motility and morphology were also low at 20% and 9%, respectively. His wife was 36 years old and suffered from PCOS and hyperthyroidism. Her cycles were irregular and often anovulatory. In addition, she had a history of one miscarriage at eight weeks. The subsequent history only describes the wife's treatment.

The wife's diagnosis was spleen-kidney dual vacuity with blood vacuity and liver depression qi stagnation. Her treatment plan included supplementing the kidney, fortifying the spleen and supplementing the qi, nourishing blood and soothing the liver.

The formula used to regulate her menstruation and promote ovulation was Tiao Jing Fang (Regulate Menstruation Formula). This contained Dang Gui (Angelicae Sinensis Radix), Bai Shao (Paeoniae Radix Alba), Chai Hu (Bupleuri Radix), Fu Ling (Poria), Shan Yao (Dioscoreae Rhizoma), Dang Shen (Codonopsis Radix), Ba Ji Tian (Morindae Officinalis Radix), Tu Si Zi (Cuscutae Semen), Shu Di Huang (Rehmanniae Radix Praeparata), Zhi Gan Cao (Glycyrrhizae Radix cum Liquido Fricta), and Xiang Fu (Cyperi Rhizoma).

Formula analysis

Dang Gui nourishes and quickens the blood; Bai Shao nourishes the blood and harmonizes the liver; Chai Hu courses the liver and rectifies the qi; and Shu Di Huang supplements kidney yin and essence and nourishes the blood. Shan Yao supplements both the spleen and kidney qi, while Fu Ling fortifies the spleen and quiets the spirit. Tu Si Zi and Ba Ji Tian supplement kidney yang and essence. Xiang Fu was added to course the liver and rectify the qi. It was also meant to help to regulate menstruation.

Her acupuncture base formula used after menstruation was ST36 (Zu San Li), SP6 (San Yin Jiao), Zi Gong (M-CA-18), LI4 (He Gu), GV20 (Bai Hui), and Yin Tang (M-HN-3). This formula supplements the qi and blood and increases the movement of blood to the lower abdominal area to improve egg quality and build uterine lining.

During menstruation, the patient took:

Wen Jing Xing Fang (Warm Menstrual Movement Formula)

Dang Gui (Angelicae Sinensis Radix)
Bai Shao (Paeoniae Radix Alba)
Shu Di Huang (Rehmanniae Radix Praeparata)
Chuan Xiong (Chuanxiong Rhizoma)
Niu Xi (Achyranthis Bidentatae Radix)
Dan Shen (Salviae Miltiorrhizae Radix)
Xiang Fu (Cyperi Rhizoma)
Gou Qi Zi (Lycii Fructus)
Xiao Hui Xiang (Foeniculi Fructus)
Gui Zhi (Cinnamomi Ramulus)

Formula analysis

Dang Gui nourishes and quickens blood; Bai Shao nourishes the blood, soothes the liver, and astringes the yin; Shu Di Huang nourishes kidney yin, essence and blood; Gou Qi Zi nourishes liver yin and blood; and Chuan Xiong, Dan Shen, and Niu Xi quicken the blood and transform stasis. Xiao Hui Xiang and Gui Zhi warm the channels and free the flow of qi. Gui Zhi also warms and frees the blood vessels.

Her acupuncture during menstruation consisted of SP6 (San Yin Jiao), SP10 (Xue Hai), CV4 (Guan Yuan), CV3 (Zhong Ji), LI4 (He Gu), and Yin Tang (M-HN-3).

Formula analysis

SP6 was used to nourish the kidney, liver, and spleen and to supplement the blood. SP10 and CV4 were used to regulate the menses and quicken the blood. CV4 and CV3 were used together to free the flow of blood downward and reduce dysmenorrhea. LI4 was used to course the liver and rectify the qi for smooth flow of blood. Finally, Yin Tang was treated to relax the mind and quiet the spirit.

Outcome

The patient received acupuncture and Chinese medicinals consistently for only two months and became pregnant naturally. She delivered a healthy baby.

Case 2: Ovarian Tumors

Ovarian tumors can be a significant factor affecting fertility. In this case, a 36-year-old woman with only 20% of her left ovary remaining wanted to try Chinese medicine. She had tried using IUI 10 times with no success. She had a history of an ovarian tumor in her right ovary which had been surgically removed and had had several dermatoid cysts in her left ovary. She had two surgeries to remove the cysts, leaving her with only 20% of her left ovary. With declining ovarian function, her FSH level was very high at 31.25, and she was unable to produce any follicles or viable eggs.

I treated this woman with both acupuncture and Chinese medicinals. She was treated to improve her ovarian function so that she would be ready for another cycle of IUI. Her diagnosis was spleen-kidney dual vacuity with blood vacuity and blood stasis as well as liver depression qi stagnation. Thus, the treatment principles were to nourish the blood and kidney, supplement the spleen, quicken the blood, and course the liver and rectify the qi. I treated this patient with three different formulas as follows.

Before menstruation, I prescribed:

Huo Jing Zhong Zi Fang (Quicken the Channels to Plant Seeds Decoction)
modified with Shu Di Huang (Rehmanniae Radix Praeparata) to nourish the
blood, liver-kidney yin and essence, and Dang Shen (Codonopsis Radix) to
strengthen the qi.

During menstruation, I prescribed:

Xing Jing Fang (Promote Menstruation Formula) modified with Yan Hu Suo
(Corydalis Rhizoma) and San Qi (Notoginseng Radix). Yan Hu Suo and San Qi
were used to quicken the blood and relieve pain during menstruation.

After menstruation, I prescribed:

Xiao Yao Fang (Relaxed Wandered Formula) modified with Dang Shen
(Codonopsis Radix), San Qi (Notoginseng Radix), Shan Zhu Yu (Corni Fructus),
and Gou Qi Zi (Lycii Fructus).

The basic acupuncture points I treated consisted of ST36 (Zu San Li), SP6 (San Yin
Jiao), zi3 gong1 xue2, LI4 (He Gu), GV20 (Bai Hui) and Yin Tang (M-HN 3). Dur-
ing menstruation, ST36 (Zu San Li), SP6 (San Yin Jiao), LR3 (Tai Chong), SP10
(Xue Hai), CV3 (Zhong Ji), CV4 (Guan Yuan), and Yin Tang (M-HN-3) were
used. To protect the possibility of pregnancy, the points KI3 (Tai Xi), ST36 (Zu San
Li), Yin Tang (M-HN-3), GV20 (Bai Hui) and ear points Shen Men, Kidney, and
Spleen were treated before menstruation.

After four months of treatment with acupuncture and Chinese medicinals, the patient conceived naturally without using any Western drugs or therapies. Her doctor
had even said her ovary was in such poor condition that it was impossible for her
to get pregnant. Even with such slim chances, this couple was able to achieve a
healthy pregnancy with the help of Chinese herbs and acupuncture.

Outcome

The patient delivered a healthy baby girl who is now three years old.

Flow for management of fertility

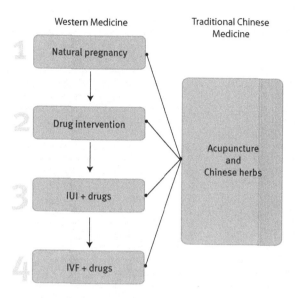

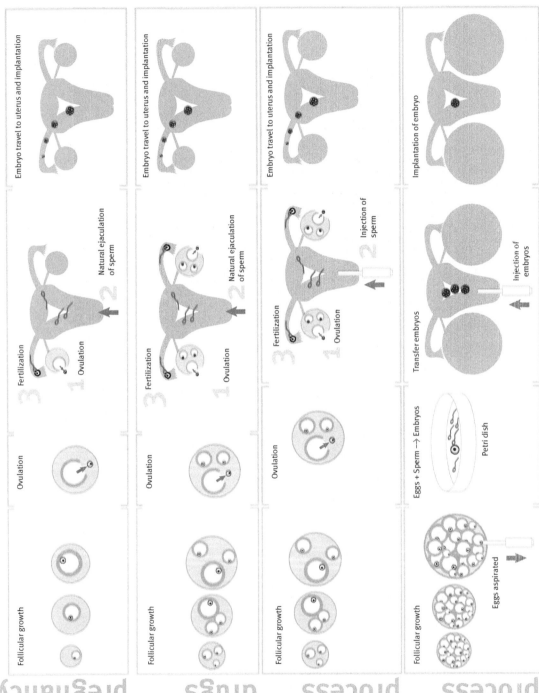

step 1 — Flow for management of fertility without Western medicine: Natural pregnancy

Stage of period	During period	After period	After ovulation	Before period
Treatment principle: TCM	Move Qi and Blood, **Nourish Blood**	Nourish K Yin, Invigorate K Yang, Supplement Blood and Qi	Nourish K Essence, Supplement Qi and Blood	Supplement Blood and Qi; Nourish K, Course LV Qi
Uterine events	Follicular growth	Ovulation; Fertilization; Natural ejaculation of sperm	Embryo travel to uterus and implantation	
Day of cycle	28 1 2 3 4 5	6 7 8 9 10 11 12 13 14 15 16 17 18	19 20 21 22 23 24	25 26 27 28
Acupuncture	SP6, SP10, Ren3, LI4, LV3	SP6, Du20, ST36, Yintang, LI4, Zigong	K3, ST36, Du20, Ear: K, SP, Shenmen	
Herbs	**Light bleeding:** Tiao Jing Xing Fang **Cramps:** Jing Tong Fang **Cold low abdomen:** Wen Jing Xing Fang	Yang Luan Fang **Yin vacuity:** Zi Ru Fang **Irregular period:** Tiao Jing Fang **If no or late ovulation:** on Day 12 of cycle (6 days of After period formula): Wen Gong Fang or Pai Luan Fang	Pai Luan Hou Fang **Low progesterone:** start Prevent miscarriage protocol	Tiao Jing Qian Fang

step 2 — Flow for management of fertility with Western medicine: Drug intervention

Stage of IUI	During period	After period and before ovulation	Ovulation	Post-ovulation
Treatment principle: Western		**Clomid:** Stimulate follicle growth Side effect: Decreases lining thickness and cervical mucus **Follistim:** Stimulate follicle growth (by increasing FSH)	Stimulate ovulation	Increase lining thickness and viscosity. Implant embryo
Treatment principle: TCM	Nourish Blood, Move Qi and Blood	Supplement K Yin and Yang, Supplement Qi and Blood, increase response to drugs (thereby increasing follicles and lining) Mitigate the Clomid side effects	Invigorate K Yang Quicken Blood to promote egg release	Supplement K Essence Fortify SP, Supplement Qi and Blood

Follicular growth · Ovulation · Fertilization · Embryo travel to uterus and implantation · Natural ejaculation of sperm

Day of cycle: 1 2 3 4 5 6 7 8 9 10 11 12 13 14 15 16 17 18 19 20 21 22 23 24 25 26 27 28

Drug:
Clomid: 50-150mg*
Follistim: 75-600 IU*
*Dosages vary by patient and doctor
● HCG injection (36 hours prior to ovulation)
Progesterone (start 3 days after ovulation)

Acupuncture:

During period	After period and before ovulation	Ovulation	Post-ovulation
SP6, SP10, Yintang, Ren3, LI4, LV3	SP6, SP10, Yintang, Ren3, LI4, LV3	SP6, K7, Du20, ST36, Yintang, LI4, Zigong	K3, ST36, Yintang, Du20, Ear: K, SP, Shenmen

Herbs:

During period	After period and before ovulation	Ovulation	Post-ovulation
Light bleeding: Tiao Jing Xing Fang **Cramps:** Jing Tong Fang **Cold low abdomen:** Wen Jing Xing Fang	Yang Luan Fang **Slow-growing follicles:** Wen Gong Fang **Fast-growing follicles:** Zi Ru Fang	Wen Gong Fang or Pai Luan Fang	**K Yin vacuity:** Zhi Tai Fang **K Yin and Yang vacuity:** Jing Tai Fang **K Yang vacuity:** Hu Tai Fang

step 3

Flow for management of fertility with Western medicine: IUI and drugs

Stage of IUI	During period	After period	Before IUI	After IUI	3 days after IUI	Pregnancy
Treatment principle: Western	Stimulate follicle growth		Encourage loosening of cervix for the uterus to better accept semen injection	Benefit embryo transfer to uterus	Benefit embryo implantation in uterus	Preserve pregnancy
Treatment principle: TCM	Nourish Blood, Move Qi and Blood	Supplement K Yin and Yang, Supplement Qi and Blood	Invigorate K Yang, Course LV Qi		Supplement K Yin, Blood, and Qi	Nourish K Essence, Supplement SP Qi and Blood
Uterine events	Follicular growth		Fertilization / Ovulation		Embryo travels to uterus and implantation	
Day of cycle	28 1 2 3 4 5 6 7 8	9 10 11 12 13	14 15 16 17	18 19 20	21 22 23 24 25 26 27 28	
Drug	Clomid: 50-150mg* / Follistim: 75-600 IU* / *Dosages vary by patient and doctor		18mm ● HCG injection (induces ovulation 36 hours later)			
Acupuncture	SP6, SP10, Yintang, Ren3, LI4, LV3	K3, ST36, SP6, Zigong, Yintang, Du14	K13, ST36, SP6, LI4, Yintang, Du20, Si Shen Cong, Ear: K, SP, Shenmen	K3, K13, ST36, Yintang, Du20, Ear: K, SP, Shenmen	K3, ST36, Du20, Yintang, Ear: K, SP, Shenmen	Du20, Yintang, Ear: K, SP, Shenmen
Herbs	**Light bleeding:** Tiao Jing Xing Fang **Cramps:** Jing Tong Fang **Cold low abdomen:** Wen Jing Xing Fang	**K Yin vacuity:** Zhi Ru Fang **Poor sleep:** Tiao Jing Hou Fang (+)stress: Yang Luan Fang (+)irregular period: Tiao Jing Fang (+)poor digestion: Jian Pi Yun Fang **K Yang vacuity:** Wen Gong Fang				**K Yin vacuity:** Zhi Tai Fang **K Yin and Yang vacuity:** Jing Tai Fang **K Yang vacuity:** Hu Tai Fang

1   2 Injection of sperm

Step 4

Flow for management of fertility with Western medicine: IVF and drugs [1]

Stage of IVF	IVF preparation	Stimulation	After retrieval	Before transfer [4]	After transfer	Confirmed pregnancy [3]
Treatment principle: Western	Supress ovaries	Encourage ovary production of follicles and thicken uterine lining	Build uterine lining, prepare embryos for implantation	Relaxation	Relaxation and help embryo implantation in uterine wall	Protect from miscarriage by encouraging embryo adhesion to uterus
	Protect ovaries quicken blood Improve egg quality					Protect from miscarriage by nourishing blood and embryo growth, relax uterus to prevent contractions
Treatment principle: TCM		Supplement SP Qi / BL, Supplement Kidney Support stimulation drug Nourish ovaries and uterus Encourage follicular growth and increase uterine lining	Nourish Blood and K Essence, increase lining, quiet spirit	Encourage loosening of cervix & relaxation of the uterus to better accept embryos, benefit sleep	Benefit embryo implantation Protect miscarriage	

Uterine events: Follicular growth → Eggs aspirated → Eggs + Sperm > Embryos (Petri dish) → Transfer embryos → Injection of embryos → Implantation of embryo

Day of cycle: 7...18...28 1 2 3 4 5 6 7 8 9 10 11 12 13 14 15 16 17 18 19 20 21 22 23 24 25 26 27 28 ...10

Drug:
- Birth control pills [2]
- Lupron [2]
- FSH: Follistim, Gonal-F
- LH (+FSH): Pergonal, Repronex, Menopur
- ● HCG injection (to promote egg development)
- Progesterone

Acupuncture	SP6, SP10, LI4, Zigong, Yintang	K3, ST36, SP6, Zigong, Yintang, Du20	K3, LI4, ST36, SP6, Yintang, Du20, Ear: K, SP, Shenmen	K3, K13, ST36, LI4, Yintang, Du20, Si Shen Cong, Ear: K, SP, Shenmen	K3, ST36, Yintang, Du20, Ear: K, SP, Shenmen	Du20, Yintang, Ear: K, SP, Shenmen
Herbs	Bei Luan Fang	**Slow follicle growth:** Wen Gong Fang **Even follicle growth:** Yang Luan Fang **Fast follicle growth:** Zhi Ru Fang	Yang Luan Fang	**Evening before and morning of transfer:** Bei Luan fang	**Heat:** Zhi Tai Fang **Neutral:** Jing Tai Fang **Cold:** Hu Tai Fang	

1 Refer to Acupuncture and IVF: Infertility chapter
2 Time for birth control use varies from 1-4 weeks, or not at all for older patients, so as not to supress ovarian function
3 Time varies from 3-5 days after retrieval, by follicular development, egg quality and MD experience
4 Typically 4 days after retrieval

Formula List

安胎方	**An Tai Fang**	Fetus-Quieting Formula
	Sang Ji Sheng	Taxilli Herba
	Xu Duan	Dipsaci Radix
	Tu Si Zi	Cuscutae Semen
	Gou Qi Zi	Lycii Fructus
	Shan Zhu Yu	Corni Fructus
	Dang Shen	Codonopsis Radix
	Bai Shao	Paeoniae Radix Alba
	Bai Zhu	Atractylodis Macrocephalae Rhizoma
八珍汤	**Ba Zhen Tang**	Eight Gem Decoction
	Shu Di Huang	Rehmanniae Radix Praeparata
	Dang Gui	Angelicae Sinensis Radix
	Bai Shao	Paeoniae Radix Alba
	Chuan Xiong	Chuanxiong Rhizoma
	Ren Shen	Ginseng Radix
	Bai Zhu	Atractylodis Macrocephalae Rhizoma
	Fu Ling	Poria
	Zhi Gan Cao	Glycyrrhizae Radix Praeparata
保阴煎	**Bao Yin Jian**	Yin-Safeguarding Brew
	Shu Di Huang	Rehmanniae Radix Praeparata
	Sheng Di Huang	Rehmanniae Radix
	Huang Qin	Scutellariae Radix
	Huang Bai	Phellodendri Cortex
	Shan Yao	Dioscoreae Rhizoma
	Gan Cao	Glycyrrhizae Radix
	Bai Shao	Paeoniae Radix Alba
	Xu Duan	Dipsaci Radix
备卵方	**Bei Luan Fang**	Prepare the Egg Formula
	Dang Gui	Angelicae Sinensis Radix
	Bai Shao	Paeoniae Radix Alba
	Chai Hu	Bupleuri Radix
	Fu Ling	Poria
	Bai Zhu	Atractylodis Macrocephalae Rhizoma
	Dan Shen	Salviae Miltiorrhizae Radix
	Zhi Ke	Aurantii Fructus
	Gan Cao	Glycyrrhizae Radix
	Shu Di Huang	Rehmanniae Radix Praeparata
	Suan Zao Ren	Ziziphi Spinosi Semen
苍附导痰丸	**Cang Fu Dao Tan Wan**	Atractylodes & Cyperus Phlegm-Abducting Pill
	Ban Xia	Pinelliae Rhizoma
	Chen Pi	Citri Reticulatae Pericarpium
	Fu Ling	Poria

	Gan Cao	Glycyrrhizae Radix
	Dan Nan Xing	Arisaema cum Bile
	Zhi Ke	Aurantii Fructus
	Cang Zhu	Atractylodis Rhizoma
	Xiang Fu	Cyperi Rhizoma
	Sheng Jiang	Zingiberis Rhizoma Recens
大宫血方	**Da Gong Xue Fang**	Major Uterine Blood Formula
	Dang Shen	Codonopsis Radix
	Huang Qi	Astragali Radix
	Xu Duan	Dipsaci Radix
	Shan Zhu Yu	Corni Fructus
	Bai Zhu	Atractylodis Macrocephalae Rhizoma
	San Qi	Notoginseng Radix
	Yi Mu Cao	Leonuri Herba
	Mo Han Lian	Ecliptae Herba
	Ai Ye	Artemisiae Argyi Folium
定经方	**Ding Jing Fang**	Stabilize the Menses Formula
	Dang Gui	Angelicae Sinensis Radix
	Bai Shao	Paeoniae Radix Alba
	Chai Hu	Bupleuri Radix
	Fu Ling	Poria
	Shan Yao	Dioscoreae Rhizoma
	Dang Shen	Codonopsis Radix
	Ba Ji Tian	Morindae Officinalis Radix
	Tu Si Zi	Cuscutae Semen
	Shu Di Huang	Rehmanniae Radix Praeparata
膈下逐瘀汤	**Ge Xia Zhu Yu Tang**	Infradiaphragmatic Stasis-Expelling Decoction
	Tao Ren	Persicae Semen
	Hong Hua	Carthami Flos
	Dang Gui	Angelicae Sinensis Radix
	Chi Shao	Paeoniae Radix Rubra
	Chuan Xiong	Chuanxiong Rhizoma
	Yan Hu Suo	Corydalis Rhizoma
	Wu Ling Zhi	Trogopteri Feces
	Mu Dan Pi	Moutan Cortex
	Xiang Fu	Cyperi Rhizoma
	Zhi Ke	Aurantii Fructus
	Wu Yao	Linderae Radix
	Gan Cao	Glycyrrhizae Radix
宫外饮	**Gong Wai Yin**	Ectopic Pregnancy Beverage
	Chi Shao	Paeoniae Radix Rubra
	Dan Shen	Salviae Miltiorrhizae Radix

	Tao Ren	Persicae Semen
	San Leng	Sparganii Rhizoma
	E Zhu	Curcumae Rhizoma
固阴煎	**Gu Yin Jian**	Yin-Securing Brew
	Ren Shen	Ginseng Radix
	Shu Di Huang	Rehmanniae Radix Praeparata
	Shan Yao	Dioscoreae Rhizoma
	Shan Zhu Yu	Corni Fructus
	Tu Si Zi	Cuscutae Semen
	Yuan Zhi	Polygalae Radix
	Wu Wei Zi	Schisandrae Fructus
	Zhi Gan Cao	Glycyrrhizae Radix Praeparata
刮宫方	**Gua Gong Fang**	Uterine-Scraping Beverage
	Ji Xue Teng	Spatholobi Caulis
	San Leng	Sparganii Rhizoma
	E Zhu	Curcumae Rhizoma
	Mu Dan Pi	Moutan Cortex
	Dan Shen	Salviae Miltiorrhizae Radix
	Chi Shao	Paeoniae Radix Rubra
	Tao Ren	Persicae Semen
	Fu Ling	Poria
	Zhi Ke	Aurantii Fructus
	Bai Zhu	Atractylodis Macrocephalae Rhizoma
	Yi Mu Cao	Leonuri Herba
	Niu Xi	Achyranthis Bidentatae Radix
刮胎方	**Gua Tai Fang**	Fetus-Removing Formula
	San Leng	Sparganii Rhizoma
	E Zhu	Curcumae Rhizoma
	Wang Bu Liu Xing	Vaccariae Semen
	Dan Shen	Salviae Miltiorrhizae Radix
	Chi Shao	Paeoniae Radix Rubra
	Xiang Fu	Cyperi Rhizoma
	Qing Pi	Citri Reticulatae Pericarpium Viride
	Hong Hua	Carthami Flos
	Yi Mu Cao	Leonuri Herba
	Niu Xi	Achyranthis Bidentatae Radix
归脾汤	**Gui Pi Tang**	Spleen-Returning Decoction
	Ren Shen	Ginseng Radix
	Bai Zhu	Atractylodis Macrocephalae Rhizoma
	Fu Shen	Poria cum Pini Radice
	Gan Cao	Glycyrrhizae Radix
	Huang Qi	Astragali Radix
	Dang Gui	Angelicae Sinensis Radix
	Long Yan Rou	Longan Arillus

	Suan Zao Ren	Ziziphi Spinosi Semen
	Yuan Zhi	Polygalae Radix
	Mu Xiang	Aucklandiae Radix
归肾丸	**Gui Shen Wan**	Kidney-Returning Pill
	Shu Di Huang	Rehmanniae Radix Praeparata
	Shan Yao	Dioscoreae Rhizoma
	Shan Zhu Yu	Corni Fructus
	Tu Si Zi	Cuscutae Semen
	Gou Qi Zi	Lycii Fructus
	Du Zhong	Eucommiae Cortex
	Dang Gui	Angelicae Sinensis Radix
	Fu Ling	Poria
固本止崩汤	**Gu Ben Zhi Beng Tang**	Root-Securing Flood-Stanching Decoction
	Dang Gui	Angelicae Sinensis Radix
	Shu Di Huang	Rehmanniae Radix Praeparata
	Ren Shen	Ginseng Radix
	Huang Qi	Astragali Radix
	Bai Zhu	Atractylodis Macrocephalae Rhizoma
	Pao Jiang	Zingiberis Rhizoma Praeparatum
	Shan Yao	Dioscoreae Rhizoma
	Sheng Ma	Cimicifugae Rhizoma
桂枝茯苓丸	**Gui Zhi Fu Ling Wan**	Cinnamon Twig and Poria Pill
	Gui Zhi	Cinnamomi Ramulus
	Fu Ling	Poria
	Tao Ren	Persicae Semen
	Chi Shao	Paeoniae Radix Rubra
	Mu Dan Pi	Moutan Cortex
活经种子丸	**Huo Jing Zhong Zi Wan**	Quicken the Channels to Plant Seeds Decoction
	Dang Gui	Angelicae Sinensis Radix
	Bai Shao	Paeoniae Radix Alba
	Chai Hu	Bupleuri Radix
	Fu Ling	Poria
	Bai Zhu	Atractylodis Macrocephalae Rhizoma
	Gan Cao	Glycyrrhizae Radix
	Zhi Ke	Aurantii Fructus
	Dan Shen	Salviae Miltiorrhizae Radix
护胎方	**Hu Tai Fang**	Fetus-Protecting Formula
	Sang Ji Sheng	Taxilli Herba
	Xu Duan	Dipsaci Radix
	Tu Si Zi	Cuscutae Semen
	Gou Qi Zi	Lycii Fructus

	Shan Zhu Yu	Corni Fructus
	Dang Shen	Codonopsis Radix
	Bai Shao	Paeoniae Radix Alba
	Bai Zhu	Atractylodis Macrocephalae Rhizoma
	Huang Qi	Astragali Radix
	Suan Zao Ren	Ziziphi Spinosi Semen
加味乌药汤	**Jia Wei Wu Yao Tang**	Supplemented Lindera Decoction
	Wu Yao	Linderae Radix
	Sha Ren	Amomi Fructus
	Mu Xiang	Aucklandiae Radix
	Yan Hu Suo	Corydalis Rhizoma
	Xiang Fu	Cyperi Rhizoma
	Bing Lang	Arecae Semen
	Gan Cao	Glycyrrhizae Radix
	Dang Gui	Angelicae Sinensis Radix
	Chuan Xiong	Chuanxiong Rhizoma
加味逍遥散	**Jia Wei Xiao Yao San**	Supplemented Free Wanderer Powder
	Dang Gui	Angelicae Sinensis Radix
	Bai Shao	Paeoniae Radix Alba
	Chai Hu	Bupleuri Radix
	Fu Ling	Poria
	Bai Zhu	Atractylodis Macrocephalae Rhizoma
	Gan Cao	Glycyrrhizae Radix
	Sheng Jiang	Zingiberis Rhizoma Recens
	Bo He	Menthae Herba
	Mu Dan Pi	Moutan Cortex
	Zhi Zi	Gardeniae Fructus
健固汤	**Jian Gu Tang**	Fortifying and Securing Decoction
	Dang Shen	Codonopsis Radix
	Bai Zhu	Atractylodis Macrocephalae Rhizoma
	Fu Ling	Poria
	Yi Yi Ren	Coicis Semen
	Ba Ji Tian	Morindae Officinalis Radix
经后方	**Jing Hou Fang**	Formula for After Menstruation
	Dang Gui	Angelicae Sinensis Radix
	Bai Shao	Paeoniae Radix Alba
	Chai Hu	Bupleuri Radix
	Fu Ling	Poria
	Bai Zhu	Atractylodis Macrocephalae Rhizoma
	Gan Cao	Glycyrrhizae Radix
	Dang Shen	Codonopsis Radix
	Shu Di Huang	Rehmanniae Radix Praeparata

	Rou Gui	Cinnamomi Cortex
	Gou Qi Zi	Lycii Fructus
经前方	**Jing Qian Fang**	Formula for Before Menstruation
	Dang Gui	Angelicae Sinensis Radix
	Bai Shao	Paeoniae Radix Alba
	Chai Hu	Bupleuri Radix
	Fu Ling	Poria
	Bai Zhu	Atractylodis Macrocephalae Rhizoma
	Gan Cao	Glycyrrhizae Radix
	Shu Di Huang	Rehmanniae Radix Praeparata
	Chen Pi	Citri Reticulatae Pericarpium
经痛方	**Jing Tong Fang**	Formula for Painful Menstruation
	Dang Gui	Angelicae Sinensis Radix
	Bai Shao	Paeoniae Radix Alba
	Chai Hu	Bupleuri Radix
	Fu Ling	Poria
	Bai Zhu	Atractylodis Macrocephalae Rhizoma
	Gan Cao	Glycyrrhizae Radix
	Xiao Hui Xiang	Foeniculi Fructus
	Gui Zhi	Cinnamomi Ramulus
	San Qi	Notoginseng Radix
	Yan Hu Suo	Corydalis Rhizoma
两地汤	**Liang Di Tang**	Rehmannia and Lycium Root Bark Decoction
	Sheng Di Huang	Rehmanniae Radix
	Di Gu Pi	Lycii Cortex
	Xuan Shen	Scrophulariae Radix
	Bai Shao	Paeoniae Radix Alba
	Mai Dong	Ophiopogonis Radix
	E Jiao	Asini Corii Colla
凉胎止血方	**Liang Tai Zhi Xue Fang**	Formula to Cool the Fetus and Stop Bleeding
	Sang Ji Sheng	Taxilli Herba
	Xu Duan	Dipsaci Radix
	Tu Si Zi	Cuscutae Semen
	Gou Qi Zi	Lycii Fructus
	Shan Zhu Yu	Corni Fructus
	Dang Shen	Codonopsis Radix
	Bai Shao	Paeoniae Radix Alba
	Bai Zhu	Atractylodis Macrocephalae Rhizoma
	Wu Wei Zi	Schisandrae Fructus
	Mo Han Lian	Ecliptae Herba
	E Jiao	Asini Corii Colla

六君子汤	**Liu Jun Zi Tang**	Six Gentleman Decoction
	Ren Shen	Ginseng Radix
	Bai Zhu	Atractylodis Macrocephalae Rhizoma
	Fu Ling	Poria
	Gan Cao	Glycyrrhizae Radix
	Chen Pi	Citri Reticulatae Pericarpium
	Ban Xia	Pinelliae Rhizoma
六味地黄丸	**Liu Wei Di Huang Wan**	Six Ingredients Rehmannia Pill
	Shu Di Huang	Rehmanniae Radix Praeparata
	Shan Zhu Yu	Corni Fructus
	Shan Yao	Dioscoreae Rhizoma
	Mu Dan Pi	Moutan Cortex
	Ze Xie	Alismatis Rhizoma
	Fu Ling	Poria
龙胆泻肝汤	**Long Dan Xie Gan Tang**	Gentian Liver-Draining Decoction
	Long Dan	Gentianae Radix
	Huang Qin	Scutellariae Radix
	Zhi Zi	Gardeniae Fructus
	Ze Xie	Alismatis Rhizoma
	Mu Tong	Akebiae Caulis
	Che Qian Zi	Plantaginis Semen
	Chai Hu	Bupleuri Radix
	Sheng Di Huang	Rehmanniae Radix
	Gan Cao	Glycyrrhizae Radix
慢盆方	**Man Pen Fang**	Formula for Chronic Pelvic Infection
	Hei Lao Hu	Kadsurae Coccineae Caulis et Folium
	Ji Gu Xiang	Crotonis Crassifolii Radix
	Fu Ling	Poria
	Dan Shen	Salviae Miltiorrhizae Radix
	Yi Yi Ren	Coicis Semen
	Bai Jiang Cao	Patriniae Herba
	Huang Qi	Astragali Radix
	Ji Xue Teng	Spatholobi Caulis
内补丸	**Nei Bu Wan**	Internal Supplementation Pill
	Lu Rong	Cervi Cornu Pantotrichum
	Tu Si Zi	Cuscutae Semen
	Sha Yuan Zi	Astragali Complanati Semen
	Rou Cong Rong	Cistanches Herba
	Rou Gui	Cinnamomi Cortex
	Huang Qi	Astragali Radix
	Ji Li	Tribuli Fructus
	Fu Zi	Aconiti Radix Lateralis Praeparata

暖胎止血方	**Nuan Tai Zhi Xue Fang**	Formula to Warm the Fetus and Stop Bleeding
	Sang Ji Sheng	Taxilli Herba
	Xu Duan	Dipsaci Radix
	Tu Si Zi	Cuscutae Semen
	Gou Qi Zi	Lycii Fructus
	Shan Zhu Yu	Corni Fructus
	Dang Shen	Codonopsis Radix
	Bai Shao	Paeoniae Radix Alba
	Bai Zhu	Atractylodis Macrocephalae Rhizoma
	Huang Qi	Astragali Radix
	Suan Zao Ren	Ziziphi Spinosi Semen
	Ai Ye	Artemisiae Argyi Folium
	E Jiao	Asini Corii Colla
排卵方	**Pai Luan Fang**	Ovulation Formula
	Dang Gui	Angelicae Sinensis Radix
	Bai Shao	Paeoniae Radix Alba
	Chai Hu	Bupleuri Radix
	Fu Ling	Poria
	Shan Yao	Dioscoreae Rhizoma
	Dang Shen	Codonopsis Radix
	Ba Ji Tian	Morindae Officinalis Radix
	Tu Si Zi	Cuscutae Semen
	Shu Di Huang	Rehmanniae Radix Praeparata
	Zhi Gan Cao	Glycyrrhizae Radix Praeparata
	Yin Yang Huo	Epimedii Herba
排卵后方	**Pai Luan Hou Fang**	Promote Ovulation Formula
	Dang Gui	Angelicae Sinensis Radix
	Bai Shao	Paeoniae Radix Alba
	Shan Zhu Yu	Corni Fructus
	Shu Di Huang	Rehmanniae Radix Praeparata
	Shan Yao	Dioscoreae Rhizoma
	He Shou Wu	Polygoni Multiflori Radix
	Gou Qi Zi	Lycii Fructus
	Tu Si Zi	Cuscutae Semen
	Dang Shen	Codonopsis Radix
	Wu Wei Zi	Schisandrae Fructus
杞菊地黄丸	**Qi Ju Di Huang Tang**	Lycium Berry, Chrysanthemum, and Rehmannia Pill
	Shu Di Huang	Rehmanniae Radix Praeparata
	Shan Zhu Yu	Corni Fructus
	Shan Yao	Dioscoreae Rhizoma
	Ze Xie	Alismatis Rhizoma
	Mu Dan Pi	Moutan Cortex
	Fu Ling	Poria

	Gou Qi Zi	Lycii Fructus
	Ju Hua	Chrysanthemi Flos
清宫方	**Qing Gong Fang**	Clear the Uterus Formula
	Dang Gui	Angelicae Sinensis Radix
	Chuan Xiong	Chuanxiong Rhizoma
	Yi Mu Cao	Leonuri Herba
	Tao Ren	Persicae Semen
	Dang Shen	Codonopsis Radix
	Niu Xi	Achyranthis Bidentatae Radix
	Xiang Fu	Cyperi Rhizoma
	San Qi	Notoginseng Radix
	Zhi Gan Cao	Glycyrrhizae Radix Praeparata
清经散	**Qing Jing San**	Clearing Menstrual Formula
	Shu Di Huang	Rehmanniae Radix Praeparata
	Di Gu Pi	Lycii Cortex
	Mu Dan Pi	Moutan Cortex
	Bai Shao	Paeoniae Radix Alba
	Qing Hao	Artemisiae Annuae Herba
	Huang Bai	Phellodendri Cortex
	Fu Ling	Poria
清热固经汤	**Qing Re Gu Jing Tang**	Heat-Clearing Menses-Securing Decoction
	Sheng Di Huang	Rehmanniae Radix
	Di Gu Pi	Lycii Cortex
	Huang Qin	Scutellariae Radix
	Gui Ban	Testudinis Plastrum
	E Jiao	Asini Corii Colla
	Ou Jie	Nelumbinis Rhizomatis Nodus
	Gan Cao	Glycyrrhizae Radix
	Mu Li	Ostreae Concha
	Zong Lu Tan	Trachycarpi Petiolus Carbonisatus
人参养荣汤	**Ren Shen Yang Rong Tang**	Ginseng Construction-Nourishing Formula
	Ren Shen	Ginseng Radix
	Bai Zhu	Atractylodis Macrocephalae Rhizoma
	Fu Ling	Poria
	Gan Cao	Glycyrrhizae Radix
	Shu Di Huang	Rehmanniae Radix Praeparata
	Dang Gui	Angelicae Sinensis Radix
	Bai Shao	Paeoniae Radix Alba
	Huang Qi	Astragali Radix
	Rou Gui	Cinnamomi Cortex
	Wu Wei Zi	Schisandrae Fructus

	Yuan Zhi	Polygalae Radix
	Chen Pi	Citri Reticulatae Pericarpium
	Sheng Jiang	Zingiberis Rhizoma Recens
	Da Zao	Jujubae Fructus
少腹逐瘀汤	**Shao Fu Zhu Yu Tang**	Lesser Abdomen Stasis-Expelling Decoction
	Dang Gui	Angelicae Sinensis Radix
	Chi Shao	Paeoniae Radix Rubra
	Chuan Xiong	Chuanxiong Rhizoma
	Xiao Hui Xiang	Foeniculi Fructus
	Gan Jiang	Zingiberis Rhizoma
	Rou Gui	Cinnamomi Cortex
	Yan Hu Suo	Corydalis Rhizoma
	Wu Ling Zhi	Trogopteri Faeces
	Pu Huang	Typhae Pollen
	Mo Yao	Myrrha
生化汤	**Sheng Hua Tang**	Engendering Transformation Decoction
	Dang Gui	Angelicae Sinensis Radix
	Chuan Xiong	Chuanxiong Rhizoma
	Tao Ren	Persicae Semen
	Pao Jiang	Zingiberis Rhizoma Praeparatum
	Zhi Gan Cao	Glycyrrhizae Radix Praeparata
圣愈汤	**Sheng Yu Tang**	Sagacious Cure Decoction
	Shu Di Huang	Rehmanniae Radix Praeparata
	Dang Gui	Angelicae Sinensis Radix
	Ren Shen	Ginseng Radix
	Huang Qi	Astragali Radix
	Tu Si Zi	Cuscutae Semen
	Sang Ji Sheng	Taxilli Herba
	Xu Duan	Dipsaci Radix
	Bai Shao	Paeoniae Radix Alba
寿胎丸	**Shou Tai Wan**	Fetal Longevity Pill
	Tu Si Zi	Cuscutae Semen
	Sang Ji Sheng	Taxilli Herba
	Xu Duan	Dipsaci Radix
	E Jiao	Asini Corii Colla
四物汤	**Si Wu Tang**	Four Substances Decoction
	Shu Di Huang	Rehmanniae Radix Praeparata
	Dang Gui	Angelicae Sinensis Radix
	Bai Shao	Paeoniae Radix Alba
	Chuan Xiong	Chuanxiong Rhizoma

胎元饮	**Tai Yuan Yin**	Fetal Origin Beverage
	Ren Shen	Ginseng Radix
	Bai Zhu	Atractylodis Macrocephalae Rhizoma
	Zhi Gan Cao	Glycyrrhizae Radix Praeparata
	Dang Gui	Angelicae Sinensis Radix
	Shu Di Huang	Rehmanniae Radix Praeparata
	Bai Shao	Paeoniae Radix Alba
	Chen Pi	Citri Reticulatae Pericarpium
	Du Zhong	Eucommiae Cortex
调肝汤	**Tiao Gan Tang**	Liver-Regulating Decoction
	Shan Yao	Dioscoreae Rhizoma
	Dang Gui	Angelicae Sinensis Radix
	Bai Shao	Paeoniae Radix Alba
	Shan Zhu Yu	Corni Fructus
	Ba Ji Tian	Morindae Officinalis Radix
	Gan Cao	Glycyrrhizae Radix
	E Jiao	Asini Corii Colla
	He Shou Wu	Polygoni Multiflori Radix
调经方	**Tiao Jing Fang**	Menstruation-Regulating Formula
	Dang Gui	Angelicae Sinensis Radix
	Bai Shao	Paeoniae Radix Alba
	Chai Hu	Bupleuri Radix
	Fu Ling	Poria
	Shan Yao	Dioscoreae Rhizoma
	Dang Shen	Codonopsis Radix
	Ba Ji Tian	Morindae Officinalis Radix
	Tu Si Zi	Cuscutae Semen
	Shu Di Huang	Rehmanniae Radix Praeparata
	Zhi Gan Cao	Glycyrrhizae Radix Praeparata
	Xiang Fu	Cyperi Rhizoma
调经后方	**Tiao Jing Hou Fang**	Menstruation-Regulating Later Formula
	Dang Gui	Angelicae Sinensis Radix
	Bai Shao	Paeoniae Radix Alba
	Chai Hu	Bupleuri Radix
	Fu Ling	Poria
	Shan Yao	Dioscoreae Rhizoma
	Dang Shen	Codonopsis Radix
	Ba Ji Tian	Morindae Officinalis Radix
	Tu Si Zi	Cuscutae Semen
	Shu Di Huang	Rehmanniae Radix Praeparata
	Zhi Gan Cao	Glycyrrhizae Radix Praeparata
	Wu Wei Zi	Schisandrae Fructus

调经前方	**Tiao Jing Qian Fang**	Menstruation-Regulating Early Formula
	Dang Gui	Angelicae Sinensis Radix
	Bai Shao	Paeoniae Radix Alba
	Shu Di Huang	Rehmanniae Radix Praeparata
	Chai Hu	Bupleuri Radix
	Fu Ling	Poria
	Bai Zhu	Atractylodis Macrocephalae Rhizoma
	Gan Cao	Glycyrrhizae Radix
	Chen Pi	Citri Reticulatae Pericarpium
	Dang Shen	Codonopsis Radix
	Suan Zao Ren	Ziziphi Spinosi Semen
调经行方	**Tiao Jing Xing Fang**	Regulate Menstrual Movement Formula
	Dang Gui	Angelicae Sinensis Radix
	Bai Shao	Paeoniae Radix Alba
	Shu Di Huang	Rehmanniae Radix Praeparata
	Chuan Xiong	Chuanxiong Rhizoma
	Niu Xi	Achyranthis Bidentatae Radix
	Dan Shen	Salviae Miltiorrhizae Radix
	Xiang Fu	Cyperi Rhizoma
	Gou Qi Zi	Lycii Fructus
	Xiao Hui Xiang	Foeniculi Fructus
	Yan Hu Suo	Corydalis Rhizoma
完带汤	**Wan Dai Tang**	Discharge-Ceasing Decoction
	Ren Shen	Ginseng Radix
	Shan Yao	Dioscoreae Rhizoma
	Bai Zhu	Atractylodis Macrocephalae Rhizoma
	Bai Shao	Paeoniae Radix Alba
	Chai Hu	Bupleuri Radix
	Cang Zhu	Atractylodis Rhizoma
	Chen Pi	Citri Reticulatae Pericarpium
	Che Qian Zi	Plantaginis Semen
	Jing Jie (Tan)	Schizonepetae Herba Carbonisatae
	Gan Cao	Glycyrrhizae Radix
温宫方	**Wen Gong Fang**	Warm the Uterus Formula
	Dang Gui	Angelicae Sinensis Radix
	Bai Shao	Paeoniae Radix Alba
	Chai Hu	Bupleuri Radix
	Fu Ling	Poria
	Shan Yao	Dioscoreae Rhizoma
	Dang Shen	Codonopsis Radix
	Ba Ji Tian	Morindae Officinalis Radix
	Tu Si Zi	Cuscutae Semen
	Shu Di Huang	Rehmanniae Radix Praeparata

	Zhi Gan Cao	Glycyrrhizae Radix Praeparata
	Rou Gui	Cinnamomi Cortex
温经汤		
	Wen Jìng Tang	Menses-Warming Decoction
	Ren Shen	Ginseng Radix
	Dang Gui	Angelicae Sinensis Radix
	Bai Shao	Paeoniae Radix Alba
	Chuan Xiong	Chuanxiong Rhizoma
	Niu Xi	Achyranthis Bidentatae Radix
	E Zhu	Curcumae Rhizoma
	Rou Gui	Cinnamomi Cortex
	Mu Dan Pi	Moutan Cortex
	Gan Cao	Glycyrrhizae Radix
温经行方	**Wen Jìng Xing Fang**	Warm the Menstrual Movement Formula
	Dang Gui	Angelicae Sinensis Radix
	Bai Shao	Paeoniae Radix Alba
	Shu Di Huang	Rehmanniae Radix Praeparata
	Chuan Xiong	Chuanxiong Rhizoma
	Niu Xi	Achyranthis Bidentatae Radix
	Dan Shen	Salviae Miltiorrhizae Radix
	Xiang Fu	Cyperi Rhizoma
	Gou Qi Zi	Lycii Fructus
	Xiao Hui Xiang	Foeniculi Fructus
	Gui Zhi	Cinnamomi Ramulus
香棱丸	**Xiang Leng Wan**	Cyperus and Sparganium Pill
	Mu Xiang	Aucklandiae Radix
	Ding Xiang	Caryophylli Flos
	Qing Pi	Citri Reticulatae Pericarpium Viride
	Chuan Lian Zi	Toosendan Fructus
	Zhi Ke	Aurantii Fructus
	San Leng	Sparganii Rhizoma
	E Zhu	Curcumae Rhizoma
	Xiao Hui Xiang	Foeniculi Fructus
小宫血方	**Xiao Gong Xue Fang**	Minor Uterine Blood Formula
	Dang Gui	Angelicae Sinensis Radix
	Bai Shao	Paeoniae Radix Alba
	Chai Hu	Bupleuri Radix
	Fu Ling	Poria
	Bai Zhu	Atractylodis Macrocephalae Rhizoma
	Gan Cao	Glycyrrhizae Radix
	Dang Shen	Codonopsis Radix
	Shan Zhu Yu	Corni Fructus
	San Qi	Notoginseng Radix

	Yi Mu Cao	Leonuri Herba
逍遥方	**Xiao Yao Fang**	Free Wanderer Formula
	Dang Gui	Angelicae Sinensis Radix
	Bai Shao	Paeoniae Radix Alba
	Chai Hu	Bupleuri Radix
	Fu Ling	Poria
	Bai Zhu	Atractylodis Macrocephalae Rhizoma
	Gan Cao	Glycyrrhizae Radix
逍遥散	**Xiao Yao San**	Free Wanderer Powder
	Dang Gui	Angelicae Sinensis Radix
	Bai Shao	Paeoniae Radix Alba
	Chai Hu	Bupleuri Radix
	Fu Ling	Poria
	Bai Zhu	Atractylodis Macrocephalae Rhizoma
	Gan Cao	Glycyrrhizae Radix
	Pao Jiang	Zingiberis Rhizoma Praeparatum
	Bo He	Menthae Herba
消症方	**Xiao Zheng Fang**	Concretion-Dispersing Formula
	Ji Xue Teng	Spatholobi Caulis
	San Leng	Sparganii Rhizoma
	E Zhu	Curcumae Rhizoma
	Mu Dan Pi	Moutan Cortex
	Dan Shen	Salviae Miltiorrhizae Radix
	Chi Shao	Paeoniae Radix Rubra
	Tao Ren	Persicae Semen
	Fu Ling	Poria
	Zhi Ke	Aurantii Fructus
	Bai Zhu	Atractylodis Macrocephalae Rhizoma
行经方	**Xing Jing Fang**	Promote Menstruation Formula
	Dang Gui	Angelicae Sinensis Radix
	Bai Shao	Paeoniae Radix Alba
	Shu Di Huang	Rehmanniae Radix Praeparata
	Chuan Xiong	Chuanxiong Rhizoma
	Niu Xi	Achyranthis Bidentatae Radix
	Dan Shen	Salviae Miltiorrhizae Radix
	Xiang Fu	Cyperi Rhizoma
	Gou Qi Zi	Lycii Fructus
血府逐瘀汤	**Xue Fu Zhu Yu Tang**	Blood Mansion Stasis-Dispelling Decoction
	Dang Gui	Angelicae Sinensis Radix
	Bai Shao	Paeoniae Radix Alba
	Sheng Di Huang	Rehmanniae Radix
	Chuan Xiong	Chuanxiong Rhizoma

	Chi Shao	Paeoniae Radix Rubra
	Tao Ren	Persicae Semen
	Hong Hua	Carthami Flos
	Chai Hu	Bupleuri Radix
	Zhi Ke	Aurantii Fructus
	Jie Geng	Platycodonis Radix
	Chuan Niu Xi	Cyathulae Radix
	Gan Cao	Glycyrrhizae Radix
养精方	**Yang Jing Fang**	Essence-Nourishing Formula
	Dang Gui	Angelicae Sinensis Radix
	Bai Shao	Paeoniae Radix Alba
	Shan Zhu Yu	Corni Fructus
	Shu Di Huang	Rehmanniae Radix Praeparata
	Shan Yao	Dioscoreae Rhizoma
	He Shou Wu	Polygoni Multiflori Radix
	Gou Qi Zi	Lycii Fructus
	Tu Si Zi	Cuscutae Semen
养胎方	**Yang Tai Fang**	Formula to Nourish the Fetus
	Tu Si Zi	Cuscutae Semen
	Shu Di Huang	Rehmanniae Radix Praeparata
	Bai Shao	Paeoniae Radix Alba
	Mai Dong	Ophiopogonis Radix
	Shan Zhu Yu	Corni Fructus
	Shan Yao	Dioscoreae Rhizoma
	Suan Zao Ren	Ziziphi Spinosi Semen
	Gan Cao	Glycyrrhizae Radix
右归丸	**You Gui Wan**	Right-Restoring Pill
	Shu Di Huang	Rehmanniae Radix Praeparata
	Shan Yao	Dioscoreae Rhizoma
	Shan Zhu Yu	Corni Fructus
	Lu Jiao Jiao	Cervi Cornus Gelatinum
	Gou Qi Zi	Lycii Fructus
	Tu Si Zi	Cuscutae Semen
	Du Zhong	Eucommiae Cortex
	Dang Gui	Angelicae Sinensis Radix
止崩方	**Zhi Beng Fang**	Check Flooding Formula
	Dang Shen	Codonopsis Radix
	Huang Qi	Astragali Radix
	Xu Duan	Dipsaci Radix
	Shan Zhu Yu	Corni Fructus
	Bai Zhu	Atractylodis Macrocephalae Rhizoma
	San Qi	Notoginseng Radix
	Yi Mu Cao	Leonuri Herba

止带汤	**Zhi Dai Tang**	Discharge-Checking Decoction
	Zhu Ling	Polyporus
	Fu Ling	Poria
	Che Qian Zi	Plantaginis Semen
	Ze Xie	Alismatis Rhizoma
植入汤	**Zhi Ru Tang**	Conception Decoction
	Shan Yao	Dioscoreae Rhizoma
	Shan Zhu Yu	Corni Fructus
	Shu Di Huang	Rehmanniae Radix Praeparata
	Fu Ling	Poria
	Mu Dan Pi	Moutan Cortex
	Ze Xie	Alismatis Rhizoma
	Bai Shao	Paeoniae Radix Alba
	Tu Si Zi	Cuscutae Semen
	Suan Zao Ren	Ziziphi Spinosi Semen
	Gan Cao	Glycyrrhizae Radix
治胎方	**Zhi Tai Fang**	Formula to Treat the Fetus
	Tu Si Zi	Cuscutae Semen
	Shu Di Huang	Rehmanniae Radix Praeparata
	Shan Zhu Yu	Corni Fructus
	Shan Yao	Dioscoreae Rhizoma
	Bai Shao	Paeoniae Radix Alba
	Mai Dong	Ophiopogonis Radix
	Suan Zao Ren	Ziziphi Spinosi Semen
	Gan Cao	Glycyrrhizae Radix
	Dang Shen	Codonopsis Radix
	Wu Wei Zi	Schisandrae Fructus
左归丸	**Zuo Gui Wan**	Left-Restoring [Kidney Yin] Pill
	Shu Di Huang	Rehmanniae Radix Praeparata
	Shan Yao	Dioscoreae Rhizoma
	Shan Zhu Yu	Corni Fructus
	Gou Qi Zi	Lycii Fructus
	Lu Jiao Jiao	Cervi Cornus Gelatinum
	Gui Ban Jiao	Testudinis Carapacis et Plastri Gelatinum
	Tu Si Zi	Cuscutae Semen
	Niu Xi	Achyranthis Bidentatae Radix

Modifications of Ding Jing Fang			
	Pathology or symptoms	Herbal modification	Formula name
Ding Jing Fang Dang gui Bai shao Chai hu Fu ling Shan yao Dang shen Ba ji tian Tu su zi Shu di	Stress	(+)Xiang fu	Tiao Jing Fang
	Ki Yang vacuity	(+)Rou gui	Wen Gong Fang
	KI Yin vacuity	(+)Shu zhu yu (+)Wu wei zi	Yang Luan Fang
	No ovulation	(+)Yin yang huo	Pai Luan Fang
	Tumors / mass	(−)Tu su zi (+)Gou qi zi	Fang Liu Yun Fang
	Poor sleep	(+)Wu wei zi	Tiao Jing Hou Fang
	Poor digestion	(−)Shu di (+)Shan zhu yu	Jian Pi Yun Fang
	Flatulence	(+)Chen pi	Ji Luan Fang

Modifications of Xiao Yao Fang			
	Pathology or symptoms	Herbal modification	Formula name
Xiao Yao Fang Dang gui Bai shao Chai hu Fu ling Bai zhu Gan cao	Stress	(+)Zhi ke (+)Dan shen (+)Shu di (+)Suan zao ren	Bei Luan Fang
	Before period	(+)Shu di (+)Chen pi (+)Dang shen (+)Suan zao ren	Tiao Jing Qian Fang
	During period with cramps	(+)Xiao hui xiang (+)Gui zhi (+)San qi (+)Yan hu suo	Jing Tong Fang
	During period with heavy bleeding and cold abdomen	(+)Dang shen (+)Shan zhu yu (+)San qi (+)Yi mu cao	Xiao Gong Xue Fang
	After period with stress, blood clots	(+)Shu di (+)Rou gui (+)Dang shen (+)Gou qi zi	Jing Hou Fang

Chinese Herbs for Gynecological Treatment

The following is a list of commonly used Chinese medicinals in gynecology. They are arranged according to how they are used in the protocols contained herein. Included are standard decoction dosages. However, the exact dose of any herb in any formula in this text is dependent on three factors:

1. The role the medicinal plays in the formula.
2. The patient's particular needs.
3. The characteristic range for the medicinal.

KIDNEY YIN SUPPLEMENTING MEDICINALS				
MEDICINAL	**NATURE & FLAVOR**	**CHANNELS ENTERED**	**ACTIONS**	**DOSAGE**
Bie Jia (Trionycis Carapax)	salty, slightly cold	Liver, Spleen	1. Enriches yin and subdues yang 2. Softens hardness and disperses binds	9-30g
Gui Ban (Testudinis Plastrum)	salty, sweet, cold	Heart, Kidney, Liver	1. Enriches yin and subdues yang 2. Boosts the kidney and fortifies the bones 3. Secures the menses and stanches bleeding 4. Nourishes the blood and supplements the heart	15-45g
Mo Han Lian (Ecliptae Herba)	sweet, sour, cool	Liver, Kidney	1. Enriches yin and boosts the kidney 2. Cools the blood and stanches bleeding	9-15g
Mai Dong (Ophiopogonis Radix)	sweet, slightly bitter, slightly cold	Heart, Lung, Spleen	1. Nourishes lung yin and clears lung heat 2. Boosts the stomach and engenders liquid 3. Clears the heart and eliminates vexation	9-15g
Nu Zhen Zi (Ligustri Lucidi Fructus)	Bitter, sweet, neutral	Liver, Kidney	1. Supplements liver and kidney yin, blackens the hair and beard and brightens the eyes	4.5-15g
Sang Ji Sheng (Taxilli Herba)	bitter, neutral	Kidney, Liver	1. Dispels wind-damp, boosts the liver and kidney, and strengthens sinew and bone 2. Quiets the fetus	12-40g
Sang Shen (Mori Fructus)	sweet, cold	Heart, Liver, Kidney	1. Enriches yin and supplements the blood 2. Engenders liquid and allays thirst 3. Moistens the intestines	6-15g
Sha Shen (Glehniae Radix)	bland, cool	Lung, Stomach	1. Nourishes yin, clears the lung, and transforms phlegm 2. Boosts the stomach and engenders liquid	9-15g
Shan Zhu Yu (Corni Fructus)	sour, slightly warm	Liver, Kidney	1. Supplements the liver and kidney 2. Secures essence and reduces urination 3. Constrains sweating and stems desertion 4. Secures the menses and stanches bleeding	4.5-9g
Zi He Che (Hominis Placenta)	sweet, salty, warm	Liver, Lung, Kidney	1. Warms the kidney and supplements essence 2. Promotes qi absorption and calms panting 3. Boosts qi and nourishes the blood	1.5-4.5g

KIDNEY YANG-SUPPLEMENTING MEDICINALS				
MEDICINAL	**NATURE & FLAVOR**	**CHANNELS ENTERED**	**ACTIONS**	**DOSAGE**
Ba Ji Tian (Morindae Officinalis Radix)	acrid, sweet, warm	Liver, Kidney	1. Supplements kidney yang 2. Strengthens sinew and bone and dispels wind-damp	9-15g
Bu Gu Zhi (Psoraleae Fructus)	acrid, bitter, very warm	Kidney, Spleen	1. Supplements the kidney and assists yang, secures essence and reduces urination 2. Warms the spleen and checks diarrhea 3. Promotes qi absorption and calms panting	3-9g
Du Zhong (Eucommiae Cortex)	sweet, slightly acrid, warm	Liver, Kidney	1. Supplements the liver and kidney; strengthens sinew and bone 2. Quiets the fetus	6-15g
Rou Cong Rong (Cistanches Herba)	sweet, salty, warm	Large Intestine, Kidney	1. Supplements kidney yang and boosts essence-blood 2. Moistens the intestines and frees the stool	9-21g
Sha Yuan Zi (Astragali Complanati Semen)	sweet, warm	Kidney, Liver	1. Supplements the kidney and secures essence 2. Nourishes the liver and brightens the eyes	6-15g
Suo Yang (Cynomorii Herba)	sweet, warm	Large Intestine, Kidney, Liver	1. Supplements kidney yang and boosts essence-blood 2. Moistens the intestines and frees the stool	4.5-15g
Tu Si Zi (Cuscutae Semen)	acrid, sweet, warm	Liver , Kidney	1. Supplements the kidney and secures essence 2. Nourishes the liver and brightens the eyes 3. Fortifies the spleen and checks diarrhea 4. Quiets the fetus	9-15g
Xu Duan (Dipsaci Radix)	bitter, acrid, slightly warm	Liver, Kidney	1. Supplements the liver and kidney, strengthens sinew and bone, treats injuries and joins bone 2. Stanches bleeding and quiets the fetus	6-24g
Yi Zhi Ren (Alpiniae Oxyphyllae Fructus)	acrid, warm	Kidney, Spleen	1. Warms the spleen, checks diarrhea, opens the stomach, and contains spittle 2. Warms the kidney, secures essence, and reduces urination	3-9g
Yin Yang Huo (Epimedii Herba)	acrid, sweet, warm	Liver, Kidney	1. Warms the kidney and invigorates yang 2. Strengthens sinew and bone 3. Dispels wind-damp	6-15g

SPLEEN QI-SUPPLEMENTING MEDICINALS				
MEDICINAL	**NATURE & FLAVOR**	**CHANNELS ENTERED**	**ACTIONS**	**DOSAGE**
Bai Zhu (Atractylodis Macrocephalae Rhizoma)	bitter, sweet, warm	Spleen, Stomach	1. Supplements qi and fortifies the spleen 2. Dries dampness and disinhibits water 3. Checks sweating 4. Quiets the fetus	4.5-15g
Da Zao (Jujubae Fructus)	sweet, warm	Spleen, Stomach	1. Supplements the center and boosts qi 2. Nourishes blood and quiets the spirit 3. Harmonizes the nature of medicinals	3-12 dates or 10-30g
Dang Shen (Codonopsis Radix)	sweet, neutral	Lung, Spleen	1. Supplements spleen and lung qi 2. Engenders liquid 3. Nourishes blood	9-30g
Fu Ling (Poria)	sweet, bland, neutral	Heart, Spleen, Lung, Kidney	1. Disinhibits water and percolates dampness 2. Fortifies the spleen 3. Quiets the spirit	9-15g
Gan Cao (Glycyrrhizae Radix)	sweet, neutral	All 12	1. Supplements heart and spleen qi 2. Dispels phlegm and relieves cough 3. Relaxes tension and relieves pain 4. Harmonizes the nature of medicinals 5. Clears heat and resolves toxin	4.5-9g
Huang Qi (Astragali Radix)	sweet, slightly warm	Lung, Spleen	1. Boosts qi and upbears yang 2. Boosts defense and secures the exterior 3. Disinhibits water and disperses swelling 4. Expresses toxin and engenders flesh	9-60g
Ren Shen (Ginseng Radix)	sweet, slightly bitter, slightly warm	Lung, Spleen	1. Greatly supplements original qi 2. Supplements lung qi 3. Supplements the spleen 4. Engenders liquid 5. Quiets the spirit and improves mental faculties	1-9g
Shan Yao (Dioscoreae Rhizoma)	sweet, neutral	Kidney, Lung, Spleen	1. Supplements the spleen, boosts qi, and nourishes yin 2. Supplements the lung and kidney 3. Secures essence and checks vaginal discharge	9-30g

BLOOD SUPPLEMENTING MEDICINALS				
MEDICINAL	**NATURE & FLAVOR**	**CHANNELS ENTERED**	**ACTIONS**	**DOSAGE**
Bai Shao (Paeoniae Radix Alba)	bitter, sour, cool	Liver, Spleen	1. Nourishes the blood and regulates menstruation 2. Emolliates the liver and relieves pain 3. Calms liver yang 4. Constrains yin and checks sweating	4.5-30g
Dang Gui (Angelicae Sinensis Radix)	sweet, acrid, warm	Heart, Liver, Spleen	1. Supplements the blood 2. Quickens the blood and relieves pain 3. Moistens the intestines	4.5-15g

Gou Qi Zi (Lycii Fructus)	sweet, neutral	Liver, Lung, Kidney	1. Supplements the liver and kidney, brightens the eyes and moistens the lung	6-18g
He Shou Wu (Polygoni Multiflori Radix)	bitter, sweet, astringent, slightly warm	Liver, Kidney	1. Supplements essence-blood (processed form) 2. Moistens the intestines and frees the stool (raw form) 3. Resolves toxin 4. Interrupts malaria	9-30g
Huang Jing (Polygonati Rhizoma)	sweet, neutral	Kidney, Lung, Spleen	1. Enriches the kidney and moistens the lung 2. Supplements kidney essence and slows aging 3. Supplements the spleen and boosts qi	9-21g
Long Yan Rou (Longan Arillus)	sweet, warm	Heart, Spleen	1. Supplements the heart and spleen, nourishes the blood, and quiets the spirit	6-15g

SECURING & ASTRINGING MEDICINALS

MEDICINAL	NATURE & FLAVOR	CHANNELS ENTERED	ACTIONS	DOSAGE
Jin Ying Zi (Rosae Laevigatae Fructus)	sour, astringent, neutral	Bladder, Kidney, Large Intestine	1. Secures essence, reduces urine, and checks vaginal discharge 2. Astringes the intestines and checks diarrhea	4.5-9g
Qian Shi (Euryales Semen)	sweet, astringent, neutral	Kidney, Spleen	1. Boosts the kidney and secures essence 2. Fortifies the spleen and checks diarrhea 3. Eliminates dampness and checks discharge	9-15g

BLOOD-QUICKENING MEDICINALS

MEDICINAL	NATURE & FLAVOR	CHANNELS ENTERED	ACTIONS	DOSAGE
Chi Shao (Paeoniae Radix Rubra)	sour, bitter, slightly cold	Liver, Spleen	1. Clears heat and cools the blood 2. Quickens the blood and transforms stasis	4.5-9g
Chuan Shan Jia (Manis Squama)	salty, cool	Liver, Stomach	1. Quickens the blood, disperses concretions, and frees the channels/menses 2. Promotes lactation 3. Disperses swelling and expels pus	3-9g
Chuan Xiong (Chuanxiong Rhizoma)	acrid, warm	Liver, Gallbladder, Pericardium	1. Quickens the blood and moves qi 2. Dispels wind and relieves pain	3-6g
Dan Shen (Salviae Miltiorrhizae Radix)	bitter, slightly cold	Heart, Pericardium, Liver	1. Quickens the blood and regulates menstruation 2. Cools the blood, clears heart, eliminates vexation, and quiets the spirit 3. Disperses welling-abscesses	6-15g

E Zhu (Curcumae Rhizoma)	bitter, acrid, warm	Liver, Spleen	1. Breaks blood and dispels stasis; moves qi and relieves pain 2. Moves qi and disperses accumulations	3-9g
Hong Hua (Carthami Flos)	acrid, warm	Heart, Liver	1. Quickens blood and frees the menses 2. Dispels stasis and relieves pain	3-9g 0.9-1.5g if used to harmonize the blood
Ji Xue Teng (Spatholobi Caulis)	bitter, sweet, warm	Heart, Liver, Spleen	1. Quickens the blood, supplements the blood, and regulates menstruation 2. Soothes the sinews and quickens the network vessels	9-15g
Lu Lu Tong (Liquidambaris Fructus)	bitter, neutral	Liver, Stomach	1. Moves qi and blood and frees the channels 2. Disinhibits urination	3-9g
Mo Yao (Myrrha)	bitter, neutral	Heart, Liver, Spleen	1. Quickens the blood and relieves pain, disperses swelling and engenders flesh	3-12g
Niu Xi (Achyranthis Bidentatae Radix)	bitter, sour, neutral	Liver, Kidney	1. Quickens the blood and frees menstruation 2. Supplements the liver and kidney and strengthens sinews and bones 3. Disinhibits urine and frees strangury 4. Conducts fire and blood downward	9-15g
Ru Xiang (Olibanum)	acrid, bitter, warm	Spleen, Heart, Liver	1. Quickens the blood, moves qi, relieves pain, and disperses swelling 2. Dispels putridity and engenders flesh	3-9g
San Leng (Sparganii Rhizoma)	bitter, acrid, neutral	Liver, Spleen	1. Breaks blood and moves qi; disperses accumulations and relieves pain	3-9g
Tao Ren (Persicae Semen)	bitter, sweet, neutral	Heart, Large Intestine, Liver, Lung	1. Quickens the blood and transforms stasis 2. Moistens the intestines and frees the stool	4.5-9g
Wang Bu Liu Xing (Vaccariae Semen)	bitter, neutral	Liver, Stomach	1. Quickens the blood and frees menstruation 2. Promotes lactation 3. Disinhibits urine and frees strangury	3-9g
Wu Ling Zhi (Trogopteri Feces)	bitter, sweet, warm	Liver, Spleen	1. Quickens the blood and relieves pain 2. Transforms stasis and stanches bleeding	3-9g
Yan Hu Suo (Corydalis Rhizoma)	acrid, bitter, warm	Heart, Liver, Lung, Stomach	1. Quickens the blood, moves qi, and relieves pain	4.5-12g
Yi Mu Cao (Leonuri Herba)	acrid, bitter, slightly cold	Heart, Liver, Bladder	1. Quickens the blood and regulates menstruation 2. Disinhibits water and disperses swelling	9-60g

			1. Quickens the blood and relieves pain, moves qi and resolves depression	
Yu Jin (Curcumae Radix)	acrid, bitter, cool	Heart, Lung, Liver	2. Clears the heart and downbears phlegm 3. Cools the blood and downbears qi 4. Disinhibits the gallbladder and abates jaundice	4.5-9g

QI-RECTIFYING MEDICINALS

MEDICINAL	NATURE & FLAVOR	CHANNELS ENTERED	ACTIONS	DOSAGE
Chen Pi (Citri Reticulatae Pericarpium)	acrid, bitter, warm, aromatic	Lung, Spleen, Stomach	1. Moves qi and fortifies the spleen 2. Dries dampness and transforms phlegm	3-9g
Li Zhi He (Litchi Semen)	sweet, astringent, warm	Liver, Stomach	1. Moves qi and disperses binds 2. Disperses cold and relieves pain	6-15g
Mu Xiang (Aucklandiae Radix)	acrid, bitter, warm	Gallbladder, Large Intestine, Spleen, Stomach	1. Moves qi, regulates the center, and relieves pain	1.5-3g
Qing Pi (Citri Reticulatae Pericarpium Viride)	bitter, acrid, warm	Gallbladder, Liver, Stomach	1. Courses the liver and breaks qi 2. Disperses accumulations and transforms stagnation	3-9g
Wu Yao (Linderae Radix)	acrid, warm	Bladder, Kidney, Lung, Spleen	1. Moves qi and relieves pain 2. Warms the kidney and disperses cold	3-9g
Xiang Fu (Cyperi Rhizoma)	acrid, slightly bitter, slightly sweet, neutral	Liver, Spleen, Triple Burner	1. Courses the liver and rectifies qi 2. Regulates menstruation and relieves pain	6-12g
Zhi Ke (Aurantii Fructus)	bitter, cool	Spleen, Stomach	1. Breaks qi and eliminates glomus 2. Transforms phlegm and disperses accumulations	3-15g

SPIRIT-QUIETING MEDICINALS

MEDICINAL	NATURE & FLAVOR	CHANNELS ENTERED	ACTIONS	DOSAGE
Bai Zi Ren (Platycladi Semen)	sweet, neutral	Heart, Kidney, Large Intestine, Spleen	1. Nourishes the heart and quiets the spirit 2. Moistens the intestines and frees the stool	6-18g
Long Gu (Mastodi Ossis Fossilia)	sweet, astringent, neutral	Heart, Kidney, Liver	1. Settles fright and quiets the spirit 2. Calms the liver and subdues yang 3. Contracts and astringes	15-30g
Mu Li (Ostreae Concha)	salty, astringent, cool	Liver, Kidney	1. Calms the liver and subdues yang 2. Softens hardness and disperses binds 3. Quiets the spirit 4. Astringes and secures	15-30g

Shu Di Huang (Rehmanniae Radix Praeparata)	sweet, slightly warm	Heart, Kidney, Liver	1. Supplements the blood 2. Enriches yin 3. Boosts essence and replenishes marrow	9-30g
Suan Zao Ren (Ziziphi Spinosi Semen)	sweet, neutral	Gallbladder, Heart, Liver, Spleen	1. Nourishes the heart and quiets the spirit 2. Constrains sweat	9-18g
Wu Wei Zi (Schisandrae Fructus)	sour, warm	Large Intestine, Liver, Lung, Spleen	1. Constrains the lung and enriches the kidney 2. Engenders liquid and constrains sweating 3. Astringes essence and checks diarrhea 4. Quiets the heart and spirit	1.5-9g
Yuan Zhi (Polygalae Radix)	bitter, acrid, slightly warm	Heart, Lung	1. Quiets the spirit and sharpens the mind 2. Transforms phlegm and opens the orifices 3. Disperses welling-abscesses and swelling	3-9g

BLOOD-STANCHING MEDICINALS				
MEDICINAL	**NATURE & FLAVOR**	**CHANNELS ENTERED**	**ACTIONS**	**DOSAGE**
Ai Ye (Artemisiae Argyi Folium)	bitter, acrid, warm	Spleen, Liver, Kidney	1. Warms the channels/menses and stanches bleeding 2. Disperses cold and regulates menstruation 3. Quiets the fetus	3-9g
Ce Bai Ye (Platycladi Cacumen)	bitter, astringent, slightly cold	Heart, Liver, Large Intestine	1. Cools the blood and stanches bleeding 2. Transforms phlegm and relieves cough	6-15g
Di Yu (Sanguisorbae Radix)	bitter, sour, slightly cold	Liver, Large Intestine, Stomach	1. Cools the blood and stanches bleeding 2. Resolves toxin and closes sores	6-15g
E Jiao (Asini Corii Colla)	sweet, neutral	Kidney, Liver, Lung	1. Supplements the blood 2. Stanches bleeding 3. Enriches yin and moistens dryness	3-15g
Huai Hua (Sophorae Flos)	bitter, cool	Liver, Large Intestine	1. Cools the blood and stanches bleeding 2. Clears liver fire	6-15g
Pu Huang (Typhae Pollen)	sweet, acrid, neutral	Liver, Heart, Spleen	1. Transforms stasis and stanches bleeding 2. Disinhibits urination and frees strangury	4.5-12g
San Qi (Notoginseng Radix)	sweet, slightly bitter, warm	Liver, Stomach, Large Intestine	1. Transforms stasis and stanches bleeding 2. Quickens the blood and settles pain	1-3g
Xue Yu Tan (Crinis Carbonisatus)	bitter, neutral	Heart, Liver, Kidney	1. Stanches bleeding and disperses stasis 2. Transforms stasis and disinhibits urination	1.5-9g

PRECIPITATING MEDICINAL				
MEDICINAL	**NATURE & FLAVOR**	**CHANNELS ENTERED**	**ACTIONS**	**DOSAGE**
Da Huang (Rhei Radix et Rhizoma)	bitter, cold	Heart, Large Intestine, Liver, Stomach	1. Drains and precipitates to attack accumulations 2. Drains fire and stanches bleeding 3. Clears heat and resolves toxin 4. Quickens the blood	3-15g

HEAT-CLEARING, FIRE-DRAINING MEDICINALS				
MEDICINAL	**NATURE & FLAVOR**	**CHANNELS ENTERED**	**ACTIONS**	**DOSAGE**
Dan Zhu Ye (Lophatheri Herba)	sweet, bland, cold	Heart, Small Intestine, Stomach	1. Clears heat and eliminates vexation 2. Frees urine	6-9g
Lu Gen (Phragmitis Rhizoma)	sweet, cold	Lung, Stomach	1. Clears heat and engenders liquid 2. Eliminates vexation and checks vomiting	6-30g
Shi Gao (Gypsum Fibrosum)	sweet, acrid, very cold	Lung, Stomach	1. Clears heat and drains fire, eliminates vexation and allays thirst 2. Absorbs dampness, closes sores, and engenders flesh	15-60g
Zhi Mu (Anemarrhenae Rhizoma)	bitter, sweet, cold	Lung, Stomach, Kidney	1. Clears heat and drains fire 2. Enriches yin and moistens dryness	6-12g
Zhi Zi (Gardeniae Fructus)	bitter, cold	Heart, Liver, Lung, Stomach, Triple Burner	1. Drains fire and eliminates vexation 2. Clears heat and disinhibits dampness 3. Cools the blood and resolves toxin 4. Disperses swelling and relieves pain	3-12g

HEAT-CLEARING, DAMPNESS-DRYING MEDICINALS				
MEDICINAL	**NATURE & FLAVOR**	**CHANNELS ENTERED**	**ACTIONS**	**DOSAGE**
Huang Bai (Phellodendri Cortex)	bitter, cold	Kidney, Bladder	1. Clears heat and dries dampness 2. Drains fire and resolves toxin 3. Abates vacuity heat	3-12g
Huang Lian (Coptidis Rhizoma)	bitter, cold	Heart, Large Intestine, Liver, Stomach	1. Clears heat and dries dampness 2. Drains fire and resolves toxin	1.5-9g
Huang Qin (Scutellariae Radix)	bitter, cold	Gallbladder, Large Intestine, Lung, Stomach	1. Clears heat and dries dampness 2. Drains fire and resolves toxin 3. Cools the blood and stanches bleeding 4. Eliminates heat to quiet the fetus	6-15g

HEAT-CLEARING, TOXIN-RESOLVING MEDICINALS

MEDICINAL	NATURE & FLAVOR	CHANNELS ENTERED	ACTIONS	DOSAGE
Bai Hua She She Cao (Oldenlandiae Diffusae Herba)	bitter, sweet, cold	Liver, Stomach, Large Intestine	1. Clears heat and resolves toxin 2. Disinhibits urine and frees strangury	15-60g
Bai Tou Weng (Pulsatillae Radix)	bitter, cold	Large Intestine, Stomach	1. Clears heat, resolves toxin, and cools the blood 2. Interrupts malaria	6-15g
Ban Zhi Lian (Scutellariae Barbatae Herba)	sweet, bland, slightly cold	Heart, Lung, Small Intestine	1. Clears heat and resolves toxin 2. Disinhibits water and disperses swelling	3-15g
Jin Yin Hua (Lonicerae Flos)	sweet, cold	Large Intestine, Lung, Stomach	1. Clears heat and resolves toxin 2. Disperses wind-heat 3. Checks dysentery 4. Treats painful swollen throat due to wind-heat or heat toxin	6-15g
Lian Qiao (Forsythiae Fructus)	bitter, slightly acrid, cool	Heart, Liver, Gallbladder	1. Clears heat and resolves toxin 2. Disperses welling-abscesses and binds	3-15g
Pu Gong Ying (Taraxaci Herba)	bitter, sweet, cold	Liver, Stomach	1. Clears heat and resolves toxin; disperses welling-abscesses and binds 2. Clears and disinhibits damp-heat; disinhibits water and frees strangury	9-30g
Yu Xing Cao (Houttuyniae Herba)	acrid, cool	Large Intestine, Lung	1. Clears heat and resolves toxin; disperses welling-abscesses and expels pus 2. Clears heat and resolves toxin; disinhibits urine and frees strangury	15-60g
Zi Hua Di Ding (Violae Herba)	acrid, bitter, cold	Heart, Liver	1. Clears heat and resolves toxin 2. Resolves snake venom	9-15g

HEAT-CLEARING, BLOOD-COOLING MEDICINALS

MEDICINAL	NATURE & FLAVOR	CHANNELS ENTERED	ACTIONS	DOSAGE
Di Gu Pi (Lycii Cortex)	sweet, cold	Lung, Liver, Kidney	1. Abates vacuity fire and steaming bone 2. Drains lung fire 3. Cools the blood	6-15g
Mu Dan Pi (Moutan Cortex)	acrid, bitter, cool	Heart, Liver, Kidney	1. Clears heat and cools the blood 2. Quickens the blood and transforms stasis 3. Abates vacuity fire	6-12g
Sheng Di Huang (Rehmanniae Radix)	sweet, bitter, cold	Heart, Kidney, Liver	1. Clears heat 2. Cools the blood 3. Nourishes yin and engenders liquid	9-30g

| Xuan Shen (Scrophulariae Radix) | salty, sweet, bitter, cold | Kidney, Lung, Stomach | 1. Clears heat and cools the blood
2. Drains fire and resolves toxin
3. Enriches yin and downbears fire | 9-30g |

HEAT-CLEARING, SUMMERHEAT-RESOLVING MEDICINAL

MEDICINAL	NATURE & FLAVOR	CHANNELS ENTERED	ACTIONS	DOSAGE
Qing Hao (Artemisiae Annuae Herba)	bitter, cold	Kidney, Liver, Gallbladder	1. Clears vacuity heat 2. Eliminates steaming bone 3. Resolves summerheat 4. Interrupts malaria	3-9g

COOL PHLEGM-TRANSFORMING MEDICINALS

MEDICINAL	NATURE & FLAVOR	CHANNELS ENTERED	ACTIONS	DOSAGE
Chuan Bei Mu (Fritillariae Cirrhosae Bulbus)	bitter, sweet, slightly cold	Heart, Lung	1. Clears heat and transforms phlegm; moistens the lung and relieves cough 2. Disperses phlegm and binds	3-12g
Dan Xing (Arisaema cum Bile)	bitter, cool	Liver, Lung, Spleen	1. Clears heat and transforms phlegm 2. Extinguishes wind and checks tetany	3-6g
Gua Lou Pi (Trichosanthis Pericarpium)	sweet, cold	Large Intestine, Lung, Stomach	1. Clears heat and transforms phlegm, loosens the chest and disperses binds	9-12g
Hai Zao (Sargassum)	bitter, salty, cold	Kidney, Liver, Lung, Stomach	1. Disperses phlegm and softens hardness 2. Disinhibits water and disperses swelling	4.5-15g
Jie Geng (Platycodonis Radix)	bitter, acrid, neutral	Lung	1. Diffuses the lung and transforms phlegm 2. Disinhibits the throat 3. Expels pus	3-9g
Kun Bu (Laminariae/Eckloniae Thallus)	salty, cold	Kidney, Liver, Stomach	1. Disperses phlegm and softens hardness 2. Disinhibits water and disperses swelling	4.5-15g
Tian Hua Fen (Trichosanthis Radix)	bitter, slightly sweet, cold	Lung, Stomach	1. Clears heat and engenders liquid 2. Clears the lung and moistens dryness 3. Resolves toxin and disperses welling-abscesses	9-15g
Zhu Ru (Bambusae Caulis in Taenia)	sweet, slightly cold	Lung, Stomach, Gallbladder	1. Clears heat and transforms phlegm 2. Clears the stomach and checks vomiting	4.5-9g

WARM PHLEGM-TRANSFORMING MEDICINAL

MEDICINAL	NATURE & FLAVOR	CHANNELS ENTERED	ACTIONS	DOSAGE
Ban Xia (Pinelliae Rhizoma)	acrid, warm, toxic	Lung, Spleen, Stomach	1. Dries dampness and transforms phlegm 2. Downbears counterflow and checks vomiting 3. Disperses swelling and relieves pain	4.5-9g

AROMATIC, DAMPNESS-TRANSFORMING MEDICINALS

MEDICINAL	NATURE & FLAVOR	CHANNELS ENTERED	ACTIONS	DOSAGE
Cang Zhu (Atractylodis Rhizoma)	acrid, bitter, warm, aromatic	Spleen, Stomach	1. Dries dampness and fortifies the spleen 2. Dispels wind-damp impediment 3. Treats external contraction of wind-cold with dampness	4.5-9g
Hou Po (Magnoliae Officinalis Cortex)	bitter, acrid, warm, aromatic	Large Intestine, Lung, Spleen, Stomach	1. Moves qi and dries dampness 2. Disperses accumulations 3. Calms panting	3-9g
Huo Xiang (Pogostemonis Herba)	acrid, slightly warm	Lung, Spleen, Stomach	1. Transforms dampness 2. Resolves summerheat 3. Checks vomiting	3-9g
Sha Ren (Amomi Fructus)	acrid, aromatic, warm	Spleen, Stomach	1. Transforms dampness and moves qi 2. Warms the center, checks vomiting, and checks diarrhea 3. Quiets the fetus	1.5-6g

DAMPNESS-PERCOLATING MEDICINALS

MEDICINAL	NATURE & FLAVOR	CHANNELS ENTERED	ACTIONS	DOSAGE
Bi Xie (Dioscoreae Hypoglaucae Rhizoma)	bitter, neutral	Bladder, Liver, Stomach	1. Disinhibits dampness and dispels turbidity 2. Dispels wind and eliminates dampness	9-15g
Che Qian Zi (Plantaginis Semen)	sweet, cold	Bladder, Kidney, Liver, Lung	1. Disinhibits water and frees strangury 2. Percolates dampness and checks diarrhea 3. Clears the liver and brightens the eyes 4. Clears the lung and transforms phlegm	4.5-9g
Dong Gua Zi (Benincasae Semen)	sweet, cold	Lung, Stomach, Large Intestine, Small Intestine	1. Clears heat and transforms phlegm, expels pus and disperses welling-abscesses 2. Clears heat and disinhibits dampness	3-12g
Mu Tong (Akebiae Trifoliatae Caulis)	bitter, cool	Bladder, Heart, Small Intestine	1. Disinhibits urine, frees strangury, and disperses swelling 2. Clears heart fire 3. Frees menstruation and promotes lactation	3-9g
Qu Mai (Dianthi Herba)	bitter, cold	Bladder, Heart, Small Intestine	1. Disinhibits urine and frees strangury 2. Quickens the blood and frees menstruation	6-12g

Tong Cao (Tetrapanacis Medulla)	sweet, bland, slightly cold	Lung, Stomach	1. Clears heat and disinhibits dampness 2. Frees qi and promotes lactation	2-4.5g
Yi Yi Ren (Coicis Semen)	sweet, bland, slightly cold	Spleen, Lung, Kidney	1. Fortifies the spleen, disinhibits water and percolates dampness 2. Eliminates impediment 3. Clears heat and expels pus	9-30g
Yin Chen (Artemisiae Scopariae Herba)	bitter, slightly cold	Liver, Spleen, Gallbladder, Stomach	1. Disinhibits the gallbladder and abates jaundice 2. Clears damp-heat	9-30g
Ze Xie (Alismatis Rhizoma)	sweet, bland, cold	Kidney, Bladder	1. Disinhibits water and percolates dampness, drains heat 2. Drains bladder heat and kidney channel vacuity fire	6-15g
Zhu Ling (Polyporus)	sweet, bland, slightly cool	Spleen, Kidney, Bladder	1. Disinhibits water and percolates dampness	6-15g

WIND-DAMP–DISPELLING MEDICINALS

MEDICINAL	NATURE & FLAVOR	CHANNELS ENTERED	ACTIONS	DOSAGE
Du Huo (Angelicae Pubescentis Radix)	bitter, acrid, warm	Kidney, Bladder	1. Dispels wind-damp and relieves impediment pain 2. Resolves the exterior 3. Also used for lesser yin headache and damp, itchy skin	3-9g
Sang Zhi (Mori Ramulus)	bitter, neutral	Liver	1. Dispels wind, frees the network vessels, and disinhibits the joints	9-15g

INTERIOR-WARMING MEDICINALS

MEDICINAL	NATURE & FLAVOR	CHANNELS ENTERED	ACTIONS	DOSAGE
Gan Jiang (Zingiberis Rhizoma)	acrid, hot	Heart, Lung, Spleen, Stomach	1. Warms the center and disperses cold 2. Returns yang and frees the pulse 3. Warms the lung and transforms rheum	3-12g
Rou Gui (Cinnamomi Cortex)	acrid, sweet, hot	Heart, Kidney, Liver, Spleen	1. Supplements fire and assists yang 2. Disperses cold and relieves pain 3. Warms the channels/menses and frees the vessels	1.5-4.5g
Wu Zhu Yu (Evodiae Fructus)	acrid, bitter, hot, slightly toxic	Liver, Spleen, Stomach	1. Disperses cold and relieves pain 2. Warms the center and checks vomiting 3. Assists yang and checks diarrhea	1.5-4.5g
Xiao Hui Xiang (Foeniculi Fructus)	acrid, warm	Liver, Kidney, Spleen, Stomach	1. Disperses cold and relieves pain 2. Rectifies qi and harmonizes the center	3-9g

WIND-EXTINGUISHING MEDICINALS

MEDICINAL	NATURE & FLAVOR	CHANNELS ENTERED	ACTIONS	DOSAGE
Gou Teng (Uncariae Ramulus cum Uncis)	sweet, slightly cold	Pericardium, Liver	1. Extinguishes wind and checks tetany 2. Clears heat and calms the liver	6-15g
Tian Ma (Gastrodiae Rhizoma)	sweet, neutral	Liver	1. Extinguishes wind and checks tetany 2. Calms liver yang 3. Dispels wind and frees the network vessels, and relieves pain	3-9g

WARM ACRID EXTERIOR-RESOLVING MEDICINALS

MEDICINAL	NATURE & FLAVOR	CHANNELS ENTERED	ACTIONS	DOSAGE
Bai Zhi (Angelicae Dahuricae Radix)	acrid, warm	Lung, Stomach	1. Resolves the exterior and disperses wind 2. Dispels wind and relieves pain 3. Disperses swelling and expels pus	3-9g
Fang Feng (Saposhnikoviae Radix)	sweet, slightly warm	Bladder, Liver, Spleen	1. Dispels wind and resolves the exterior 2. Overcomes dampness and relieves pain 3. Resolves tetany 4. Also used for patterns of liver qi exploiting the spleen or liver-stomach disharmony, manifesting in diarrhea with abdominal pain that is relieved by defecation	3-9g
Gui Zhi (Cinnamomi Ramulus)	acrid, sweet, warm	Heart, Lung, Bladder	1. Promotes sweating and resolves the exterior 2. Warms and frees the channels 3. Warms and assists yang qi 4. Treats yang vacuity and congealing cold in the kidney and bladder with impaired qi transformation	3-9g
Jing Jie Sui (Schizonepetae Flos)	acrid, aromatic, slightly warm	Lung, Liver	1. Dispels wind and resolves the exterior 2. Out-thrusts papules and relieves itching 3. Disperses sores 4. Stanches bleeding	3-9g
Qiang Huo (Notopterygii Rhizoma et Radix)	acrid, bitter, aromatic, warm	Bladder, Kidney	1. Disperses wind-cold 2. Dispels wind-damp and relieves pain	6-15g
Sheng Jiang (Zingiberis Rhizoma Recens)	acrid, warm	Lung, Spleen, Stomach	1. Promotes sweating and resolves the exterior 2. Warms the center and checks vomiting 3. Warms the lung and relieves cough	3-9g
Xi Xin (Asari Radix)	acrid, warm	Lung, Kidney	1. Dispels wind and disperses cold 2. Relieves pain 3. Warms the lung and transforms rheum 4. Opens the orifices	1-3g

COOL ACRID EXTERIOR-RESOLVING MEDICINALS

MEDICINAL	NATURE & FLAVOR	CHANNELS ENTERED	ACTIONS	DOSAGE
Bo He (Menthae Herba)	acrid, aromatic, cool	Lung, Liver	1. Disperses wind-heat 2. Clears and disinhibits the head and eyes 3. Disinhibits the throat 4. Outthrusts papules 5. Courses the liver and moves qi	1.5-6g
Chai Hu (Bupleuri Radix)	acrid, bitter, cool	Gallbladder, Liver, Pericardium, Triple Burner	1. Harmonizes and resolves the exterior and abates heat 2. Courses the liver and resolves depression 3. Uplifts yang qi	3-9g
Ju Hua (Chrysanthemi Flos)	sweet, bitter, slightly cold	Liver, Lung	1. Disperses wind-heat 2. Clears the liver and drains fire; brightens the eyes 3. Calms liver yang 4. Clears heat and resolves toxin	4.5-15g
Niu Bang Zi (Arctii Fructus)	Acrid, bitter, cold	Lung, Stomach	1. Disperses wind-heat and disinhibits the throat 2. Outthrusts papules 3. Resolves toxin and disperses swelling	3-9g
Sang Ye (Mori Folium)	sweet, bitter, slightly cold	Liver, Lung	1. Disperses wind-heat 2. Clears the liver and brightens the eyes	4.5-15g

COUGH-RELIEVING MEDICINALS

MEDICINAL	NATURE & FLAVOR	CHANNELS ENTERED	ACTIONS	DOSAGE
Kuan Dong Hua (Farfarae Flos)	acrid, warm	Lung	1. Moistens the lung, transforms phlegm, and relieves cough	4.5-9g
Xing Ren (Armeniacae Semen)	bitter, slightly warm, slightly toxic	Large Intestine, Lung	1. Relieves cough and calms panting 2. Moistens the intestines and frees the stool	3-9g
Zi Wan (Asteris Radix)	acrid, bitter, slightly warm	Lung	1. Moistens the lung, transforms phlegm, and relieves cough	5-9g

FOOD-DISPERSING MEDICINALS

MEDICINAL	NATURE & FLAVOR	CHANNELS ENTERED	ACTIONS	DOSAGE
Gu Ya (Setariae Fructus Germinatus)	sweet, neutral	Spleen, Stomach	1. Disperses food and harmonizes the center 2. Fortifies the spleen and opens the stomach	9-15g
Mai Ya (Hordei Fructus Germinatus)	sweet, neutral	Liver, Spleen, Stomach	1. Disperses food and harmonizes the center 2. Terminates lactation 3. Courses the liver and resolves depression	6-15g
Shan Zha (Crataegi Fructus)	sour, sweet, slightly warm	Liver, Spleen, Stomach	1. Disperses food and transforms accumulation 2. Quickens the blood and disperses stasis 3. Moves qi	9-15g

TCM Nutrition

China has a long history of promoting life through food therapy. Chinese culture established a complete theory of food therapy that is based on Chinese medicine. In the modern day, knowledge about nutrition is integrated into food therapy as well.

Below are some dietary guidelines for a variety of gynecological diseases:

Outline:
Advanced Menstruation
Delayed Menstruation
Irregular Menstruation
Profuse Menstruation (Menorrhagia)
Menstrual Block (Amenorrhea)
Painful Menstruation
Abnormal Vaginal Discharge
Threatened Abortion and Habitual Miscarriage
Perimenopausal Symptoms

Food Therapy

A. Advanced Menstruation

Congee with celery and beef (for blood heat)
Ingredients: Celery 120g, rice 100g, cooked beef 25g
Actions: Clears heat, cools the blood, and supplements vacuity

Stir-fried chives with lamb's liver (for liver and kidney vacuity)
Ingredients: Chives 150g, lamb's liver 200g
Actions: Nourishes the liver and warms the kidney

B. Delayed Menstruation

Donkey hide gelatin beef stew
Ingredients: Donkey hide gelatin (E Jiao) 15g, beef 150g, rice wine 20g, fresh ginger (appropriate amount)
Actions: Supplements yang, nourishes the blood, warms the center

Motherwort jujube tea (for vacuity cold)
Ingredients: Motherwort (Yi Mu Cao) 20g, jujube (Hong Zao) 100g, red sugar 20g
Actions: Warms the channels, nourishes the blood, warms the center and fortifies the spleen

Fermented black beans lamb stew (for cold congealing)
Ingredients: Fermented black beans 100g, lamb 500g, fresh ginger (appropriate amount)
Actions: Warms the channels and disperses cold
(This stew is taken daily for 3 to 5 days, starting 10 days before menstruation.)

C. Irregular Menstruation

1. Motherwort pork stew
Ingredients: Motherwort (Yi Mu Cao) 15g, lean pork 150g
Actions: Supplements the center, boosts qi, quickens the blood, regulates menstruation, and nourishes the blood

2. Ginseng astragalus lotus seed congee
Ingredients: Rice 60g, ginseng (Ren Shen) 5g, astragalus (Huang Qi) 30g, jujube (Hong Zao) 15 pieces, lotus seed (Lian Zi) 15g
Actions: Supplements qi, warms the center, and regulates menstruation

D. Profuse Menstruation (Menorrhagia)

1. Oyster shell calcium pork stew
Ingredients: Fresh oyster shell (Mu Li) 250g, lean pork 100g
Actions: Nourishes yin, boosts qi, and nourishes the blood

2. Cuttlefish bone chicken stew
Ingredients: Chicken 200g, cuttlefish bone (Wu Zei Gu) 30g (broken into powder), Chinese angelica (Dang Gui) 30g
Actions: Astringes to stop bleeding and supplements the blood

3. Ligusticum and Chinese angelica soup

Ingredients: Chuan Xiong (Chuanxiong Rhizoma) 8g, Dang Gui (Angelicae Sinensis Radix) 12g, E Jiao (Asini Corii Colla) 20g, Ai Ye (Artemisiae Argyi Folium) 12g, Sheng Di Huang (Rehmanniae Radix) 20g, Bai Shao (Paeoniae Radix Alba) 16g, half a black hen, lean pork 200g, fresh ginger 2 pieces, water 15 bowls

Actions: Warms the channels, supplements vacuity, quickens the blood, and stanches bleeding

E. Menstrual Block (Amenorrhea)

1. Stir-fried squid and chives

Ingredients: Squid 250g, chives 100g

Actions: Warms the kidney and frees the channels

2. Squid with walnuts stew

Ingredients: Squid 300g, walnuts 10 pieces

Actions: Supplements yin and blood, quickens the blood and frees the channels

F. Painful Menstruation

1. Chinese angelica and astragalus steamed chicken (for qi and blood vacuity)

Ingredients: Chinese angelica (Dang Gui) 20g, astragalus (Huang Qi) 10g, 1 whole hen

Actions: Supplements qi and nourishes the blood

2. Grilled tilapia with aged tangerine peel and nutmeg (for qi and blood stagnation)

Ingredients: 1 whole tilapia, nutmeg (Rou Dou Kou), aged tangerine peel (Chen Pi), corydalis (Yan Hu Suo) 6g, fresh ginger (Sheng Jiang) 12g

Actions: Moves qi and blood and relieves pain

3. Codonopsis root and lamb belly soup (for qi and blood vacuity)

Ingredients: Lamb meat 250g, lamb belly 150g, Chinese angelica (Dang Gui) 15g, cistanches (Rou Cong Rong) 10g, fermented black bean 10g

Actions: Warms the channels, nourishes the blood, and relieves pain

4. Eucommia pork kidney (for liver-kidney vacuity)

Ingredients: Eucommia bark (Du Zhong) 20g, pork kidney 300g, cooking wine 12g, red sugar 12g

Actions: Supplements the liver and kidney, strengthens sinew and bone

Preparation: First cook the eucommia bark into a concentrated decoction, then add the decoction while stir-frying the pork kidney.

G. Abnormal Vaginal Discharge

1. Chinese wild yam, lotus seed, and Chinese barley congee
Ingredients: Chinese yam (Shan Yao) 30g, lotus seed (Lian Zi) 30g, Chinese barley (Yi Yi Ren) 30g, water 500 ml
Actions: Fortifies the spleen and checks vaginal discharge

2. Stir-fried snow peas with fresh Chinese yam
Ingredients: Snow peas 200g, fresh Chinese yam (Shan Yao) 200g
Actions: Supplements the spleen and kidney to check vaginal discharge

3. Lily bulb, jujube, gingko, and beef soup
Ingredients: Lily bulb (Bai He) 40g, jujube (Hong Zao) 10 pieces, gingko nut (Yin Xing) 40g, lotus seed (Lian Zi) 40g, beef 240g, fresh ginger 2 pieces
Actions: Benefits the skin, generates flesh, supplements qi and blood, and checks vaginal discharge

4. Chinese angelica, codonopsis, black hen stew
Ingredients: Chinese angelica (Dang Gui) 20g, codonopsis (Dang Shen) 30g, 1 whole black hen
Actions: Supplements the liver and kidney, supplements qi and blood, and boosts liquid

5. Lotus seed and pork belly stew
Ingredients: Lotus seed 40 pieces, 1 whole pork belly
Actions: Supplements vacuity, nourishes the heart and kidney, and fortifies the spleen and stomach

6. Fresh Chinese yam and pig's feet stew
Ingredients: Pig's feet (trotters) 500g, fresh Chinese yam 50g
Actions: Warms the kidney, fortifies the spleen, and checks vaginal discharge

H. Threatened Abortion and Habitual Miscarriage

1. Fresh Chinese yam and sesame congee
Ingredients: Rice 60g, fresh Chinese yam 15g, black sesame 120g, fresh milk 200g, rock sugar 120g
Actions: Nourishes yin, supplements the kidney and spleen, lubricates the intestines and quiets the fetus

2. Lotus seed glutinous rice congee
Ingredients: Glutinous rice 100g, lotus seed 50g, red sugar (to taste)

Actions: Supplements the center and boosts qi, clears heart heat, and quiets the fetus

3. Stir-fried egg with fish
Ingredients: Salmon 250g, 4 whole eggs
Actions: Nourishes yin and blood, quiets the fetus
This recipe is especially beneficial for pregnant women with a history of early miscarriage. It quiets the fetus and strengthens the body, and is also beneficial to the development of the central nervous system and the bone system.

4. Jujube and astragalus codfish stew
Ingredients: 1 whole codfish, astragalus (Huang Qi) 25g, jujube (Hong Zao) 8 pieces, fresh ginger (to taste)
Actions: Supplements qi, nourishes yin, and quiets the fetus
This recipe treats restless fetus.

I. Perimenopausal Symptoms

1. Chilled jellyfish
Ingredients: Jellyfish 100g, bok choy 100g, black sesame 30g
Actions: Nourishes the liver and subdues yang
This recipe is used for yin vacuity with ascending hyperactivity of liver yang.

2. Fresh Chinese yam and goji berry stir-fried shredded pork
Ingredients: Goji berry (Gou Qi Zi) 30g, Chinese yam (Shan Yao) 100g, lean pork 150g
Actions: Supplements the spleen, liver, and kidney, and brightens the eyes
This recipe is suitable for liver-kidney yin vacuity.

3. Fresh Chinese yam with lily bulb and rabbit meat stew
Ingredients: Rabbit meat 300g, Chinese yam (Shan Yao) 30g, fresh ginger 2 pieces
Actions: Clears heart heat, quiets the spirit, supplements the kidney, and astringes essence
This recipe is for patients with chronic diarrhea, chronic dysentery, and frequent urination due to vacuity of the lung, spleen, and kidney.

4. Goji berry steamed halibut
Ingredients: Halibut 450g, goji berry (Gou Qi Zi) 15g, chicken broth 1,000g, cooking wine (to taste)
Actions: Supplements the liver and kidney
This recipe is suitable for cases of liver-kidney yin vacuity.

Recipes

Spring Wood element—taste sour

Eat plenty of tofu, millet, mung beans, aduki beans, watercress, dark grapes, blackberries, rasberries, black strap molasses, young beets, and spring greens. All of these are harmonizing and nourish blood in the spring. Dulse flakes instead of salt are a great source of vitamin B12 (important for mothers and nursing mothers).

Aduki Bean and Hawthorne Berry Soup

Marjoram pinch
Hawthorne berries 3
Organic carrots 5
Satsuma white sweet potato 1 medium chopped small cubes
Aduki beans 1 cup (soaked the night before and rinsed well before using)
Yellow onion 1 cup diced
Vegetable broth 5 cups
Sea salt pinch
Chicken breast with skin (2)
Brown chicken breast in pan and put aside.

Sautee onions, carrots, sweet potato, and marjoram until onions are translucent. Add aduki beans and chicken breasts, bring to a boil and simmer for 1½ hours. Serve with steamed beets and young spinach. Using dulse flakes instead of salt on food is a wonderful source of B12 which is an important blood and immune builder for pregnant and nursing mothers.

Summer Fire element—taste is bitter

Enjoy summer foods such as brightly colored summer fruits and vegtables. Cook lightly and steam or simmer foods for a shorter period of time. Enjoy salads, cucumber, tofu, mint and chamomile tea, watermelon, lemons, limes, oatstraw tea, and celery as a crunchy snack or juice. Try fresh squeezed limes with mint and water, sweetened with sucanat or agave for a summer drink. Also watermelon blended with water as a cold soup. Have steamed spinach sprinkled with dulse flakes (high in vitamin B12 and wonderful for pregnant and nursing mothers) and grilled vegetables.

Mint Lime Refresher Drink

Spring water 1 liter
Myer lemons or key limes 6 squeezed
Agave raw 3 tbs.
Sea salt 1 pinch

Mix together and refrigerate; serve with fresh mint sprig.

Watermelon Soup

Spring water 4 cups
Watermelon ½ of melon (remove seeds)
Sea salt 1 pinch

Blend together in blender.

Late Summer Earth—taste sweet

Late summer brings mildly sweet foods like yellow or golden color fruits and vegetables. Golden yellow corn on the cob is delicious this time of year. There is a wide variety of fresh carrots, cabbage, garbanzo beans, squash, yams, tofu sweet rice, rice and amaranth. Prepare mild and simple meals. Eat small frequent meals and chew well.

Fresh tofu salad sprinkled with green scallion and drizzled with soy sauce. Pair it with grilled sweet corn, and a crunchy cabbage salad.

Fresh tofu cut into cubes and piled onto serving dish, chop fresh green onion and place on top, drizzle tamari or soy sauce just before serving.

Organic cabbage sliced very thin, three organic carrots shredded, and toasted almonds tossed in your favorite salad dressing. Sprinkle top with remaining toasted almond slivers.

Grill sweet white or yellow corn, or boil and brown up on the stove top flame (if gas stove) Squeeze sweet key lime and sprinkle dulse flakes instead of salt just before serving.

Fall Metal Element—taste pungent

Sourdough bread, sauerkraut, olives in small amounts, tempeh, spinah, barley, millet, pear, plum, apple, loquat, almond, pinenut, honey, eggs, pork, fennel, watercress, and ginger, chard.

Winter Element Water—taste salty

Winter welcomes small dark beans, hearty soups, and steamed winter greens. Cook foods longer and at lower temperature. Watercress, endive, escarole, turnip, celery, asparagus, black beans, potato, small amounts of eggs, and cheese. Nettle tea.

Pork and Black Bean Soup

Country pork (boneless) 2 cubed
Onion 1 chopped
Parsnip 1 chopped
Celery 2 stalks chopped
Kombucha squash 2 cups cubed
Black beans 1 cup (soaked overnight with 1 strip Kombu) rinse well before
using remove Kombu
Water 3 cups
Chicken broth 3 cups
Coriander and cumin ½ tbs. each
Dash of sake

Sautee onion, parsnip, celery, squash, black beans, and spice; add pork, cook until onions are translucent. Add a dash of sake, let alcohol steam off and add water and stock, bring to a boil and simmer for 3 hours. Serve with rice and steamed or boiled kale with drizzled tamari.

Winter – Water Element—taste salty

Winter is the quietest time of year. You can prepare warm robust soups and stews, roasted nuts, miso soup, and green lettuces. It is a good idea to alternate between millet, rolled barley flake, and oats for a hot breakfast cereal with blackstrap molasses to sweeten. Almond milk is very good for mother and child and can be used to sweeten cream cereal. Black bean soup, and kidney bean chili are yummy and nourishing. Try walnut pesto. AVOID coffee, alcohol and lamb, cinnamon, and overeating.

Walnut Pesto

Spinach (1 bunch) rinsed well

Walnuts organic a handful toasted just before using
Parsley organic ½ a bunch rinsed well
Olive oil 1 cup
Parmasean 1 cup
1 pinch sea salt

Blend all of these in a food processor and serve over rice with ground turkey.

Mejool Dates

Soak dates in clarified butter for three days and serve as dessert with warm barley tea, and winter oranges. Ghee soaked dates are very nourishing to mother and child. Limit two dates per serving.

You can make fresh ghee or buy it in a health food store. Melt ghee in saucepan and place dates in glass mason jar. Fill jar with dates and pour melted ghee over them and place lid on for 3 days.

Barley Breakfast Cereal

Rolled barley flakes 1cup
Butter 1 tbs.
Goji berris ½ cup
Water 2 cups

Toast barley in pan until brown and smells nutty. Add to boiling water with butter and berries. Simmer for five minutes and cover for 10 minutes. Serve with almond milk and agave to sweeten. The same recipe can be prepared with roled oats.

Millet

Millet needs to be soaked overnight and requires three cups water. Bring water to a boil with a pinch of sea salt and simmer for 30 minutes. Serve with almond milk. Suitable for kidney yin vacuity type of perimenopausal syndrome.

General Index

A

Abdominal distention, 31, 73, 75, 85, 120, 121
Abdominal pain, 28, 29, 46, 68, 79, 84, 85, 132, 144, 152, 156, 160, 187, 190, 193, 201, 202, 206, 207
Abnormal uterine bleeding, 57, 59, 61, 63-65, 67, 69, 155, 203, 205
Abnormal vaginal discharge, 43, 181, 185, 187, 189, 191, 193, 195, 197, 199, 293, 296
Abortion, 25, 125, 128-130, 139, 144, 158, 293, 296
Adenoma, 24, 40
Adhesions, 85, 94, 126, 143, 150, 194, 211, 212, 218, 223, 240
Adnexa, 201
Adrenal, 8, 118, 166
After menstruation, 36, 52, 77, 78, 80, 81, 87, 88, 92-95, 98-101, 226, 234, 252, 254
Aldosterone, 8
Amenorrhea, 17-19, 24, 39, 41-49, 51, 53, 55, 128, 144, 166, 217, 293, 295
Amenorrhea, primary, 39
Amenorrhea, secondary, 39
Amniocentesis, 7, 126, 127, 129
Amniotic cavity, 6
Anatomical abnormalities, 39, 83
Androgens, 40
Anemia, 26, 40, 59

Anorexia nervosa, 24
Anovulation, 12, 25, 57, 63, 202, 218, 228, 239
Anovulatory, 222, 251
Antibiotics, 25, 127, 165, 178, 186, 189, 195, 196
Antidepressants, 104
anxiety, 12, 17, 72, 73, 79, 81, 84, 104, 105, 115, 140, 160, 234, 250
Anxiousness, 105
ART, 235, 239
Assisted Reproductive Technology, 235
Ascendant liver yang hyperactivity, 18, 73-76, 110, 171
Atherosclerosis, 12
Atresia, 4
Atrophic vaginitis, 177, 186, 187, 189

B

Backache, 9, 52, 114
Bacterial vaginosis, BV, 181, 185, 186
Balanced diet, 105
Basal body temperature, 25
Before menstruation, 19, 35, 51, 76, 78, 79, 81, 88, 89, 97, 99, 100, 235, 253, 254, 294
Binding depression of the liver qi, 31, 173
Blastocyst, 6
Bleeding, 10, 16-18, 20, 23-29, 31, 33, 34, 36-38, 41, 57-70, 87, 91, 98-101, 123, 125,

127-141, 144-148, 155-161, 185, 187, 188, 202, 203, 205, 208, 209, 211, 218, 224, 234, 294, 295
Blighted ovum, 126
Bloating, 17, 42, 79, 85, 104, 113, 123, 124, 182, 193, 198, 206
Blood heat, 62, 63, 67, 132-134
Blood coagulation, 156
Blood cold, 21
Blood loss, 4, 23, 136, 148, 155-158, 165
Blood stagnation, 212
Blood stasis, 20, 42, 44, 61-68, 70, 87, 88, 91-93, 97, 99, 100, 146, 149, 150, 152, 158, 159, 161, 170, 191, 194, 195, 207-214, 221, 223, 253
Blood vacuity, 20, 29, 30, 32-34, 37, 42, 44, 46, 48, 52, 68, 74, 77-81, 88, 93, 99, 109, 115, 130, 132-134, 152, 157-159, 168-170, 173, 181, 182, 219, 223, 233, 251, 253, 295
Body, 1, 3, 5, 8-10, 12, 15-18, 20, 25, 26, 35, 40, 44, 45, 52, 60-62, 74, 75, 80, 81, 97, 98, 106, 111, 113, 114, 122, 127, 134, 135, 139, 145, 148, 150, 157, 158, 171, 172, 179, 197, 202, 206, 209, 211, 212, 218, 236, 241, 244, 248, 297
Body aches, 74, 106

Body temperature, 5, 25
Breast cancer, 13, 104, 203
Breast distention, 42, 73, 74, 81, 85, 98, 99
Breast pain, 77, 79, 173
Breast tenderness, 18, 31, 72, 144, 203, 221
Breastfeeding, 10, 11, 40, 165
Burning urination, 67, 186
Butoconazole/Femstat, 189
BV, 181, 185, 186, 188, 189

C
Calcium, 12, 41, 84, 105
Cancer, 13, 58, 59, 103, 104, 187, 188, 201, 203, 251
Candida vaginitis, 186
Cardiovascular disease, 41, 104, 105
Cell division, 245
Centrifugation, 246
Cervical os, 85, 127-129
Cervicitis, 25
Cervix, 1, 9, 10, 57, 63, 92, 126, 127, 129, 130, 138, 143, 148, 156, 157, 159, 185, 188, 201, 209, 219, 222, 223, 239, 240, 246, 249, 250
Cesarean, 155, 166, 173
Changeable stools, 99
chemotherapy, 26, 40, 103, 189
Chills, 73, 103, 127
Chlamydia, 143, 145, 177, 186-188, 218, 219
Chromosomal abnormalities, 125-127, 129
Cilia, 1
Climacteric, 103
Clomid, 48, 236, 240
Clotrimazole/Gyne-lotrimin, 189
Clotting disorders, 25, 126
Clotting, 25, 67, 126
Clots, 23, 27, 30, 31, 61, 66, 68, 83, 85, 86, 98, 99, 139, 158-160, 207
Cold extremities, 106, 146
Cold in the uterus, 34
Complete miscarriage, 125, 129, 130
Conception, 6, 110, 115, 127-

129, 134, 147, 172, 217, 220, 221, 227, 228, 230, 236, 239, 241, 245, 246, 248
Condom, 178, 186, 189
Confusion, 156
Congenital (problems), 44
Constant midline dull ache, 125
Constipation, 8, 47, 72, 80, 81, 83, 98, 104, 109, 158, 160, 208, 214
Contractions, 8, 9, 83-85, 124, 128, 135-137, 139, 141, 235, 239, 250, 251
Coronary artery disease (CAD), 12
Corpus luteum, 3, 5, 8, 25, 202, 246
Corpus luteum cysts, 202
Cortisol, 8, 163
Cramping, 20, 21, 34, 63, 76, 83, 85, 91, 92, 101, 123, 125, 127-130, 138, 157, 158, 187, 225
Cryopreserved, 246
CT, 25, 204, 205
computerized tomography, 25
Cyst, 3, 164, 202, 204, 210

D
D & C, 26, 63, 127-129, 158, 161
Damp stagnation in all three burners, 197
Damp-heat, 152, 153, 171, 180-182, 190, 193, 196, 210
Damp-heat toxin, 190
Dehydration, 117, 118, 121
Delayed menstruation, 28, 33, 37, 152, 207, 293, 294
Depression, 12, 17, 18, 27, 31, 37, 52, 63, 72, 73, 75, 77-80, 85, 89, 90, 92, 93, 99, 101, 103-105, 108, 114, 115, 120, 121, 123, 139, 140, 167-169, 171-174, 182, 197, 206, 212-215, 221, 223, 225, 247, 251, 253
Dermoid cysts, 202
diabetes, 8, 40, 118, 126, 177, 186, 187
Diabetes, 8, 40, 118, 126, 177, 186, 187

Diaphragm, 9, 178, 186
Diarrhea, 17, 19, 72-75, 77, 78, 80, 83, 84, 90, 91, 106, 107, 112, 120, 192, 239, 297
Difficulty concentrating, 74
Digestive problems, 76, 99, 243
Digestive disorders, 42
Distention, 31, 42, 43, 73-75, 77, 79, 81, 85, 98, 99, 101, 120, 121, 147, 168, 173
Dizziness, 19, 33, 37, 41, 42, 52, 73, 74, 77, 79, 87, 88, 98, 99, 106, 108, 110, 123, 128, 144, 152, 153, 156, 157, 160, 161, 203
Dry skin, 42, 167, 219
Du, 15, 29, 41, 61, 106, 112, 130, 132, 190, 191, 220
governing vessel, 15
Dysfunctional uterine bleeding, 24, 25, 57
Dysmenorrhea, 18, 83-85, 87-91, 93-95, 97, 99, 101, 170, 206, 221, 253
Dysuria, 177, 185, 187

E
Early PPH, 155
Eclampsia, 19
Ectopic pregnancy, 20, 128, 129, 143-153, 187, 194, 203, 218
Ectopic pregnancies, 143, 146, 148, 151
Ectopic pregnancy—blood stasis, 146
blood stasis, 20, 42, 44, 61-68, 70, 87, 88, 91-93, 97, 99, 100, 146, 149, 150, 152, 158, 159, 161, 170, 191, 194, 195, 207-214, 221, 223, 253
Edema, 8, 17, 43, 106, 113, 188
Embryo, 5-7, 126, 127, 129, 147, 148, 195, 217-219, 235, 241, 244, 246, 247, 249, 251
Embryonic period, 7
Emotional changes, 85, 105
Emotional issues, 76
Emotions, 101, 113, 120, 174
Endocrine, 35, 36, 44, 51, 52,

63, 160, 227, 229

Endometrial cancer, 13, 187, 188

Endometrial hyperplasia, 104

Endometrial lining, 1, 4, 5, 234, 251

Endometrial polyps, 25, 218

Endometriosis, 20, 57, 58, 84, 94, 98, 144, 145, 202, 208, 218, 223

Endometritis, 25

Endometrium, 24, 185, 217, 223

Episiotomy, 156

Essence, jing, 17, 135

Estradiol, 5, 11, 189, 223

Estradiol vaginal creams, 189

Estrogen, 3-5, 8, 11-13, 23, 25, 26, 40, 44, 58, 63, 71, 92, 103-105, 113, 117, 166, 178, 185-187, 189, 204, 205, 208, 217, 224, 229, 245

Estrogen replacement therapy (ERT), 12

Estrogen rings, 189

Exercise, 12, 24, 40, 57, 72, 84, 105, 127, 128, 203, 218

F

Fallopian tubes, 1, 19, 48, 143-148, 151, 153, 194, 201, 218, 222, 223, 239

fat cells, 40

Fatigue, 37, 41-43, 63, 68, 72, 73, 76, 83, 88, 99, 104, 106, 118, 123, 157, 160, 167, 219

Fatty liver disease, 118

Female reproductive anatomy, 1, 3, 5, 7, 9, 11, 13

Fertile cervical mucus, 4

Fertilization, 4-6, 52, 217, 244-246

Fetal heart motion, 246

Fetal heartbeat, 126-128

Fetal sac, 246

Fetus, 1, 7-9, 16, 64, 66, 121, 122, 125, 126, 128, 130, 132, 134-137, 139-141, 144, 147, 168, 173, 232, 233, 235, 238, 244, 249, 296, 297

Fibroid, 1, 85, 204, 205, 208-210, 218

Fibroids, 1, 20, 25, 58, 59, 126, 204-209, 211, 213-215, 218

Fimbria, 3, 5

Flagyl, 189

Follicle, 3-5, 11, 103, 201, 202, 245, 246

Follicle-stimulating hormone, (FSH), 3, 4, 219

Follicles, 3, 4, 11, 38, 48, 104, 204, 223, 236, 237, 239, 244, 245, 247, 248, 250, 253

Follicular cysts, 201

Follicular phase, 3, 4

Follistim, 236, 245

Follitropin-alpha (Gonal-F), 245

Follitropin-beta (Follistim), 245

Frequent urination, 52, 83, 99, 104, 112, 140, 144, 197, 198, 205, 214, 297

FSH, 3-5, 11, 23, 36, 40, 44, 58, 98, 103, 217, 218, 223, 234, 240, 244, 245, 250, 253

G

Galactorrhea, 19, 168

Gardnerella vaginalis, 177, 185, 186

Gas, 104, 123, 124, 182, 193

Genetic defects, 40

genetic factors, 39

Gestational diabetes, 8

GNRH, 3-5, 23, 40, 104, 218

Gonadotropin-releasing hormone (GnRH), 3, 4

Gonal-F, 245

Gonorrhea, 145, 177, 186-188, 219

Granulosa cells, 245

H

HCG trigger, 239

Headache, 74, 75, 77, 79, 81, 83, 90, 103, 108, 110, 114, 168, 171

Headaches, 12, 19, 42, 72, 73, 76, 80, 81, 84, 104, 108, 114

Heart blood vacuity, 68, 77, 79, 109, 115

Heart palpitations, 8, 66, 68, 78, 80, 92, 104, 106, 109, 114, 115, 152, 160, 167

Heart yin & blood vacuity, 80

Heart yin vacuity, 77, 79, 90

Heart yin-blood vacuity, 75

Heavy bleeding, 17, 18, 24, 26, 28, 57, 59-63, 65, 68, 87, 91, 98, 101, 128, 158, 159, 209

Heavy uterine bleeding, 20, 68, 218

Hemophilia, 25

Hemorrhage, 20, 91, 143, 144, 149, 155, 157, 159, 161, 165

Hemorrhagic cysts, 202

Hirsutism, 40

hormonal imbalances, 24, 39, 57, 203

Hormonal therapy, 40

Hormone replacement therapy (HRT), 13, 41, 104, 113

Hormone therapy, 24, 57, 205

Hormones, 3-6, 8, 10, 15, 23, 35, 40, 44, 45, 94, 126, 128, 143, 163, 178, 204, 218, 224, 234, 239, 245, 250

Hot flashes, 12, 17, 67, 72, 103-106, 110, 115, 116, 213, 214

HRT, 13, 41, 104, 113

Human chorionic gonadotropin hormone (hCG), 4

Hymen, 39

Hymen, closed, 39

Hyperemesis gravidarum, 117, 118

Hyperparathyroidism, 117

Hyperthyroid, 26

Hyperthyroidism, 26, 118, 251

Hypoglycemia, 71, 166

Hypomenorrhea, 24, 26, 36

Hypothalamic insufficiency, 26

Hypothalamus, 3-5, 40, 163, 218

Hypothyroid, 26

Hypothyroidism, 24-26, 40, 166, 218

Hysterectomy, 63, 204, 205

Hysterosalpingogram (HSG), 144, 151, 153

Hysterosalpingography, 25

Hysteroscopy, 25, 205

I

Implantation, 5, 6, 143, 147,

217, 218, 232, 241, 246, 251
Incomplete miscarriage, 63,
125, 128, 130, 149
Incontinence, 104, 106, 187
Increased heart rate, 156, 165,
166
Incubation, 245, 246
Inevitable abortion, 125, 129,
130
Inevitable miscarriage, 125,
128, 129
Infection, 126, 127, 143, 147,
148, 151, 153, 165, 171,
177, 178, 180-182, 185-187,
192-196, 218, 223
Infertility, 15, 17-21, 40, 143,
145, 187, 194, 203, 205,
217-219, 221-225, 227, 229,
231, 233, 235, 237, 239-241,
243, 245, 247, 249, 251,
253, 255, 257, 259
Inflammation, 25, 143, 145,
151, 178, 186, 187, 196, 218
Insemination, 52, 239, 240,
246
Insomnia, 12, 66, 72-78, 80,
87, 93, 104, 105, 108, 109,
111, 114-116, 133, 136, 213,
214
Insufficient lactation, 18-20,
163-165, 167-171, 173, 175
Insulin, 8, 40, 163
Insulin resistance (IR), 40
Intensive exercise, 40
Internal stirring of liver wind,
18, 74
Intramural fibroids, 204
Intrauterine devices, 23, 58,
143
Irregular menstruation, 23-27,
29-35, 37, 94, 217, 221, 222,
242, 293, 295
Isthmus, 1
IUD, 25, 85, 145, 178, 186
IVF transfer, 250, 251

J
Jing, 17, 26-32, 34, 37, 45, 46,
48-51, 53, 54, 62, 66, 69, 70,
77, 78, 81, 91-96, 100, 112,
132, 133, 135, 161, 170,
179, 181-184, 191, 198, 210,

220, 224-227, 229, 231-233,
236, 238, 242-244, 247-249,
252, 254

K
Karyotyping, 40
Ketoconazole/Nizoral, 189
Kidney qi vacuity, 17, 140, 173
Kidney vacuity, 31, 41, 44, 46,
63, 65, 76, 108, 123, 124,
131, 133, 161, 173, 195,
196, 219, 293
Kidney yang vacuity, 17, 31,
37, 41, 46-48, 52, 60, 61, 65,
67, 68, 93, 99, 100, 106,
108, 111, 114, 131, 132,
134, 136, 170, 191, 197,
219, 223, 238, 244, 249
Kidney yin vacuity, 17, 31, 46,
47, 60, 65, 67, 80, 81, 93,
105, 107, 108, 110, 111,
115, 116, 130, 131, 134,
136, 138, 214, 215, 220,
223, 228, 233, 238, 241,
244, 249

L
Lactation, 18-20, 163-175
Lactobacillus, 189
Laparoscopy, 203, 205, 245
Late PPH, 155
Leukemia, 25
Leukorrhea, 177, 180, 182,
185, 186
LH, 3-5, 8, 11, 23, 218, 234,
239, 245
LH surge, 4, 5, 11, 239
Light-headedness, 74, 144
Liver assailing the spleen, 80,
197
Liver blood vacuity, 80
Liver cirrhosis, 25
Liver depression qi stagnation,
17, 31, 37, 73, 75, 77-80, 89,
90, 93, 99, 101, 108, 114,
115, 139, 140, 197, 212-215,
247, 251, 253
Liver depression qi stagnation,
severe, 73, 77-79
Liver depression transforming
heat, 18, 27, 168
Liver disease, 58, 118

Liver fire flaming upward, 74,
75
Liver heat, 67
Liver qi assailing the spleen, 74
Liver qi depression & binding,
73, 85, 108, 172, 221
Liver qi depression and binding,
108, 121, 123, 169, 173
Liver wind stirring internally,
110
Low back pain, 41, 98, 99, 111
Low estrogen levels, 11, 26
Lower abdominal pain, 28, 29,
68, 79, 84, 85, 132, 144,
152, 160, 187, 190, 193
Lung-spleen qi vacuity, 197
Luteal phase, 5, 71
Luteinizing hormone (LH), 3-5,
23

M
Malar flushing, 67, 167
Membrane rupture, 125, 129
Menarche, 3, 23, 41
Menopausal syndrome, 103,
105, 107-109, 111, 113, 115
Menopause, 3, 11-13, 17, 19,
39, 40, 58, 63, 103-105, 108-
111, 113, 114, 185, 187,
188, 205
Menopur, 245
Menorrhagia, 24, 25, 57, 58,
293, 294
Menstrual blood, 16, 41, 83
Menstrual cycle, 1, 3-5, 11, 16,
18, 26, 28, 33, 34, 44, 71,
72, 79, 84, 168, 201, 202,
236
Menstrual flow, 4, 26, 44, 46,
52, 58, 85
Menstruation, 3, 4, 11, 16-21,
23-39, 41-49, 51-54, 59, 63,
73, 76-81, 83-95, 97-101,
103-105, 108, 127, 144, 152,
188, 202, 203, 205, 207,
209, 217, 219, 221, 222,
224-227, 229, 231, 232, 234-
236, 242, 243, 247, 248,
252-254, 293-295
Metaphase II eggs, 245
Methimasole, 26
Methyltrexate, 145, 148, 150

Metrorrhagia, 25, 57, 58, 62-64, 67
Miconazole/Monistat, 189
Migraine, 74
Migraines, 19, 42
Miscarriage, 7, 17, 19-21, 63, 121, 125, 127-131, 133-139, 141, 149, 217, 232, 233, 241, 251, 293, 296, 297
Missed abortion, 125, 128
Molar pregnancy, 126
Mood swings, 8, 12, 18, 73, 89, 93, 99, 214
Moodiness, 42, 79, 120, 121, 221
Morning sickness, 19, 117
Motility, 240, 251
Moxa, 67, 69, 114, 122
MRI, 25, 40, 201, 204, 205

N
Nails, 42, 219
Nausea, 7, 19, 68, 83, 84, 98, 99, 117-120, 122, 124, 131, 132, 144, 168, 203, 239
Nervousness, 105, 135
Night sweats, 12, 41, 104, 105, 110, 114, 167
No appetite, 109
Nonsteroidal anti-inflammatory drugs (NSAIDs), 72

O
obesity, 40, 57, 204
OCP, 44
Oocyte, 245, 246
Oocyte aspiration, 245
Oocytes, 3, 244
oral contraceptive pills, 23, 44, 244
Oral contraceptive pills, 23, 44, 244
Oral estrogen, 25, 186, 189
osteoporosis, 12, 13, 41, 104, 105, 112, 113
Ova, 3, 229
Ovary, 3, 6, 11, 24-26, 143, 144, 202, 204, 218, 245, 253, 254
Ovulation, 3-5, 10, 11, 24, 35, 36, 48-50, 57, 59, 63, 73, 84, 103, 145, 185, 201, 202,

204, 217, 218, 223, 227-231, 234, 235, 237, 239, 243-245, 250, 252
Ovulatory cycles, 25, 38, 58
Ovulatory phase, 3, 5
Oxytocin, 9, 10, 128, 157, 163, 166

P
Pain, 9, 12, 16, 20, 21, 28, 29, 33, 34, 37, 40-42, 46, 61, 62, 66-68, 72-75, 77, 79, 83-91, 93, 96-101, 111, 112, 119, 125, 127, 131-133, 138-140, 144, 146, 148-152, 156-160, 165, 168, 169, 173, 177, 187-195, 201-203, 205-207, 212, 218, 219, 221, 225, 254, 295
Palpitations, 8, 12, 66, 68, 78, 80, 90, 92, 104-106, 109, 114, 115, 152, 160, 167
Pancreatitis, 117, 144
Pelvic inflammatory disease, 25, 85, 143, 193, 218
Pelvic sonography, 25
Pergonal, 245
Perimenopause, 11, 12, 24, 58, 103
Perineum, 156, 157
Period, 3, 4, 6, 7, 11, 44, 45, 48, 52, 66, 70, 103, 116, 147, 157, 164, 299
Pheochromocytoma, 118
Phlegm damp obstruction, 19, 43, 44
Phlegm-damp stagnation, 213
PID, 85, 143-146, 187, 193-196, 203, 218
pituitary abnormalities, 40
pituitary adenoma, 24, 40
Pituitary gland, 3-5, 9, 11, 24, 51, 218
Pituitary hormone, 163, 218
Placenta, 6, 8, 10, 41, 126, 155, 157-159, 161
Polycystic ovary syndrome (PCOS), 24, 218
polymenorrhea, 24, 57, 59
Poor memory, 74, 104, 105
Postpartum, 20, 155, 157-161, 165, 166

Postpartum hemorrhage, 20, 155, 157, 159, 161, 165
Potassium deficiency, 117
PPH, postpartum hemorrhage, 155
Predictor kit, 239
Preeclampsia, 156
Pregnancy, 1, 5-8, 17, 19-21, 39, 57-59, 83, 110, 117-130, 134, 139, 141, 143-153, 158-160, 168, 173, 185, 187, 188, 194, 201, 203, 205, 217, 218, 224, 232, 234, 235, 238, 239, 244, 246, 249, 251, 254, 299
Premature menopause, 11
Premature ovarian failure, 11, 103
Premenstrual syndrome (PMS), 71, 73, 75, 77, 79, 81
Premiscarriage, 125, 127, 130
Progesterone, 3-6, 8, 9, 11, 23-25, 40, 44, 58, 63, 71, 72, 103, 104, 126, 144, 217, 218, 223, 224, 229, 232, 246
Progestin, 13, 40, 44, 166
Prolactin, 10, 24, 40, 58, 71, 72, 163, 165, 166, 218
Propylthiouracil, 26
Puberty, 3

Q
Qi and blood vacuity, 33, 44, 52, 134, 158, 159, 168, 169, 223
Qi stagnation, 17, 18, 20, 30-32, 34, 36, 37, 42, 44, 47, 52, 73, 75-80, 88-90, 93, 99, 101, 108, 114, 115, 139, 140, 152, 161, 168, 170, 183, 193, 195, 197, 198, 206, 208, 212-215, 221, 223, 225, 229, 247, 251, 253
Qi stagnation and blood stasis, 44, 214
Qi vacuity, 17, 19, 20, 28, 32, 33, 46, 48, 52, 59, 63, 65, 68, 70, 78, 80, 81, 99, 100, 123, 130, 131, 133-135, 137, 139, 140, 152, 153, 168, 173, 182, 190, 197, 212, 223
Quiet the spirit, 36, 52, 66, 68,

69, 74, 75, 79, 91, 94, 97, 98, 101, 106, 114, 124, 135, 139, 141, 211, 228, 233, 235, 241, 242, 249-251, 253

R
Radiation, 26, 103
Rash, 181, 182, 185
Red eyes, 67
Replete cold, 21, 28
Replete heat, 21, 26, 66, 132
Reproductive tract, 24, 25
Repronex, 245
Restlessness, 17, 66, 73, 74, 250
Retained placenta, 155
Rhythmic cramping, 125, 127

S
Salpingitis, 218
Scanty menses, 24
Secondary sexual characteristics, 39
Secretory phase, 3
Selective estrogen receptor modulators (SERMS), 13
Septic abortion, 128
Shock, 144, 146, 148, 155, 156, 203
Shortness of breath, 156
Sonohysterography, 25
Sore lower back, 31, 105, 191, 197, 198
Sperm, 5, 6, 147, 218, 219, 234, 239, 240, 244-246, 251
Sperm count, 240, 251
Spleen qi vacuity, 19, 48, 59, 63, 65, 68, 70, 80, 81, 99, 100, 123, 134, 139, 140, 152, 173, 182, 190, 197
Spleen yang vacuity, 19, 78
Spleen-kidney yang vacuity, 75, 77, 80, 99
Spontaneous abortion, 125, 129
Stenosis, 219
Stiffness, 114
Stop bleeding, 33, 34, 59-62, 65-69, 127, 145, 160
stress, 24, 35-37, 40, 57, 84, 115, 117, 119, 160, 166, 173, 174, 182, 185-187, 197, 215, 223, 243, 247, 249

Stroke, 13, 104
Submucosal fibroids, 204, 209
Surgery, 26, 40, 59, 63, 72, 85, 94, 143, 145, 148, 150, 152, 153, 157, 189, 195, 205, 208-211, 214, 215
Surgical damage, 103

T
T3, 40
T4, 40
Thiamin, 117
Thinning of the skin, 104
Thrombocytopenia, 156
Thyroid, 8, 26, 40, 57, 58, 126, 218
Thyroid gland, 8, 218
Thyroid hormones, 40
Tioconazole/Vagistat, 189
Trauma, 25, 129, 143, 156, 157, 211
Trichomoniasis, 186-189
Tumor, 24, 118, 166, 204, 253
Tumors, 19, 20, 25, 40, 58, 149, 178, 204, 206, 218, 253
Turner's Syndrome, 40

U
Ultrasonography, 40, 246
Uncontrolled diabetes, 186, 187
Unformed bowel movements, 52, 68, 93, 104, 106, 118, 123, 124, 157
Unstable vital signs, 156
Urinary incontinence, 104
Uterine atony, 155
Uterine corpus, 1
Uterine fibroids, 1, 20, 58, 126, 206, 208, 213
Uterine inversion, 156, 157
Uterine lining, 4, 5, 20, 23, 44, 48, 63, 84, 94, 128, 129, 204, 218, 224, 235, 236, 250-252
Uterine myoma, 223
Uterine prolapse, 17, 19, 20
Uterine rupture, 156
Uterine wall, 6, 127, 129, 209
Uterus, 1, 3, 5-11, 15-17, 19-21, 34-36, 40, 48, 49, 52, 57, 63-65, 67, 69, 70, 84, 85, 91, 92, 97, 98, 101, 111, 122, 124-126, 128, 129, 136, 138,

141, 144, 145, 147, 149, 153, 155-161, 201, 204, 205, 208, 209, 212, 213, 218-220, 223, 228, 230, 232, 234-237, 239-242, 244, 246, 247, 250, 251

V
Vacuity cold, 21, 29, 32, 37, 69, 132, 197, 294
Vacuity heat, 17, 21, 27, 65, 81, 115, 116, 132, 136, 171, 172, 215, 234
Vagina, 10, 40, 156, 157, 177, 178, 181, 185, 186, 188, 223, 240, 245
Vaginal discharge, 17-19, 21, 43, 177, 178, 181, 182, 184-189, 191, 193, 195, 197-199, 293, 296
Vaginal dryness, 12, 104
Vaginal estrogens, 105
Vaginal spotting, 125, 127
Vaginal yeast infection, 185, 186
Vaginitis, 177, 178, 185-189
Vitamin B-6 deficiency, 71
Vitamin B-complex deficiency, 186
Vitamin D, 105
Vitamin K, 117, 163
Vomiting, 84, 117-124, 131, 132, 139, 144, 187, 203, 239
Vulvovaginitis, 25, 177

W
Water swelling, 19, 75, 107, 112, 113
Weakness, 19, 41, 83, 84, 112, 123, 140, 144, 156, 203
Weight change, 24, 40
Weight gain, 12, 104, 164, 203
Weight loss, 117
Wind-damp, 75

Y
Yang supplementation, 75
Yeast overgrowth, 185
Yolk sac, 6

Z
Zygote, 3, 6

Formula Index

A

An Tai Fang, 安胎方, 134-136, 138

B

Ba Zhen Tang, 八珍汤, 42
Bao Yin Jian, 保阴煎, 132
Bei Luan Fang, 备卵方, 211, 247, 249
Bei Xie Sheng Shi Tang, 萆解胜湿汤, 178

C

Cang Fu Dao Tan Wan, 苍附导痰丸, 43
Chang Ning Tang, 肠宁汤, 158

D

Da Gong Xue Fang, 大宫血方, 65, 68, 69
Da Ying Jian, 大营煎, 29
modified Ding Jing Fang, 定经方, 32, 37, 54, 70, 78, 112, 226, 229, 232, 236, 242, 247, 248

E

Er Chen Tang, 二陳汤, 92, 183
Er Xian Tang, 二仙汤, 107

G

Ge Xia Zhu Yu Tang, 膈下逐瘀汤, 86
Gong Wai Yin, 宫外孕, 146
Gong Xue Fang, 宫血方, 64, 65, 67-69
modified Gu Ben Zhi Beng Tang, 固本止崩汤, 60

Gu Yin Jian, 固阴煎, 31
Gua Gong Fang, 刮宫方, 150
Gua Tai Fang, 刮胎方, 148, 149
Gui Pi Tang, 归脾汤, 28
Gui Shen Wan, 归肾丸, 41
Gui Zhi Fu Ling Wan, 桂枝茯苓丸, 207

H

Hu Tai Fang, 护胎方, 135, 232, 233, 238, 244, 249
Huo Jing Zhong Zi Fang, 活精种子方, 94, 96, 254

J

Ji Luan Fang, 激卵方, 243
Jia Wei Wu Yao Tang, 加味乌药汤, 30
Jia Wei Xiao Yao San, 加味逍遥散, 27, 90
Jian Gu Tang, 健固汤, 75
Jing Hou Fang, 经后方, 70, 77, 81, 92, 94, 95, 100
Jing Tai Fang, 静胎方, 135, 233, 238, 244, 249
Jing Tong Fang, 经痛方, 91, 94-96, 100, 225

K

Kai Yu Zhong Yu Tang, 开郁种玉汤, 221

L

Liang Di Tang, 两地汤, 27
Liu Jun Zi Tang, 凉胎止血方, 118, 120, 123, 124, 195, 196
Liu Wei Di Huang Wan, 六味地黄丸, 110, 116, 228, 231,

234, 242
modified Long Dan Xie Gan Tang, 龙胆泻肝汤, 192, 193

M

modified Man Pen Fang, 清热固经汤, 147, 148, 151, 153

N

Nei Bu Wan, 内补丸, 191
modified Nuan Tai Zhi Xue Fang 暖胎止血方, 138

P

Pai Luan Fang, 排卵方, 230, 237
Pai Luan Hou Fang, 排卵后方, 50, 230, 231

Q

Qi Gong Wan, 启宫丸, 222
Qi Ju Di Huang Wan, 杞菊地黄丸, 74
modified Qing Gong Fang, 清宫方, 159, 161
Qing Jing San, 清经散, 27
modified Qing Re Gu Jing Tang, 清热固经汤, 62

R

Ren Shen Yang Ying Tang, 人参养营汤, 29

S

Shao Fu Zhu Yu Tang, 少腹逐瘀汤, 86
Sheng Hua Tang, 生化汤, 158
Sheng Mai San, 生脉散, 120-122

Sheng Yu Tang, 圣愈汤, 88, 133
modified Shi Xiao San, 失笑散, 61, 91, 100
Shou Tai Wan, 寿胎丸, 131
Si Jun Zi Tang, 四君子汤, 47, 120, 227, 229
Si Shen Wan, 四神丸, 107, 192
modified Si Wu Tang, 四物汤, 45, 46, 61, 172, 225, 231
Su Ye Huang Lian Tang, 苏叶黄连汤, 119

T
Tai Yuan Yin, 胎元饮, 130
Tiao Gan Tang, 调肝汤, 87
modified Tiao Jing Fang, 调经方, 45, 46, 48, 49, 53, 54, 161, 227, 242, 243, 252
Tiao Jing Hou Fang, 调经后方, 70, 77, 81
Tiao Jing Qian Fang, 调经前方, 49, 50, 210, 231, 232
Tiao Jing Xing Fang, 调经行方, 49, 50, 224, 226
Tong Ru Dan, 通乳丹, 167

W
Wan Dai Tang, 完带汤, 190, 198
Wen Gong Fang, 温宫方, 48, 49, 111, 228, 230, 236, 237, 242, 247
Wen Jing Tang, 温经汤, 29
Wen Jing Xing Fang, 温经行方, 49, 51, 225, 252
Wu Zi Zhong Zi Wan, 五子种子丸, 220

X
Xiang Leng Wan, 香棱丸, 206
Xiang Sha Liu Jun Zi Tang, 香砂六君子汤, 118
Xiao Yao Fang, 逍遥方, 76, 81, 89-91, 93-96, 99, 108, 170, 174, 211, 247, 249, 254
Xiao Yao San, 逍遥散, 27, 31, 67, 73, 89, 90, 94, 100, 109, 168, 170
modified Xiao Zheng Fang, 消症方, 94, 96, 209, 214
modified Xing Jing Fang, 行经方, 45, 53, 254

Xue Fu Zhu Yu Tang, 血府逐瘀汤, 42, 87

Y
Yang Luan Fang, 养卵方, 226, 236, 243, 248
Yang Tai Fang, 养胎方, 136, 137, 233, 238
modified You Gui Wan, 右归丸, 61, 106
Yu Lin Zhu, 毓鳞珠, 219

Z
Zeng Ru Fang, 增乳方, 169
Zeng 十 Tang, 增液汤, 120, 121
Zhi Bai Di Huang Wan, 知柏地黄丸, 180
Zhi Beng Fang, 止崩方, 65, 159
Zhi Dai Tang, 止带汤, 190
modified Zi Ru Fang, 滋育方, 115, 228
Zi Tai Fang 滋胎方, 139, 235, 240
modified Zuo Gui Wan, 左归丸, 60
Zuo Gui Yin, 左归饮, 105

OTHER BOOKS ON CHINESE MEDICINE AVAILABLE FROM:
BLUE POPPY PRESS
Colorado: 1990 North 57th Court, Unit A, Boulder, CO 80301
For ordering 1-800-487-9296 PH. 303-447-8372 FAX 303-245-8362
California: 1725 Monrovia Ave. Unit A4, Costa Mesa, CA 92627
For ordering 1-800-293-6697 PH. 949-270-6511 FAX 949-335-7110
Email: info@bluepoppy.com Website: www.bluepoppy.com

ACUPOINT POCKET REFERENCE
by Bob Flaws
ISBN 0-936185-93-7
ISBN 978-0-936185-93-4

ACUPUNCTURE & IVF
by Lifang Liang
ISBN 0-891845-24-1
ISBN 978-0-891845-24-6

ACUPUNCTURE FOR STROKE REHABILITATION
Three Decades of Information from China
by Hoy Ping Yee Chan, *et al.*
ISBN 1-891845-35-7
ISBN 978-1-891845-35-2

ACUPUNCTURE PHYSICAL MEDICINE:
An Acupuncture Touchpoint Approach to the Treatment of
Chronic Pain, Fatigue, and Stress Disorders
by Mark Seem
ISBN 1-891845-13-6
ISBN 978-1-891845-13-0

AGING & BLOOD STASIS:
A New Approach to TCM Geriatrics
by Yan De-xin
ISBN 0-936185-63-6
ISBN 978-0-936185-63-7

AN ACUPUNCTURISTS GUIDE TO MEDICAL RED
FLAGS & REFERRALS
by Dr. David Anzaldua, MD
ISBN 1-891845-54-3
ISBN 978-1-891845-54-3

BETTER BREAST HEALTH NATURALLY
with CHINESE MEDICINE
by Honora Lee Wolfe & Bob Flaws
ISBN 0-936185-90-2
ISBN 978-0-936185-90-3

BIOMEDICINE: A TEXTBOOK FOR PRACTITIONERS OF
ACUPUNCTURE AND ORIENTAL MEDICINE
by Bruce H. Robinson, MD
ISBN 1-891845-38-1
ISBN 978-1-891845-38-3

THE BOOK OF JOOK:
Chinese Medicinal Porridges
by Bob Flaws
ISBN 0-936185-60-6
ISBN 978-0-936185-60-0

CHANNEL DIVERGENCES
Deeper Pathways of the Web
by Miki Shima and Charles Chase
ISBN 1-891845-15-2
ISBN 978-1-891845-15-4

CHINESE MEDICAL OBSTETRICS
by Bob Flaws
ISBN 1-891845-30-6
ISBN 978-1-891845-30-7

CHINESE MEDICAL PALMISTRY:
Your Health in Your Hand
by Zong Xiao-fan & Gary Liscum
ISBN 0-936185-64-3
ISBN 978-0-936185-64-4

CHINESE MEDICAL PSYCHIATRY
A Textbook and Clinical Manual
by Bob Flaws and James Lake, MD
ISBN 1-845891-17-9
ISBN 978-1-845891-17-8

CHINESE MEDICINAL TEAS: Simple, Proven, Folk
Formulas for Common Diseases & Promoting Health
by Zong Xiao-fan & Gary Liscum
ISBN 0-936185-76-7
ISBN 978-0-936185-76-7

CHINESE MEDICINAL WINES & ELIXIRS
by Bob Flaws   Revised Edition
ISBN 0-936185-58-9
ISBN 978-0-936185-58-3

CHINESE MEDICINE & HEALTHY WEIGHT
MANAGEMENT
An Evidence-based Integrated Approach
by Juliette Aiyana, L. Ac.
ISBN 1-891845-44-6
ISBN 978-1-891845-44-4

CHINESE PEDIATRIC MASSAGE THERAPY: A Parent's &
Practitioner's Guide to the Prevention & Treatment of
Childhood Illness
by Fan Ya-li
ISBN 0-936185-54-6
ISBN 978-0-936185-54-5

CHINESE SELF-MASSAGE THERAPY:
The Easy Way to Health
by Fan Ya-li
ISBN 0-936185-74-0
ISBN 978-0-936185-74-3

THE CLASSIC OF DIFFICULTIES:
A Translation of the *Nan Jing*
translation by Bob Flaws
ISBN 1-891845-07-1
ISBN 978-1-891845-07-9

A CLINICIAN'S GUIDE TO USING GRANULE
EXTRACTS
by Eric Brand
ISBN 1-891845-51-9
ISBN 978-1-891845-51-2

A COMPENDIUM OF CHINESE MEDICAL
MENSTRUAL DISEASES
by Bob Flaws
ISBN 1-891845-31-4
ISBN 978-1-891845-31-4

CONCISE CHINESE MATERIA MEDICA
by Eric Brand and Nigel Wiseman
ISBN 0-912111-82-8
ISBN 978-0-912111-82-7

CONTEMPORARY GYNECOLOGY: An Integrated
Chinese-Western Approach
by Lifang Liang
ISBN 1-891845-50-0
ISBN 978-1-891845-50-5

CONTROLLING DIABETES NATURALLY WITH
CHINESE MEDICINE
by Lynn Kuchinski
ISBN 0-936185-06-3
ISBN 978-0-936185-06-2

CURING ARTHRITIS NATURALLY WITH
CHINESE MEDICINE
by Douglas Frank & Bob Flaws
ISBN 0-936185-87-2
ISBN 978-0-936185-87-3

CURING DEPRESSION NATURALLY WITH
CHINESE MEDICINE
by Rosa Schnyer & Bob Flaws
ISBN 0-936185-94-5
ISBN 978-0-936185-94-1

CURING FIBROMYALGIA NATURALLY WITH
CHINESE MEDICINE
by Bob Flaws
ISBN 1-891845-09-8
ISBN 978-1-891845-09-3

CURING HAY FEVER NATURALLY WITH
CHINESE MEDICINE
by Bob Flaws
ISBN 0-936185-91-0
ISBN 978-0-936185-91-0

CURING HEADACHES NATURALLY WITH
CHINESE MEDICINE
by Bob Flaws
ISBN 0-936185-95-3
ISBN 978-0-936185-95-8

CURING IBS NATURALLY WITH CHINESE
MEDICINE
by Jane Bean Oberski
ISBN 1-891845-11-X
ISBN 978-1-891845-11-6

CURING INSOMNIA NATURALLY WITH
CHINESE MEDICINE
by Bob Flaws
ISBN 0-936185-86-4
ISBN 978-0-936185-86-6

CURING PMS NATURALLY WITH CHINESE
MEDICINE
by Bob Flaws
ISBN 0-936185-85-6
ISBN 978-0-936185-85-9

DISEASES OF THE KIDNEY & BLADDER
by Hoy Ping Yee Chan, et al.
ISBN 1-891845-37-3
ISBN 978-1-891845-35-6

THE DIVINE FARMER'S MATERIA MEDICA
A Translation of the Shen Nong Ben Cao
translation by Yang Shouz-zhong
ISBN 0-936185-96-1
ISBN 978-0-936185-96-5

DUI YAO: THE ART OF COMBINING
CHINESE HERBAL MEDICINALS
by Philippe Sionneau
ISBN 0-936185-81-3
ISBN 978-0-936185-81-1

ENDOMETRIOSIS, INFERTILITY AND
TRADITIONAL CHINESE MEDICINE:
A Layperson's Guide
by Bob Flaws
ISBN 0-936185-14-7
ISBN 978-0-936185-14-9

THE ESSENCE OF LIU FENG-WU'S GYNECOLOGY
by Liu Feng-wu, translated by Yang Shou-zhong
ISBN 0-936185-88-0
ISBN 978-0-936185-88-0

EXTRA TREATISES BASED ON INVESTIGATION &
INQUIRY: A Translation of Zhu Dan-xi's Ge Zhi Yu Lun
translation by Yang Shou-zhong
ISBN 0-936185-53-8
ISBN 978-0-936185-53-8

FIRE IN THE VALLEY: TCM Diagnosis & Treatment of
Vaginal Diseases
by Bob Flaws
ISBN 0-936185-25-2
ISBN 978-0-936185-25-5

FULFILLING THE ESSENCE:
A Handbook of Traditional & Contemporary Treatments
for Female Infertility
by Bob Flaws
ISBN 0-936185-48-1
ISBN 978-0-936185-48-4

FU QING-ZHU'S GYNECOLOGY
trans. by Yang Shou-zhong and Liu Da-wei
ISBN 0-936185-35-X
ISBN 978-0-936185-35-4

GOLDEN NEEDLE WANG LE-TING: A 20th Century
Master's Approach to Acupuncture
by Yu Hui-chan and Han Fu-ru, trans. by Shuai Xue-zhong
ISBN 0-936185-78-3
ISBN 978-0-936185-78-1

A HANDBOOK OF CHINESE HEMATOLOGY
by Simon Becker
ISBN 1-891845-16-0
ISBN 978-1-891845-16-1

A HANDBOOK OF TCM PATTERNS
& THEIR TREATMENTS   Second Edition
by Bob Flaws & Daniel Finney
ISBN 0-936185-70-8
ISBN 978-0-936185-70-5

A HANDBOOK OF TRADITIONAL
CHINESE DERMATOLOGY
by Liang Jian-hui, trans. by Zhang Ting-liang
& Bob Flaws
ISBN 0-936185-46-5
ISBN 978-0-936185-46-0

A HANDBOOK OF TRADITIONAL
CHINESE GYNECOLOGY
by Zhejiang College of TCM, trans. by Zhang Ting-liang
& Bob Flaws
ISBN 0-936185-06-6 (4th edit.)
ISBN 978-0-936185-06-4

A HANDBOOK of TCM PEDIATRICS
by Bob Flaws
ISBN 0-936185-72-4
ISBN 978-0-936185-72-9

THE HEART & ESSENCE OF DAN-XI'S
METHODS OF TREATMENT
by Xu Dan-xi, trans. by Yang Shou-zhong
ISBN 0-926185-50-3
ISBN 978-0-936185-50-7

HERB TOXICITIES & DRUG INTERACTIONS:
A Formula Approach
by Fred Jennes with Bob Flaws
ISBN 1-891845-26-8
ISBN 978-1-891845-26-0

IMPERIAL SECRETS OF HEALTH & LONGEVITY
by Bob Flaws
ISBN 0-936185-51-1
ISBN 978-0-936185-51-4

INSIGHTS OF A SENIOR ACUPUNCTURIST
by Miriam Lee
ISBN 0-936185-33-3
ISBN 978-0-936185-33-0

INTEGRATED PHARMACOLOGY: Combining Modern
Pharmacology with Chinese Medicine
by Dr. Greg Sperber with Bob Flaws
ISBN 1-891845-41-1
ISBN 978-0-936185-41-3

INTRODUCTION TO THE USE OF
PROCESSED CHINESE MEDICINALS
by Philippe Sionneau
ISBN 0-936185-62-7
ISBN 978-0-936185-62-0

KEEPING YOUR CHILD HEALTHY WITH
CHINESE MEDICINE
by Bob Flaws
ISBN 0-936185-71-6
ISBN 978-0-936185-71-2

THE LAKESIDE MASTER'S STUDY OF THE PULSE
by Li Shi-zhen, trans. by Bob Flaws
ISBN 1-891845-01-2
ISBN 978-1-891845-01-7

MANAGING MENOPAUSE NATURALLY WITH
CHINESE MEDICINE
by Honora Lee Wolfe
ISBN 0-936185-98-8
ISBN 978-0-936185-98-9

MASTER HUA'S CLASSIC OF THE CENTRAL VISCERA
by Hua Tuo, trans. by Yang Shou-zhong
ISBN 0-936185-43-0
ISBN 978-0-936185-43-9

THE MEDICAL I CHING: Oracle of the Healer Within
by Miki Shima
ISBN 0-936185-38-4
ISBN 978-0-936185-38-5

MENOPAIUSE & CHINESE MEDICINE
by Bob Flaws
ISBN 1-891845-40-3
ISBN 978-1-891845-40-6

MOXIBUSTION: A MODERN CLINICAL HANDBOOK
by Lorraine Wilcox
ISBN 1-891845-49-7
ISBN 978-1-891845-49-9

MOXIBUSTION: THE POWER OF MUGWORT FIRE
by Lorraine Wilcox
ISBN 1-891845-46-2
ISBN 978-1-891845-46-8

A NEW AMERICAN ACUPUNTURE By Mark Seem
ISBN 0-936185-44-9
ISBN 978-0-936185-44-6

POCKET ATLAS OF CHINESE MEDICINE
Edited by Marne and Kevin Ergil
ISBN 3-131416-11-7
ISBN 978-3-131416-11-7

POINTS FOR PROFIT: The Essential Guide to Practice
Success for Acupuncturists 4rd Edition
by Honora Wolfe, Eric Strand & Marilyn Allen
ISBN 1-891845-25-X
ISBN 978-1-891845-25-3

PRINCIPLES OF CHINESE MEDICAL ANDROLOGY: An
Integrated Approach to Male Reproductive and Urological
Health by Bob Damone
ISBN 1-891845-45-4
ISBN 978-1-891845-45-1

PRINCE WEN HUI's COOK: Chinese Dietary Therapy
By Bob Flaws & Honora Wolfe
ISBN 0-912111-05-4
ISBN 978-0-912111-05-6

THE PULSE CLASSIC:
A Translation of the Mai Jing
by Wang Shu-he, trans. by Yang Shou-zhong
ISBN 0-936185-75-9
ISBN 978-0-936185-75-0

THE SECRET OF CHINESE PULSE DIAGNOSIS
by Bob Flaws
ISBN 0-936185-67-8
ISBN 978-0-936185-67-5

SECRET SHAOLIN FORMULAS FOR THE TREATMENT
OF EXTERNAL INJURY
by De Chan, trans. by Zhang Ting-liang & Bob Flaws
ISBN 0-936185-08-2
ISBN 978-0-936185-08-8

STATEMENTS OF FACT IN TRADITIONAL
CHINESE MEDICINE   Revised & Expanded
by Bob Flaws
ISBN 0-936185-52-X
ISBN 978-0-936185-52-1

STICKING TO THE POINT: A Step-by-Step Approach to
TCM Acupuncture Therapy
by Bob Flaws & Honora Wolfe   2 Condensed Books
ISBN 1-891845-47-0
ISBN 978-1-891845-47-5

A STUDY OF DAOIST ACUPUNCTURE
by Liu Zheng-cai
ISBN 1-891845-08-X
ISBN 978-1-891845-08-6

THE SUCCESSFUL CHINESE HERBALIST
by Bob Flaws and Honora Lee Wolfe
ISBN 1-891845-29-2
ISBN 978-1-891845-29-1

THE SYSTEMATIC CLASSIC OF ACUPUNCTURE &
MOXIBUSTION
A translation of the Jia Yi Jing
by Huang-fu Mi, trans. by Yang Shou-zhong & Charles Chace
ISBN 0-936185-29-5
ISBN 978-0-936185-29-3

THE TAO OF HEALTHY EATING: DIETARY
WISDOM ACCORDING TO CHINESE MEDICINE
by Bob Flaws   Second Edition
ISBN 0-936185-92-9
ISBN 978-0-936185-92-7

TEACH YOURSELF TO READ MODERN
MEDICAL CHINESE
by Bob Flaws
ISBN 0-936185-99-6
ISBN 978-0-936185-99-6

TEST PREP WORKBOOK FOR BASIC TCM THEORY
by Zhong Bai-song
ISBN 1-891845-43-8
ISBN 978-1-891845-43-7

TEST PREP WORKBOOK FOR THE NCCAOM BIO-
MEDICINE MODULE: Exam Preparation & Study Guide
by Zhong Bai-song
ISBN 1-891845-34-9
ISBN 978-1-891845-34-5

TREATING PEDIATRIC BED-WETTING WITH
ACUPUNCTURE & CHINESE MEDICINE
by Robert Helmer
ISBN 1-891845-33-0
ISBN 978-1-891845-33-8

TREATISE on the SPLEEN & STOMACH: A Translation
and annotation of Li Dong-yuan's
Pi Wei Lun
by Bob Flaws
ISBN 0-936185-41-4
ISBN 978-0-936185-41-5

THE TREATMENT OF CARDIOVASCULAR DISEASES
WITH CHINESE MEDICINE
by Simon Becker, Bob Flaws &
Robert Casañas, MD
ISBN 1-891845-27-6
ISBN 978-1-891845-27-7

THE TREATMENT OF DIABETES MELLITUS WITH
CHINESE MEDICINE
by Bob Flaws, Lynn Kuchinski &
Robert Casañas, M.D.
ISBN 1-891845-21-7
ISBN 978-1-891845-21-5

THE TREATMENT OF DISEASE IN TCM, Vol. 1:
Diseases of the Head & Face, Including Mental &
Emotional Disorders   New Edition
by Philippe Sionneau & Lü Gang
ISBN 0-936185-69-4
ISBN 978-0-936185-69-9

THE TREATMENT OF DISEASE IN TCM, Vol. II:
Diseases of the Eyes, Ears, Nose, & Throat
by Sionneau & Lü
ISBN 0-936185-73-2
ISBN 978-0-936185-73-6

THE TREATMENT OF DISEASE IN TCM, Vol. III:
Diseases of the Mouth, Lips, Tongue, Teeth & Gums
by Sionneau & Lü
ISBN 0-936185-79-1
ISBN 978-0-936185-79-8

THE TREATMENT OF DISEASE IN TCM, Vol IV:
Diseases of the Neck, Shoulders, Back, & Limbs
by Philippe Sionneau & Lü Gang
ISBN 0-936185-89-9
ISBN 978-0-936185-89-7

THE TREATMENT OF DISEASE IN TCM, Vol V: Diseases
of the Chest & Abdomen
by Philippe Sionneau & Lü Gang
ISBN 1-891845-02-0
ISBN 978-1-891845-02-4

THE TREATMENT OF DISEASE IN TCM, Vol VI:
Diseases of the Urogential System & Proctology
by Philippe Sionneau & Lü Gang
ISBN 1-891845-05-5
ISBN 978-1-891845-05-5

THE TREATMENT OF DISEASE IN TCM, Vol VII:
General Symptoms
by Philippe Sionneau & Lü Gang
ISBN 1-891845-14-4
ISBN 978-1-891845-14-7

THE TREATMENT OF EXTERNAL DISEASES WITH
ACUPUNCTURE & MOXIBUSTION
by Yan Cui-lan and Zhu Yun-long, trans. by Yang Shou-zhong
ISBN 0-936185-80-5
ISBN 978-0-936185-80-4

THE TREATMENT OF MODERN WESTERN
MEDICAL DISEASES WITH CHINESE MEDICINE
by Bob Flaws & Philippe Sionneau
ISBN 1-891845-20-9
ISBN 978-1-891845-20-8

UNDERSTANDING THE DIFFICULT PATIENT: A Guide
for Practitioners of Oriental Medicine
by Nancy Bilello, RN, L.ac.
ISBN 1-891845-32-2
ISBN 978-1-891845-32-1

WESTERN PHYSICAL EXAM SKILLS FOR
PRACTITIONERS OF ASIAN MEDICINE
by Bruce H. Robinson & Honora Lee Wolfe
ISBN 1-891845-48-9
ISBN 978-1-891845-48-2

YI LIN GAI CUO (Correcting the Errors in the Forest of
Medicine)
by Wang Qing-ren
ISBN 1-891845-39-X
ISBN 978-1-891845-39-0

70 ESSENTIAL CHINESE HERBAL FORMULAS
by Bob Flaws
ISBN 0-936185-59-7
ISBN 978-0-936185-59-0

160 ESSENTIAL CHINESE READY-MADE MEDICINES
by Bob Flaws
ISBN 1-891945-12-8
ISBN 978-1-891945-12-3

630 QUESTIONS & ANSWERS ABOUT CHINESE
HERBAL MEDICINE:
A Workbook & Study Guide
by Bob Flaws
ISBN 1-891845-04-7
ISBN 978-1-891845-04-8

260 ESSENTIAL CHINESE MEDICINALS
by Bob Flaws
ISBN 1-891845-03-9
ISBN 978-1-891845-03-1

750 QUESTIONS & ANSWERS ABOUT ACUPUNCTURE
Exam Preparation & Study Guide
by Fred Jennes
ISBN 1-891845-22-5
ISBN 978-1-891845-22-2